Self Assessment & Review of NEUROSCIENCES

Nayil Khursheed MS MCh (Neurosurgery) [NIMHANS]
Fellowship Cerebrovascular Surgery [SCTIMST]

Additional Professor

Department of Neurosurgery,
Sher-i-Kashmir Institute of Medical Sciences,
Soura, Srinagar, Jammu & Kashmir, India

Rumana Makhdoomi MD (Pathology)
Fellowship Oncopathology [KMIO]
Fellowship Neuropathology [NIMHANS]

Additional Professor

Department of Pathology,
Sher-i-Kashmir Institute of Medical Sciences,
Soura, Srinagar, Jammu & Kashmir, India

Forewords

Altaf Umar Ramzan

Suresh Nair

Donlin M Long

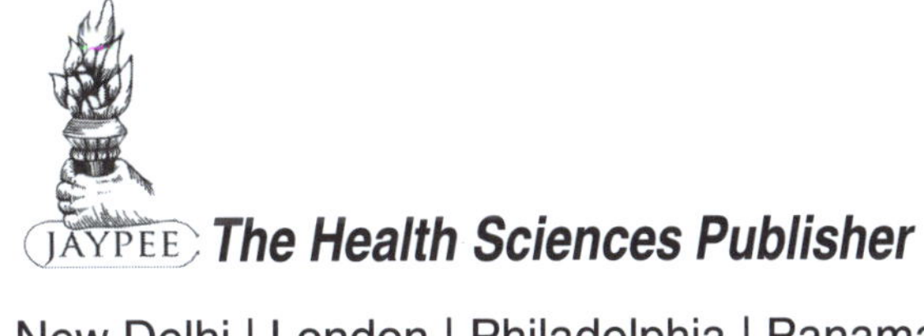

New Delhi | London | Philadelphia | Panama

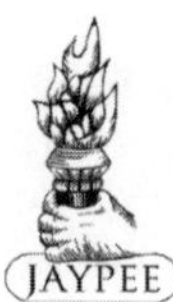

Jaypee Brothers Medical Publishers (P) Ltd

Headquarters
Jaypee Brothers Medical Publishers (P) Ltd.
4838/24, Ansari Road, Daryaganj
New Delhi 110 002, India
Phone: +91-11-43574357
Fax: +91-11-43574314
E-mail: jaypee@jaypeebrothers.com

Overseas Offices
J.P. Medical Ltd.
83, Victoria Street, London
SW1H 0HW (UK)
Phone: +44-20 3170 8910
Fax: +44(0)20 3008 6180
E-mail: info@jpmedpub.com

Jaypee-Highlights Medical Publishers Inc.
City of Knowledge, Bld. 235, 2nd Floor, Clayton
Panama City, Panama
Phone: +1 507-301-0496
Fax: +1 507-301-0499
E-mail: cservice@jphmedical.com

Jaypee Medical Inc.
325 Chestnut Street
Suite 412
Philadelphia, PA 19106, USA
Phone: +1 267-519-9789
E-mail: support@jpmedus.com

Jaypee Brothers Medical Publishers (P) Ltd.
17/1-B, Babar Road, Block-B, Shaymali
Mohammadpur, Dhaka-1207
Bangladesh
Mobile: +08801912003485
E-mail: jaypeedhaka@gmail.com

Jaypee Brothers Medical Publishers (P) Ltd.
Bhotahity, Kathmandu, Nepal
Phone: +977-9741283608
E-mail: kathmandu@jaypeebrothers.com

Website: www.jaypeebrothers.com
Website: www.jaypeedigital.com

Self Assessment & Review of Neurosciences

First Edition: **2013**
Second Edition: **2017**
ISBN: 978-93-86150-43-1
Printed at Rajkamal Electric Press, Plot No. 2, Phase-IV, Kundli, Haryana.

Dedicated to

The residents of Neurosciences

Foreword to the Second Edition

Dr Nayil and Dr Rumana's book on Neurosciences has proved to be a very useful companion to the aspirants of a career in Neurosciences. In my personal experience, I have found it to be a complete book, which has a great acceptance and readership among residents. The book is well thought of and provides a concept-based readership. It discourages rote learning. Very challenging case histories are outlined, which compel a resident to think hard before arriving at a diagnosis. Most of the standard texts in Neurosciences have been consulted to frame questions. No wonder the book is very popular among residents and examiners, who frame questions for entrance examinations. I wish the book serves the purpose for which it has been created.

Altaf Umar Ramzan MS MCh
Professor and Head
Department of Neurosurgery
Sher-i-Kashmir Institute of Medical Sciences (SKIMS)
Soura, Srinagar, Jammu and Kashmir, India

Foreword to the First Edition

He chose the path less trodden....

Nayil Khursheed has been a revelation and an inspiration for me and I have always been enamored by his passion for Neurosurgery and his jest for life.

He was never blessed with the best of conditions but he has mastered the ability to make the best of conditions. His passion for Neurosurgery saw him come down to our institute from all the way north travelling the entire length of India. His love for Neurosurgery is obvious by the number of international publications he has already authored during his short Neurosurgical career.

Through this book, Dr Khursheed has displayed yet another facet of his personality—the desire to teach. At the time and phase of life when he could have easily been lured by the materialistic prospects of a flourishing Neurosurgical career, he chose the less trodden path of academics of teaching and learning through teaching. His desire to spread wisdom beyond the confines of the institute where he is employed has borne fruits in the form of this book.

I have always felt that it is much easier to write an essay than answer a multiple-choice question. The latter requires a precise and in-depth knowledge of the subject. Similarly, answering an MCQ is much easier than preparing one, a fact which I have painfully realized in my long teaching career.

Khursheed is laudable and I am sure this is an act which is unlikely to be duplicated in the near future. Neurosurgery textbooks we may have in plenty—but an MCQ book is extremely unlikely.

Khursheed and Rumana have compiled an excellent collection of questions and answers, rich in information and based on practical wisdom. Such an informative book was the need of the hour and both the authors deserve unlimited praise and applause. I strongly recommend this book not only to all Neurosurgery residents, but all faculty members as well. To all Neurosurgeons and to all Neurosurgeons in the making—this is a must-read.

Suresh Nair
Professor (Senior Grade) and Head
Department of Neurosurgery
Sree Chitra Tirunal Institute for
Medical Sciences & Technology (SCTIMST)
Thiruvananthapuram, Kerala, India

Foreword to the First Edition

Nayil Khursheed has presented a book which should be of real value to the trainees in the Neurosciences. The book is authored by Dr Nayil Khursheed and Dr Rumana Makhdoomi. It covers all the important disciplines which constitute the Neurosciences. It serves several functions for the students in the field. It can be a quick reference to gain a rapid overview of a topic. It can be utilized as a basic first study guide for comprehensive view of the Neurosciences, which then can be expanded by detailed study of the selected areas. It also serves as a self-test, a mechanism allowing the student to examine his/her own information on most of the topics important to the Clinical Neurosciences.

The major function of the book comes from the detailed questions about its contents. These offer the student an opportunity to assess the knowledge gained or obtained from this and other sources. Anyone who can answer these questions correctly has a reasonable fundamental understanding of the Neurosciences and their application. The questions are comprehensive and valuable. I suggest that anyone who wants to use the book should first try to answer all the questions. Then the study of the book supplemented by other sources, when obviously needed, should be followed by repeating the examination. I have not examined every question compared to the content of the book, but for all those representative questions I reviewed, the answers were to be found within the book itself. I think this is a valuable resource for the students in the Neurosciences. It has an outline of the basic information one needs in the Neurosciences and then offers the reader an opportunity to test whether that information has been assimilated into a personal databank. I think this will be a useful resource for the students in the Neurosciences and an excellent self-test mechanism to be taken and repeated as the training continues.

Donlin M Long MD
Distinguished Service Professor of Neurosurgery
Department of Neurosurgery
Johns Hopkins Hospital
Baltimore, USA

Preface to the Second Edition

After the success of the first edition and after proving to be of great help to those residents who want to pursue their career in Neurosciences, we have added the recent advances in all fields of Neurosciences. We have also endeavored to make the book more elaborate by adding explanatory notes of most of the questions. All the sections have been updated and the number of questions in each section has been increased keeping in view the recent advances and updates. Sections have been relaid and made easy to comprehend. The book has been given a major facelift.

Nayil Khursheed
Rumana Makhdoomi

Preface to the First Edition

The book has been designed to suit the needs of the residents of Neurosciences, who wish to plunge further and deeper into Neurosciences. It aims at presenting the basic concepts of Neurosciences in a manner which is easy to comprehend and follow. It stresses on developing proficiency in problem-solving. The book will benefit those who wish to appear for various entrance tests for MCh in Neurosurgery, DM in Neurology, DM in Neuroradiology and Postdoctoral course in Neuropathology. The questions are based on sound knowledge of the topic rather than pure rote. Besides questions, most of the topics have been discussed in a crisp manner to accommodate almost everything that is expected of a candidate sitting for competitive exams in Neurosciences in National-level institutions. The book is handy and will serve as a quick review for the consultants practicing Neurosurgery and Neurology. Also other health care personnel who deal with neurological patients shall be benefitted by this book. The residents who are pursuing doctoral courses in Neurosciences will be benefited by the summaries of various cases presented in the book and an overview of basic sciences presented in it. Neuropathology and Neuroradiology come in separate sections to cater to the demands of those interested to pursue further courses in these subspecialties and to those who are already pursuing.

Nayil Khursheed
Rumana Makhdoomi

Acknowledgments

I would like to express my sincere thanks to the faculty and residents of Neurosurgery, Sher-i-Kashmir Institute of Medical Sciences (SKIMS), Soura, Srinagar, Jammu and Kashmir, India for acting as a stimulus for me to write the book. I am thankful to my family members for supporting me all through the writing and compilation of the book. My wife and co-author Rumana needs to be thanked for her support and help. My parents need to be thanked for their kind blessings and care. My daughters kept me going with their smiles and love.

My teachers—Professor Suresh Nair, Professor Indra Devi and Dr Altaf Umar Ramzan—have been of great help and support. I thank Professor Donlin M Long, Distinguished Service Professor of Neurosurgery, Johns Hopkins Hospital, Baltimore, USA, and editor of *Neurosurgery Quarterly* for reading my manuscript and writing the foreword.

The editorial staff of Jaypee Brothers Medical Publishers, New Delhi are to be thanked for making this book a reality.

From the Publisher's Desk
We request all the readers to provide us their valuable suggestions/errors (if any)
at: jppgmee@gmail.com
so as to help us in further improvement of this book in the subsequent edition(s).

Abbreviations

Adams—Principles of Neurology by Adams and Victor, 7th ed, International edition, McGraw-Hill, New York, 2001.

Al-Mefty—Meningiomas by Al-Mefty O, Raven Press, New York, 1991.

AJR—American Journal of Radiology.

AJNR—American Journal of Neuroradiology.

AO Spine—AO Spine Manual; Principles and Techniques by Aebi M, Arlet V, Webbs K, 2007, Thieme, Stuttgart.

Brain Pathology—Brain Pathology by Clayton Wiley published by the International Society of Neuropathology, Pittsburgh, PA 15213, USA.

Bickerstaff—Bickerstaff's Neurological Examination in Clinical Practice, 6th ed, 1997, Blackwell Science, Birmingham.

Craniovertebral junction anomalies—Craniovertebral Junction Anomalies—The Indian Experience by Jain VK, Behari S, SGPGI, Lucknow, India.

Greenberg—Handbook of Neurosurgery by Mark S Greenberg, 4th ed, 1997, Greenberg's Graphics Inc.

JNNP—Journal of Neurology, Neurosurgery and Psychiatry.

Kleihause—World Health Organization's Classification of Tumors; Pathology and Genetics: Tumors of the Nervous System by Kleihause P and Cavenee WK. IARC Press, Lyon, 2000.

Medically Refractory Epilepsy—Medically Refractory Epilepsy by Radhakrishnan K; Sree Chitra Tirunal Institute for Medical Sciences & Technology, 1st ed, 1999.

Movement Disorders—Movement Disorders by Fahn S, Jankovic J. Principles and Practice of Movement Disorders. 2008, Elsevier, Philadelphia.

Midroni—Biopsy Diagnosis of Peripheral Neuropathy by Midroni G, Bilbao J, Butterworth-Heinemann, 1995, Washington Street, Boston, Massachusetts, USA.

Neurosurgery Clinics—Neurosurgery Clinics of North America by Mayberg MR, Winn HR, WB Saunders, Philadelphia, Vol. 9, No. 3, 1998.

Osborn—Diagnostic Imaging Brain by Anne and Osborn, 1st edition, 2005, Amirsys Inc, Salt Lake City, Utah, USA.

Osborn Angiography—Diagnostic Cerebral Angiography by Osborn A, 1st ed, 2000, Lippincott Williams and Wilkins.

Patten—Neurological Differential Diagnosis by Patten J, 2nd ed, 1998, Springer, London.

Schmidek and Sweet—Operative Neurosurgical Techniques: Indications, Methods and Results by Schmidek and Sweet, 4th ed, 2000, WB Saunders, Philadelphia.

Snell's Neuroanatomy—Clinical Neuroanatomy for Medical Students; 3rd ed, 1992, Little-Brown, Boston, Massachusetts, USA.

Thieme—Controversies in Pediatric Neurosurgery by Jallo GI, Kothbauer KF, Pradilla G. Thieme Medical Publishers, 1st ed, 2010, New York, USA.

Youmans—Youmans Neurological Surgery, 5th ed, 2004, Saunders, New York, USA.

Contents

Contents

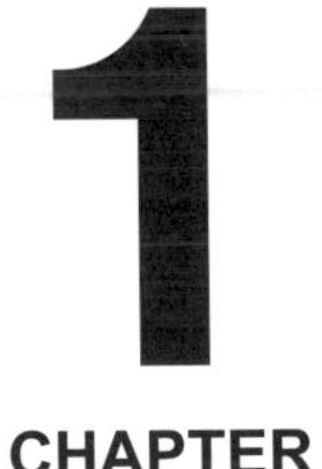

CHAPTER

Head Injury

Nayil Khursheed, Irfan Bhat

IMPORTANT THEORY

BIOMECHANICS OF CLOSED HEAD INJURY

In accidents, head is a part of a collision that results in an impact that generally lasts between 5 and 200 ms.

There are 3 Types of Loads

Impacts (duration of impact <50 ms). Impulsive loads (duration of impact 50–200 ms). Static loads (duration of impact >200 ms).

When a head suffers sudden mechanically-induced load, two different types of motions can be induced—translation and rotation.

Translation: Head's center of gravity moves along a straight line.

Rotation: Head moves around its center.

Rotational (angular) acceleration induces most devastating forces that affect the brain.

Ommaya's Centripetal Theory

"That the distribution of damaging diffuse strains induced by inertial loading would decrease in magnitude from the surface to the center of the approximately spheroidal brain mass".

As a result, the higher the magnitude of the injury force, the deeper the functional and structural damage of brain structures – that is traumatic unconsciousness develops only when the magnitude of the tensile and shear strains reach the upper brainstem.

Classification of Head Injury

Two main types:

1. Primary damage occurring at the moment of injury that takes the form of surface contusions and lacerations, diffuse axonal injury or diffuse vascular injury.
2. Secondary damage produced by complicating processes that are initiated at the moment of injury but do not present clinically until later which includes intracranial hemorrhage, brain swelling, raised ICP, hypoxic brain damage.

Diffuse vascular injury: Multiple small petechial hemorrhages are seen, common in frontal lobes and rostral part of 4th ventricle. Pathogenesis of these lesions seems to be acceleration/deceleration forces.

Other types of primary brain injury include cranial nerve injury especially I, II, VIII. Damage to pituitary gland and hypothalamus. Pituitary stalk can get occasionally torn and massive infarction can occur.

Diffuse Axonal Injury (DAI)

Occurs in 50% of severely head injured patients and accounts for 35% of all deaths from head injury.

Triad

Lesion in corpus callosum.

Lesion in dorsolateral quadrant of brainstem.

Axonal rolling of white matter.

The corpus callosum (CC) is preferentially affected because of the relative immobilization of brain hemispheres by the falx and because of its relatively greater mobility when inertial forces are generated.

Grading DAI

i. Microscopic axonal damage in the white matter, corpus callosum (CC), brainstem or cerebellum without any macroscopic evidence.
ii. Macroscopic or microscopic focal lesions in the CC + diffuse axonal damage.
iii. Macroscopic or microscopic focal injury to CC + dorsolateral quadrant of rostral brainstem.

Pathogenesis of DAI

Four stages can be defined:

Stage I: *Axonal membrane injury and alteration in ionic fluxes:* Weakest part of axon is node of Ranvier and the paranodal region. At a strain of 5% ionic influx changes and causes a temporary failure in the generation and propagation of action potentials. The most significant alteration at this stage is an increase in cytosolic free Ca^{++}.

Stage II: *Reversible cytoskeletal damage:* When the stretch is 5–10%, ionic disturbances are greater and frequently associated with local swelling of the axon as well as abnormalities in the axoplasmic transport. These abnormalities result in axonal viscosities, but not axonal disconnection. Restitution of axonal structure and function can generally be expected.

Stage III: If strain is 15–20% on axons, severe alterations in ionic fluxes are produced first which evolve to structural abnormalities that end in axontmesis. The influx of Ca^{++} causes activation of proteases and phospholipases. Proteases cause degradation of cytoskeletal protein such as spectrin, neurofilaments and microtubule associated proteins. Phospholipases attack membrane fatty acids activating free-radical species and various inflammatory mediators. If the process leading to secondary or delayed axotomy can be interrupted, then perhaps reparative mechanism can rescue the axon from permanent destructive damage.

Stage IV: *Primary axotomy:* This is the most severe form of DAI, consists of tearing of axons provoked by severe strains immediately on impact, occurs when strain is >20%.

Mechanoporation: By inducing a transient structural microdefect in the cell membrane, abnormal ionic fluxes occur, which lead to increase in intracellular Ca^{2+}, Na^{+}, Cl^{-} and leakage of K^{+} from the cell. The increased calcium load in mitochondrial matrix produces mitochondrial permeability transition pore which increases the permeability of inner mitochondrial membrane to various solutes and causes mitochondrial failure. The lack of energy disturbs the homeostasis of the axolemma and provokes further increase in calcium influx, which leads to secondary axotomy.

Brain Ischemia and Ischemic Penumbra

One of the most frequent causes of brain tissue hypoxia in head injuries is ischemia when oxygen delivery is significantly reduced, the normal ionic gradients through the cell membrane cannot be maintained and it leads to depolarization which leads to activation of pre-synaptic voltage-dependent Ca^{++} channels and massive release of excitotoxic amino acids into the extracellular space.

Because of energy failure, the extracellular space is not effectively cleared by the glial cells which contributes to the toxic levels of extracellular glutamate found after ischemia.

Furthermore excitatory amino acids activate postsynaptic NMDA (N-methyl-D-aspartate) and metabotropic receptors, which induces calcium overload of the postsynaptic neurons. An additional effect of hyperactivated NMDA receptors is an excessive influx of Na^{+} and inside the cells, with water passively following it and contributing to cytotoxic edema. With edema there is microcirculatory compression by the swollen tissue and an increase in the diffusion distance of oxygen between RBC and the tissue.

Final event in ischemia is increase in cytosolic Ca^{++} that activates proteases and phospholipases causing degradation of actin, spectrin as well as extracellular matrix proteins such as laminin. Activation of phospholipases and cycloxygenases generates oxygen derived free radicals that contribute to neural tissue damage.

EDH

Commonest in temporal region. Associated with fracture in 90% adults. Source is middle meningeal artery, sometimes venous sinuses. Unusual for EDH <30 ml to cause neurological signs. Small EDH liquefies, reabsorbs and disappears by 6- weeks.

SDH

Rupture of bridging veins or small tear in a cortical artery. 72% of SDHs are caused by fall or assault and 28% by road traffic accident. The high incidence of SDH in assault or fall is because of very high rates of acceleration or deceleration. Acute SDH is the most common type of intracranial injury found in infants subjected to non-accidental injury.

Brain Swelling

Three main types of brain swelling:

Swelling of the brain adjacent to contusions is due to physical disruption of the tissue with damage to blood brain barrier and loss of normal physiologic regulation of arterioles. Water and electrolytes leak into the brain tissue (vasogenic edema).

Diffuse swelling of one cerebral hemisphere: Most often seen in association with ipsilateral acute SDH. When this is evacuated, the brain simply expands to occupy the space, it is because of engorgement of a nonreactive vascular bed.

Diffuse swelling of both cerebral hemispheres: Usually seen in young adults, brain is swollen and ventricles are small and symmetric. The pathogenesis is supposed to be loss of vasomotor tone and consequent vasodilatation. Reduced intracranial compliance due to failure of CSF absorption has also been proposed.

New Concepts in Brain Swelling

Cells use organic osmolytes for volume regulation.

In mammalian CNS, the main osmolytes are myoinositol and the amino acid taurine.

Organic osmolytes enter and leave the cell through a volume sensitive organic osmolyte/anion channel (VSOAC).

Disturbance of these channels cause brain edema.

Aquaporins: A new family of water channel molecules.

Marshall's CT Classification of Diffuse Injury

1.	Diffuse injury I (no visible pathology)	No visible Intracranial pathology seen on CT scan
2.	II	Cisterns are present with midline shift 0–5 mm, no high or mixed density lesion >25 cc; may include bone fragments and foreign bodies
3.	III (swelling)	Cisterns compressed or absent with midline shift 0–5 mm; no high or mixed density lesion >25 cc
4.	IV (shift)	Midline shift >5 mm, no high or mixed density lesion >25 cc
5.	Evacuated mass lesion	Any lesion surgically evacuated
6.	Non-evacuated mass lesion	High or mixed density lesion >25 cc; not surgically evacuated

General Facts About Head Injury

Initial CT examinations demonstrate abnormalities in approximately 90% of patients with severe head injury.

The prognosis in patients with severe head injury with demonstrable pathology on initial CT examination is less favorable than when CT scan is normal.

In patients with normal CT on admission, outcome is primarily related to concomitant extra cranial injuries.

The absence of abnormalities on CT at admission does not preclude the occurrence of increased ICP and significant new lesions may develop in 40% of patients.

Compressed or absent basal cisterns indicate a three-fold risk of raised ICP.

The status of basal cistern is related to outcome.

Mortality is increased two to three fold in the presence of compressed or absent basal cistern.

Presence of mass lesions in patients over 45-years of age carries a positive predictive value (PPV) of 79% for poor outcome.

Mortality is higher in acute SDH than in EDH.

Presence of midline shift is inversely related to prognosis.

Positive predictive value [PPV] of 78% for poor outcome in the presence of shift >5 mm.

Morality is twice in patients >65 years than in patients <65 years.

Children <5 years – good outcome than older children.

Adults with initial clinical findings of transtentorial herniation – 18% functional recovery compared to 55% in children and adolescents.

Positive alcohol screen – bad outcome.

Associated injuries causing hypotension and hypoxia – bad outcome. Hypotension (<90 mmHg systolic) – twice is the mortality.

82% with GCS >11 have good outcome. 87% with GCS of 3 will die.

Abnormalities of pupillary function and extraocular movements (EOM), posturing predict poor outcome. Only 10% of patients with bilateral impaired pupillary responses and EOM have functional recovery.

Poor outcome is seen in 85% of patients who on imaging have absent basal cisterns, 64% – compressed cisterns, 44% – normal cisterns.

If midline shift is disproportionate to the extent of focal lesion – poor prognosis.

If MRI reveals lesions of white matter and brainstem – poor prognosis.

Persistently elevated or uncontrollable ICP – poor outcome. 78% with normal ICP – good outcome. All patients with uncontrollable ICP – die.

Increased catecholamine levels – poor outcome.

Increased CSF creatinine kinase BB isoenzyme – poor outcome.

Increased α-2 plasmin-inhibitor plasmin complex (>15 μg/ml)-poor outcome Increased D-dimer (>5 μg/ml) – poor outcome.

Intracranial Pressure Monitoring

Indications

A. Patients with GCS 3–8 after cardiopulmonary resuscitation with abnormal CT scan.

B. Patients with GCS 3–8, with normal CT scan but if two or more of the following features are noted at admission i.e.

   a. Age >40 years.

   b. Unilateral or bilateral motor posturing.

   c. Systolic BP <90 mm Hg.

Less than 3% of patients with GCS – 13–15 and 10% with GCS 9–12, will progress to coma and be classified as severe head injury.

Patients with normal ICP have the best prognosis whereas those with uncontrollable ICP do the worst.

ICP monitoring helps in early detection of intracranial mass lesion.

ICP monitoring limits the indiscriminate use of potentially harmful therapies to control ICP.

Intracranial pressure treatment threshold—Current data support 20 mm Hg as an upper threshold above which treatment to lower ICP should generally be initiated.

Cerebral perfusion pressure should be maintained at a minimum of 70 mm Hg.

Management of Raised ICP

Headend elevation

Sedation – commonest agent IV Fentanyl.

ICP refractory to analgesia and sedation demands neuromuscular blockade.

Mannitol

Dose: 0.25 g/Kg–1 g/Kg

Immediate effect – plasma expanding effect – reduces blood viscosity, increased CBF and increases cerebral oxygen delivery.

Delayed (15–30 min) – osmotic effect – effect persists up to 6 hours.

Mannitol is known to cause "opening" of the blood brain barrier, meaning that mannitol may pass and accumulate in the brain. The accumulation of mannitol is most marked when it is given as continuous infusion. Thus it is recommended that mannitol should be administered as repeated boluses.

Side effects – acute tubular necrosis, especially if serum osmolality is 320 m Osm/Kg or more.

Frusemide causes super-additive lowering effect which may be useful when the response to Mannitol is unsatisfactory.

Barbiturate coma

Mechanism: Depression of metabolic activity which indirectly decreases CBF (Coupling).

Dose: Loading dose of 10 mg/Kg of Pentobarbital over 30 min, then infusion of 5 mg/Kg/hour for next 3 hours, then 1 mg//Kg/hour. The dose can be increased to 2–3 mg/Kg (Eisenberg's protocol).

Goal: Burst suppression of EEG and ICP control. In cases burst suppression has been attained but ICP is increased, high dose of barbiturates are given even to cause electrocerebral silence. Serum level of 3–4 mg%. When adequate ICP control has been obtained for 24-48 hours high dose barbiturate therapy is maintained and tapered under cover of analgesia and sedation.

Side Effect

Hypotension, Infection (immunologic anergy).

Contraindication: Hypotension.

Hypothermia for ICP Control

Temperature of 32–34°C is maintained for at least 48 hours and is to be started within 8 hours of head injury. K^+ supplements to be given as it causes hypokalemia.

S/E: Immunologic anergy, Coagulopathy.

Contraindications: Extracranial injuries as it can induce diffuse bleeding.

Alternate Treatment Philosophies in TBI Management

CPP-based therapy (Rosner et al).

ICP does not need treatment as long as CPP is maintained at 70 mm Hg or higher.

Hypervolemia be maintained.

Pressors be liberally used to maintain increased CPP. However, no randomized control trial (RCT) to support it.

Critics say that effect of elevating CPP may simply be the avoidance of hypotensive episodes and not related to increased CBF at all.

Lundh Method of ICP Management

Based on Starlings model of vasogenic edema.

To increase hydrostatic and osmotic forces favoring maintenance of fluid within the vascular compartment. Use β-blockers and central α-agonists to maintain CPP, in range of 70 mm Hg. Negative fluid balance to increase serum osmolality. Na^+ levels up to 150 meq/L. Liberal use of albumin and plasma for fluid resuscitation. Dihydroergotamine for decreasing hydrostatic forces. However, there is no randomized controlled trial supporting it.

Metabolic derangements in head injury:

Increased catecholamines, insulin, glucagon, cortisol. IL-1, IL-6 are increased in ventric CSF and serum. Increased urinary N_2 losses. Hyperglycemia (diabetes of stress). Experimental evidence that increased blood sugar causes secondary neuronal damage by cerebral acidosis.

75% of patients with (TBI) traumatic brain injury with admission albumin levels of d 2.5 g% had unfavorable outcome while only 38% with >2.5% albumin had unfavorable outcome (McClean), cause being increased vascular permeability of albumin secondary to acute phase reactants (IL-1, IL-6). Zn^{++} decreases vascular permeability, So Zn^{++} is added to increase albumin levels. Patients who are started on nutrition earlier have better outcome than when it is started late.

Goals of Nutritional Therapy

Blood sugar <150 mg%

Prevention of catabolic state by aiming for a positive N_2 balance (2 g/Kg/day).

Maintenance of serum mineral levels (Zn, Fe).

Antiseizure Prophylaxis

Risk factors for post-traumatic seizures include

GCS <10, contusion, depressed fracture, SDH, intracerebral hematoma. Seizure within 24 hours of injury.

Early seizures – phenytoin and carbamazepine reduces the incidence of early seizures.

Late seizures – no drug is effective.

If late post-traumatic seizures occur patients should be managed in accordance with standard approaches to patients with new onset seizures.

MULTIPLE CHOICE QUESTIONS

1. **Following names are synonymous with growing skull fracture, except:**
   a. Craniocerebral erosion
   b. Expanding skull fracture
   c. Traumatic ventricular cyst
   d. Lukenschadle

   Ref. Greenberg, 4th/e, p726

2. **The commonest site for growing skull fractures is:**
   a. Frontal bone
   b. Parietal bone
   c. Temporal bone
   d. Occipital bone

   Ref. Greenberg, 4th/e, p726

3. **All the following entities can mimic shaking impact syndrome, except:**
   a. Coagulopathies
   b. Glutaricaciduria
   c. Osteogenesis imperfecta
   d. Myoclonic seizures

   Ref. Youmans, 5th/e, p3500

4. **Burst lobe is defined as:**
   a. Complex of subdural hematoma and damaged and necrotic brain
   b. Complex of subdural and epidural hematoma
   c. Complex of epidural hematoma and compound depressed fracture
   d. None of the above

   Ref. Youmans, 5th/e, p5044

5. **All the following about diffuse axonal injury are true, except:**
   a. It was first described by Strich
   b. there is diffuse degeneration of white matter
   c. It is also referred to as shearing injury of brain
   d. It is usually associated with lucid interval

   Ref. Greenberg, 4th/e, p690

6. **In which of the following head injuries axonal rolling is a feature:**
   a. Diffuse axonal injury
   b. Diffuse axonal injury
   c. Concussion injury
   d. Multiple contusions

   Ref. Youmans, 5th/e, p5045

7. **The commonest lesion in a head injured patient is:**
   a. Fracture
   b. Contusion
   c. Extradural hematoma in temporal region
   d. Traumatic SAH

   Ref. Youmans, 5th/e, p5041

8. **The centripetal theory of Ommaya states that:**
   a. Lesion depth is dependent on the force of injury
   b. Lesion depth is independent of the force of injury
   c. Lesion number is dependent on the force of injury
   d. None of the above

   Ref. British Journal of Neurosurgery 2002; 16(3):220-42

9. **The minimum volume of epidural hematoma in infratentorial compartment which needs evacuation in adults is:**
   a. 10 ml
   b. 20 ml
   c. 30 ml
   d. 40 ml

   Ref. Acta Neurochir (Wien) 1994;126:124-7

10. **The volume of epidural hematoma (ml) is calculated by:**
    a. $4\pi^2$
    b. $4/3\pi^2$
    c. axbxc
    d. axbxc/2

    Ref. Neurocritical Care 2010;12(1):30-4

ANSWERS

1. d **2.** b **3.** d **4.** a **5.** d **6.** b **7.** b **8.** a **9.** a **10.** d

11. Dementia Pugilistica occurs in:

a. Rugby footballers b. Boxers
c. Gymnasts d. Scuba divers

Ref. Greenberg, 4th/e, p746

12. All the following statements about ossified posterior longitudinal ligament (OPLL) are true, except:

a. Predominant mechanism of injury is vascular
b. Commonest location is cervical
c. OPLL starts predominantly at C5/C6 level
d. It causes myelopathy

Ref. Youmans, 5th/e, p4475

13. The incidence of bleed in subdural space is more than in subarachnoid space because:

a. There are more crossing veins in the subdural space than in the subarachnoid space
b. The bridging veins in the subarachnoid space are supported by the arachnoid trabeculae
c. The subdural space is more capacious than the subarachnoid space
d. All the above

Ref. World Journal. of Neurosurgery 2012; 77(1):103-10

14. Which of the following statements is/are correct:

a. Contusions are common in frontal and temporal lobes
b. A combination of contusion and hematoma qualifies for a burst lobe
c. If the blood constitutes at least 50% of the total volume of the traumatic brain lesion, it qualifies for an intracerebral hematoma
d. Gliding contusions occur beneath the depressed bone fragment

Ref. Youmans, 5th/e, p5041-2

15. Which of the following descriptions best describes moderate diffuse axonal injury (DAI):

a. Coma lasting >24 hours without decerebrate posturing
b. Coma lasting >24 hours with decerebrate posturing
c. Coma lasting >48 hours without decerebrate posturing
d. Coma lasting >48 hours with decerebrate posturing

Ref. Youmans, 5th/e, p5045

16. All the following are indications for ICP monitoring, except:

a. GCS score of ≤ 8 with abnormal CT scan findings
b. GCS score of ≤ 8 with normal CT scan and age >40 years
c. GCS score of ≤ 8 with normal CT scan but systolic BP of 90 mm Hg or lower
d. GCS score of ≤ 10 with abnormal CT scan

Ref. Greenberg, 4th/e, p706

17. The normal lower limit of cerebral perfusion pressure is:

a. 18 mm Hg b. 25 mm Hg
c. 50 mm Hg d. 80 mm Hg

Ref. Greenberg, 4th/e, p706

18. All the following are signs of skull base fracture, except:

a. Battle sign b. Racoon sign
c. CSF rhinorrhoea d. Kernohans notch

Ref. Greenberg, p692, 4th/e, p722, Youmans 5th/e, p5090

19. A pedestrian was hit by a motor cycle following which he had loss of consciousness for 10–15 minutes. He recovered and went home. About 1 week later, he reports to the emergency room with history of headache and diplopia. On examination, he is conscious, coherent and ambulant. He has papilledema and bilateral 6th nerve palsy. CT scan reveals hyperdensity below the bone at the vertex. He is further evaluated with an MRI brain which shows an extradural hematoma at the vertex with mass effect. The most likely mechanism which can explain his papilledema and bilateral 6th nerve palsy is:

a. Partial blockage of sagittal sinus by EDH with decreased venous return and increased ICP
b. Thrombosis of SSS with consequent raised ICP
c. Complete blockage of SSS by EDH with raised ICP features
d. All the above

Ref. Turkish Journal of Neurosurgery 2011; 22(2):257-60

ANSWERS

11. b	**12.** c	**13.** b	**14.** a	**15.** a	**16.** d	**17.** c	**18.** d	**19.** d

20. Which of the following criteria on CT scan is/are indications for treating an extradural hematoma conservatively?

a. Clot volume of <30 ml
b. Clot thickness of <15 mm
c. Midline shift of <5 mm
d. All the above

Ref. Surgical Neurology 2007;68:155-8

21. Which of the hematoma sites is most likely to present early?

a. 15 ml temporal extradural hematoma (EDH)
b. 15 ml frontal EDH
c. 15 ml posterior fossa EDH
d. 15 ml parietal EDH

Ref. Neurosurgery 1985;16(5):602-6

22. Which of the following terms describes features of hypotension and tachycardia in posterior fossa ICSOL?

a. Cushing's response
b. Reverse Cushing's response
c. Inverted Cushing's response
d. Cushing's variant response

Ref. Youmans, 5th/e, p5090

23. Which of the following statements about diffuse axonal injury (DAI) is/are correct?

a. It was first described by Strich
b. In grade III DAI, there are lesions in cerebral peduncle
c. It is usually caused by sagittal acceleration injury
d. 'a' and 'b'

Ref. Youmans, 5th/e, p5045

24. All the following statements regarding carotid artery injury are true, except:

a. Type II injuries occur after hyperextension of the neck
b. Type III injuries occur more in adults
c. Type IV injuries can lead to intracranial bleed
d. None of the above

Ref. Youmans, 5th/e, p1669-70

25. About apnea test, all the following are correct, except:

a. Preoxygenation for 10 minutes with 100% oxygen
b. Disconnect the ventilator and given oxygen by tracheal cannula
c. Wait for 10 minutes and if there are respiratory efforts during this period, the patient is not brain dead
d. During the disconnection if ABG reveals PCO_2>40 mm Hg and there are no respiratory efforts, the patient is brain dead there are no respiratory efforts, the patient is brain dead

Ref. Youmans, 5th/e, p398

26. A cut-off value which divides a low-velocity missile injury to brain from a high velocity injury is:

a. 1000 feet/sec
b. 1500 feet/sec
c. 2000 feet/sec
d. 2500 feet/sec

Ref. Greenbergs, 4th/e, p739

27. All the following statements regarding fractures of temporal bone are correct, except:

a. Longitudinal petrous temporal bone fractures have more incidence of Battles sign than transverse fractures
b. Facial nerve palsy is common in longitudinal fractures than in transverse fractures
c. CSF rhinorrhea is commoner in transverse fractures than in longitudinal fracture
d. Longitudinal fractures are common than transverse fractures

Ref. Youmans, 5th/e, p5275-84

28. A young motor-cyclist sustained an accident and started complaining of neck pain. His neurological examination was normal. X-ray cervical spine showed overhang of C_1 lateral masses which measured 7.1 mm, the most likely diagnosis is:

a. Type II odontoid fracture
b. Atlanto-occipital subluxation
c. Jeffersons fracture
d. Hangman's fracture

Ref. Youmans, 5th/e, p4934

ANSWERS

20. d **21.** c **22.** d **23.** d **24.** b **25.** d **26.** b **27.** b **28.** c

29. A teen-ager received a blow on her neck. About 4 hours later, she started with weakness of one side of her body. Examination also revealed Horner's syndrome on the side of blow. The most likely diagnosis is a

a. Carotid artery injury
b. Vertebral artery injury
c. Cervical spine fracture with cord compression
d. Cervical spine epidural hematoma

Ref. Youmans, 5th/e, p1669-70

30. Which of the following procedures is not helpful to treat CSF otorrhea?

a. Mannitol therapy
b. Lumbar drainage
c. Eustachian tube ligation
d. Trendlenberg's position

Ref. Youmans, 5th/e, p5265-70

31. Hearing loss after head injury is because of

a. Tympanic membrane perforation
b. Ossicular chain disruption
c. Cochlear concussion
d. All the above

Ref. Youmans, 5th/e, p5280

32. Persistent vertigo after head injury is usually because of:

a. Brainstem contusion
b. Atlantoaxial subluxation
c. Perilymph fistula
d. Basilar artery thrombosis

Ref. Youmans, 5th/e, p2903-4

33. The term coning refers to:

a. Subfalcine herniation
b. Uncal herniation
c. Tonsillar herniation
d. None of the above

Ref. Youmans, 5th/e, p1504-5

34. The hypodensity in extradural hematomas seen on CT scan is known as:

a. Swirl sign
b. Edge effect
c. Aliasing
d. Shine-through effect

Ref. Journal of Neurosurgery 2011;8:417-21

35. The commonest cause of loss of olfaction is:

a. Local nasal disease
b. Head injury
c. Olfactory groove meningioma
d. Esthesioneuroblastoma

Ref. Greenberg, 4th/e, p722

Answers

29. a **30.** a **31.** d **32.** c **33.** c **34.** a **35.** a

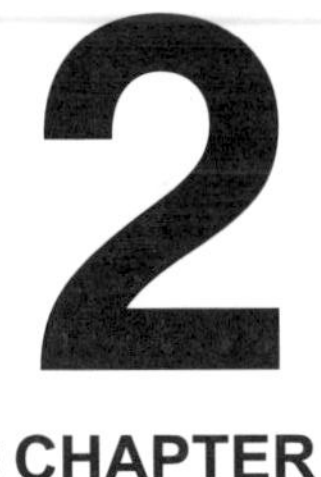

CHAPTER

Brain Tumors

Muhammad Sultan, Rumana Makhdoomi, Nayil Khursheed

IMPORTANT THEORY

PINEAL GLAND

Histology

Pineocytes are type I and type II. Type I – S100 positive and neuron-specific-enolase (NSE) negative. Type II – S100 negative and NSE positive. At birth, type I cells predominate. By age 1 year, type II cells outnumber. Pineocytes constitute about 90% of the parenchyma. The cells belong to the APUD cells. Pineocytes are considered 'paraneuronal cells.

Classification of Pineal Tumors

Germ cell origin	Parenchymal cell origin
Germinoma (Seminoma, dysgerminoma, atypical teratoma)	Pineoblastoma
Endodermal sinus tumor	Pineocytoma
Choriocarcinoma	Tumors of glial and other cell origin
Teratoma	Non-neoplastic cysts and masses
Embryonal cell carcinoma – tumor of totipotential cells	

Germinomas

Most common germ cell tumor (80%). Constitutes 5.6–9% of intracranial tumors in Japan. Extremely malignant but highly radiosensitive. With therapy, 2/3rd of patients survive >5 years.

Spinal cord metastasis seen in 14%. Tumor is light gray, granular solid. Hemorrhage, necrosis, cystic areas are uncommon. Microscopically- islands of large cells with well defined cytoplasmic membranes, cytoplasm is clear or eosinophilic. Cells are separated by fibrovascular stroma infiltrated by T-lymphocytes.

Embryonal Cell Carcinoma

Tumor arises from most primitive cells. Cuboidal or columnar cells in a glandular or papillary pattern.

Endodermal Sinus Tumor

Most infrequent tumor of the group. Reticular arrangement of primitive epithelial cells. Communicating cavities and channels. Papillary structures and solid areas. Schiller-Duval body is the histopathological hallmark.

Choriocarcinoma

Extra embryonic differentiation of totipotential cells. Most often is a component of another malignant germ cell tumor. Highly vascular, composed of cords of large, round cytotrophoblastic cells with clear cytoplasm surrounded by multinucleated synctiotrophoblastic cells.

Teratoma

Occurs mainly in young males especially in first decade. Contains derivatives of all three layers.

Immature teratomas are more common. Behave usually in a malignant manner and may disseminate. Mature teratomas remain well localized. Cut surface is variegated and areas of cartilage, bone, teeth are seen.

Tumors of Pineal Parenchyma

Constitute about 20% of pineal tumors. 2/3rd of patients are males. Arise from pineocytes. 50% of these tumors – pineoblastomas, 25% – pineocytomas, 25% – pineal parenchymal tumors with intermediate differentiation.

Pineoblastomas

Median age is 18 years. Malignant by nature. Invade locally and disseminate also. Highly cellular, small round oval nucleus. High mitosis and ill-defined cytoplasm. Resembles medulloblastoma. Homer-Wright Rosettes – common. Occasionally Fleurettes and Flexner-Wintersteiner (FW) rosettes are seen. These represent abortive attempts at photoreceptor development. Fleurettes – more advanced – semicircular arrangement of columnar cells with terminal membranes. FW rosettes are more primitive and are characterized by a circular arrangement of columnar cells.

Pineocytoma

Median age is 36 years. Most differentiated pineal tumor. Slow growth. Localized, noninvasive.

Consists of small rounded cells. Cells sometimes form pineocytomatous rosettes. Mitotic figures are absent.

Pineal Parenchymal Tumors with Intermediate Differentiation

Median age of presentation – 12 years. Mitotic figures may or may not be present. Dissemination through CSF pathways is less frequent. No specific immunohistochemical stain for pineal parenchymal cells exist, however expression of non-specific enolase and synaptophysin has been demonstrated in pineocytomas. S-antigen (arrestin) reactivity may be seen in pineal parenchymal tumors.

Tumors of Glial and Other Cell Origin

Astroblastoma, astrocytoma, glioblastoma, ependymoma, oligodendroglioma, choroid plexus papilloma, Medullo-epithelioma, paraganglioma, hemangiopericytoma, hemangioma, lipoma, arachnoid cysts, tuberculomas, cysticercosis, sarcoid, syphilitic gumma.

Management of Hydrocephalus Associated with Pineal Region Tumors

90% of patients have hydrocephalus secondary to aqueductal compression

Options

a. VP shunt
b. External ventricular drainage
c. Endoscopic third ventriculostomy (ETV)
d. Aqueductoplasty.

Management of Tumor

For tissue diagnosis, options available are:

a. Stereotactic biopsy
b. Neuroendoscopic biopsy
c. Open biopsy

Stereotactic Biopsy

Not feasible because of:

High chances of bleeding, sufficient specimen for histologic examination may not be available, high rate of mixed histologies particularly those of germ cell origin poses another difficulty.

In a French trial, 370 STB of pineal tumors:

Diagnostic yield – 94%, Mortality – 1.3%, morbidity – 1%

Other uses of stereotaxy are:

Aspiration of cysts, brachytherapy.

Endoscopic Management

Endoscopic third ventriculostomy (ETV) and biopsy of the lesion is possible.

Open Biopsy

Major advantage: It allows resection at the same time, however it has a mortality of 10% and morbidity of 10%.

Management of Hydrocephalus

a. VP shunt, other than risks of routine complications tumor dissemination is an added risk.
b. EVD—Avoids the need for a permanent shunt.
c. Aqueductoplasty is another option. In this procedure a Silastic stent is put along the aqueduct which maintains the patency and this procedure avoids the risk of opening the floor of 3rd ventricle.
d. ETV—It allows biopsy of the tumor, in addition avoids complications of EVD and shunt.

Need for Tissue Diagnosis Versus Tumor Markers

If tumor markers provide enough information to base treatment – then?

Is cytoreduction advantageous?

Various retrospective studies show – lack of correlation between extent of surgery and outcome for both germinomas and malignant non-germinomatous germ cell tumors (NGGCT's)

In tumors with negative markers, surgery has a role.

If tumor is metastatic – biopsy, radiochemotherapy.

No evidence of metastasis, e.g. pineal cell tumors or malignant gliomas radical resection – RT/CT

Benign tumors – radical resection.

Only non-metastatic tumor in marker negative category for which radical resection is not needed is germinoma.

If tumor markers are positive, i.e. biopsy is not needed, assume malignant germ cell tumor and start chemotherapy and craniospinal radiotherapy.

Consider resection in case of residual lesion.

Pineal Meningiomas

These tumors constitute 6–8% of pineal tumors and 0.3% of intracranial meningiomas. These arise from velum interpositum. Average age 28 years, less than for other sites. M:F – 7:4 (contrast to other meningiomas).

Metastases

Lung is the commonest primary, followed by breast, melanoma, stomach, kidney, gallbladder. Metastatic small cell carcinoma of lung needs to be differentiated from pineoblastoma. In one of the trials with radiosurgery complete response was seen in 8 cases (26.7%) and the response rate was 73.3%, however tumor progression was seen in 8 cases (26.7%) of whom 7 (23.3%) died. Germinomas and pineocytomas showed higher response and control rates (100%).

ORBITAL TUMORS

Optic Nerve Gliomas

Seen in first decade of life. Signs and symptoms—visual loss and proptosis CT appearance—globular, expanded, enhancing suprasellar mass. MRI demonstrates the intracanalicular portion of optic nerve better and also delineates the intracranial extension better. On MRI it is hypo on T_1W and hyper on T_2W. Enhancement is intense despite them being as low grade astrocytomas (Pilocytic.) Vascular encasement is not a feature of these tumors. Histologically – Pilocytic astrocytoma (low grade). Decision to operate depends on progression of tumor. If visual acuity is normal –observe, no vision-surgery and radiotherapy, progressive visual loss-surgery. Surgical approach is transcranial.

Orbital Meningiomas

Arise from meningothelial cells of dura or pia-arachnoid. Common in females.

Trimodal presentation:

a. Subdural – visual loss, papilledema, secondary optic atrophy
b. Extradural – proptosis
c. Combined – originate from arachnoid and burst through the dura to become exophytic causing proptosis

Management is dependent on the status of vision and the size of tumor. Vision intact – irrespective of the site – observe. Progressive visual loss – if tumor is located in the middle or anterior compartment of the orbit – lateral orbitotomy, if located in the apex of the orbit – radiotherapy. Complete loss of vision – surgery. Intracranial extension – transcranial approach.

Cavernous Hemangioma

Commonest benign tumor in adults. It is seen in 2nd and 4th decade. Painless proptosis, enlarges during pregnancy. Ocular movements are full. Encapsulated tumor, good cleavage. Large cavernous spaces, filled with blood. Treatment is lateral orbitotomy.

Neurofibroma

Solitary – seen in adults, chronic painless proptosis, visual loss is minimal, tumor is usually superior and posterior in the orbit, causing upward gaze palsy, tumor is well encapsulated, firm and easy to dissect.

Multicentric – seen in children as disfiguring proptosis and visual loss. Treatment is total orbital exenteration, recurrence is the rule.

Dermoid/Epidermoid

Most frequent developmental cyst of orbit, most common orbital tumor in children, occurs in superior portion of orbit, causes little amount of proptosis. Occasionally it may erode the bone and extend intracranially. Treatment is lateral orbitotomy, in case of intracranial extension – transcranial approach.

Osteoma

Commonest bony tumor of orbit. Arises from frontal or ethmoid sinus. CT scan is confirmatory.

Presents as hard non-tender swelling, causing proptosis. Treatment is excision. Recurrence is common if excision is incomplete.

Hemangiopericytoma

Very rare tumor, presents as chronic painless proptosis. Grossly red or reddish blue and appears to be encapsulated. Histologically is of benign, borderline and malignant subtypes. Metastasizes in 15%.

Fibrous Dysplasia

Non-neoplastic lesion of childhood/adolescence. When involving the orbit, the bones involved are sphenoid, ethmoid, maxilla, zygomatic bone, frontal bone. Painless proptosis, if maxillary bone is involved predominantly. Visual loss if sphenoid bone is involved. There is arrest of immature woven bone into mature lamellar bone. Orange rind appearance is a characteristic feature.

Treatment: If there is optic nerve compression, trancranial approach is used. Radiation is contraindicated.

Mucoceles

Secondary to impacted mucus in a sinus. Proptosis, ophthalmoplegia, headache are common symptoms. Mucocele of posterior ethmoid – causes relapsing and remitting visual loss (mimicking ophthalmoplegic migraine). Sometimes V1, V2 sensory loss.

Diagnosis is by CT, MRI. Treatment is surgical.

Metastasis

In elderly males – Carcinoma lung is a frequent cause and in females – carcinoma breast is a frequent cause. In children– neuroblastoma is a common cause, may be bilateral with sudden exophthalmos and ecchymosis, bone destruction especially of lateral orbital wall. Testicular tumors/leukemias are also seen in children presenting as metastasis.

Pseudotumor

Idiopathic orbital inflammation. Orbital pain, edema of lids and conjunctiva. Diffuse hyperplasia of orbital tissues. Treatment is steroids and radiotherapy.

Lymphoid Tumors

Average age 60 years, painless proptosis. External ocular movements are full. Orbital lymphoid tumors are soft, friable, lack connective tissue. These tumors mould to the globe. 40% involve lacrimal gland. Usually NHL, B-cell lymphomas. D/D – lymphocyte infiltration of Grave's disease. In Grave's disease, lymphocytic infiltrate involves the muscle and spares the tendon.

Rhabdomyosarcoma

Malignant tumor in children. Histologic subtypes are alveolar, botyroid and pleomorphic.

Fibrous Histiocytoma

Most common mesenchymal tumor in adults. May undergo malignant transformation

Lymphangioma

Enlargement may occur secondary to sudden hemorrhage which may lead to formation of chocolate cysts. Infiltrative nature hence difficult to extirpate.

Lacrimal Gland Tumors

10–15% of orbital tumors. 50% of epithelial tumors of lacrimal gland are pleomorphic adenomas and half are malignant. Adenoid cystic carcinoma is the commonest malignant tumor of lacrimal gland. Perineural invasion is common. Mucoepidermoid carcinoma – good prognosis. Lacrimal sac tumors include exophytic and inverted papilloma.

Primary Osteosarcoma

It is a late complication of radiotherapy to eye.

Imaging Findings in Orbital Tumors

Meningioma

Fusiform widening of the nerve/sheath complex. Globular/Sleeve like calcification. Central enhancement. MRI, fat suppression technique – enhancing on contrast, demonstrates intracranial extension.

Optic Nerve Gliomas

Widening of the nerve itself. Associated UBOs (unidentified bright objects) in basal ganglia, brainstem, cerebral and cerebellar white matter. Importance of these lesions – unknown. These lesions can be seen in optic tracts and should not be assumed to necessarily represent extension of optic gliomas.

Cavernous Hemangioma

Because of large blood flow contrast gets diluted, so enhancement is mild. MRI – mixed intensity lesion. Hyperintensity – methemoglobin. Hypointensity – Hemosiderin.

Schwannomas/Neurofibroma-Hypo to iso on T_1W, hyper on T_2W.

Dermoid-Hyper in both T_1W and T_2W, as it contains fat. No enhancement unless inflammation is present.

Hemangiopericytoma-Enhancing on contrast. Lots of flow voids

Rhabdomyosarcoma-CT scan – well circumscribed enhancing mass. MRI – isointense to muscle on T_1W and hyper on T_2W.

Orbital pseudotumor-Hypo on T_1W, Hypo to iso on T_2W. Lymphoma is hyper on T_2W, this feature distinguishes it from pseudotumors. If in doubt, trial of steroids – no improvement – biopsy. Bilateral pseudotumor is seen in Wegner's granulomatosis, sarcoidosis, polyarteritis nodosa. On CT scan – both lymphoma/pseudotumor –are seen as homogenous masses that have irregular margins and enhance an contrast. Both infiltrate the orbital muscle. Lymphoma tends to coat the globe.

Lymphangiomas

Because of bleeds, MRI shows cysts containing hypo and hyper intense signals. Characteristic of blood of different ages producing a "Bubbly" appearance. Calcification may be seen.

Simpson's Grading of Meningioma Excision

i. Macroscopically complete removal with excision of dural attachment and abnormal bone (including sinus resection when involved)
ii. Macroscopically complete excision with diathermy of dural attachment
iii. Macroscopically complete excision without diathermy of dural attachment or of its extradural extensions (e.g. hyperostotic bone)
iv. Partial removal, leaving some tumor in situ
v. Biopsy

Parasagittal Meningiomas (Hakuba Modification of Bonnal and Brotchi)

i. Outer surface of lateral wall of sinus is involved
ii. Recess of sinus is involved
iii. Full lateral wall is involved
iv. Roof is partially involved
v. Lumen is occluded
vi. Sinus is totally occluded

Cavernous Sinus Meningiomas

Grade	Internal carotid artery	Cavernous sinus
i.	Not involved	One area only involved
ii.	Displaced/partially encased	Multiple areas involved
iii.	Total encasement	Multiple areas involved
iv.	Encased and narrowed	Unilateral invasion
v.	Encased with or without narrowing	Bilateral invasion

Clinoidal Meningioma

i. Arises inferior to anterior clinoid. No arachnoid investment between tumor and carotid
ii. Arises from the superior aspect of anterior clinoid. Arachnoid investment present.
iii. Arises from the optic foramen and extends into the optic canal and to the tip of the anterior clinoid. Arachnoid investment may or may not be present.

Tuberculum Sella Meningioma

Olfactory groove and planum sphenoid meningioma depress the anterior visual pathways while as tuberculum sella elevates it. Morbidity and mortality is more if tumor is >3 cm. Recurrence is 10%, Pterional craniotomy and excision is the usual surgical approach. Advantage of pterional craniotomy over subfrontal craniotomy is that olfactory nerve is not at risk.

Sphenoid Wing Meningioma

Divided into clinoidal, alar and pterional. The ICA supplies the tumor through recurrent meningeal artery (a branch of ophthalmic artery) and through the cavernous branches of ICA.

Glomus Jugulare

These are the commonest tumors of the temporal bone. These are usually seen in females on left side and may be familial. These are slow growing, benign chemodectomas. Presentation is hearing loss and tinnitus. A bruit may be heard over the mastoid bone. Otoscopy may reveal a fleshy mass. Presence of Horner's syndrome suggests involvement of carotid artery. Papilledema suggests sigmoid sinus/internal jugular vein block. Erosion of the jugular foramen is best seen on CT scan (bone windows). Contrast MRI is the investigation of choice. MRA demonstrates status of the carotid arteries. A secretory tumor may raise VMA levels in urine. The feeding artery of the tumor is ascending pharyngeal artery. Presurgical embolization may help reduce the vascularity of the tumor. Tumor is removed by lateral skull base approach or infratemporal fossa approach. Facial nerve re-routing is an important surgical step. Tumors ≤ 3 cm are amenable to radiosurgery. The commonest complication of surgery is lower cranial nerve palsy.

Epidermoids and Dermoids

These lesions are essentially benign lesions and arise secondary to defects in gastrulation. The common sites of epidermoids are cerebellopontine angle and parasellar regions. Dermoids can be present both intracranially and in spine. Signs and symptoms depend on the location of the tumors. Epidermoids are commoner than dermoids. Chemical meningitis is usually a feature of epidermoids. Both the lesions are commoner in females. Dermoids occur at a younger age than epidermoids. On CT scan, both the lesions are non-enhancing hypodense lesions. On MRI, epidermoids are hypointense on T_1 weighted sequence and hyperintense on T_2-weighted. On FLAIR (fluid-attenuated-inversion-recovery), the lesion does not invert with CSF, while as arachnoid cyst inverts on FLAIR. Dermoids are hyperintense on both T_1 and T_2-weighted sequences. Dermoids of skull cause lytic bone defects. Epidermoids contain keratin, cholesterol and desquamated epithelium while as hair follicles and sebaceous glands are contents of dermoids. Both the lesions are dealt by surgery. Recurrence is common in epidermoids.

Carcinomatous Meningitis

This leptomeningitic process occurs usually secondary to leukemia/lymphoma. Though solid tumors of body can also rarely manifest like this. The usual symptoms and signs are headache, confusion, visual disturbances and polyradiculopathy. Centrifuging the CSF may yield neoplastic cells. Contrast craniospinal MRI may reveal sugar coating appearance of the leptomeninges. Treatment is palliative and overall prognosis is poor.

Transtemporal Approaches to the Posterior Cranial Fossa

Temporal bone approaches:

a. Middle cranial fossa
   Extended middle cranial fossa
   Middle cranial fossa transtentorial
b. Posterior approach
   Retrolabyrinthine – presigmoid
   Retrolabyrinthine – retrosigmoid

Retrolabyrinthine – transsigmoid
Transotic
Translabyrinthine
Infralabyrinthine
Transcochlear

c. Combined approaches
Petrosal
Infratemporal fossa

Middle Fossa Approach

House's technique identifies greater superficial petrosal nerve (GSPN) – Follows it to the geniculate ganglion, and then proceeds along the labyrinthine segment of the facial nerve to the internal auditory canal (IAC).

Fisch uses the superior semicircular canal (SSC) as the primary landmark.

Garcia – Begins the dissection at the bisection of the angle between GSPN and the arcuate eminence

Indications – Lesions situated lateral within the IAC that have limited extension into the CPA (<1 cm) and where hearing preservation is the goal. Tumors that are medial in position and do not extend to the fundus of the IAC are best approached by posterior approaches (e.g. retrosigmoid approach).

The middle fossa approach gives access to the labyrinthine segment of the facial nerve without sacrificing hearing, thus decompression of the facial nerve in traumatic facial nerve palsy is possible. Selective sectioning of vestibular nerve fibers for Menieres disease, advanced otosclerosis, nerve section for tinnitus, facial nerve repair, repair of middle fossa encephaloceles and CSF leaks through tegmen are also indications for this approach.

Subtemporal Craniotomy

Dura is opened from posterior to anterior direction, it helps to avoid inadvertent elevation of GSPN and subsequent traction injury to the geniculate ganglion and facial nerve. Several landmarks before bone removal can begin over the IAC are:

a. Middle meningeal artery (MMA)
b. Arcuate eminence
c. GSPN
d. Facial hiatus

The foramen spinosum through which the MMA travels, marks the anterior limit of dural elevation. GSPN serves as a landmark for the lateral margin of the horizontal segment of the petrous carotid. Arcuate eminence is drilled till the superior semicircular canal (SSC) is visualized (blue line). In 15%, arcuate eminence is absent. In 50%, it is rotated in relation to the SSC. Localization of the IAC using 2 angles:

GSPN – SSC (120°)

SSC – IAC (60°)

Once the IAC is identified, exposure proceeds from lateral to medial until the entire IAC is exposed along its superior surface. A safer technique is to begin medially exposing first the porus acousticus and then working laterally. At the fundus of IAC, vertical crest (Bill's bar) separates the superior vestibular nerve and 7th nerve is identified. Finally dura over the IAC is opened, first posteriorly over the superior vestibular nerve.

Complications

CSF leak, retraction injury to temporal lobe, seizures, hemiparesis

Extended Middle Fossa Approach – Anterior Petrosectomy

Indications: Anterior petrosectomy provides access to petrous apex and clivus, providing access to the posterior fossa past the carotid artery and 5th, 7th cranial nerves. It is a hearing preservation approach. It can provide additional exposure in the posterior fossa by sacrificing superior semicircular canal (SCC) and labyrinth.

Meningioma and chordoma of the anterior cerebellopontine angle and clivus can be resected through this approach as well as lesions of the petrous apex. Lesions of petrous carotid artery, posterior cavernous sinus, basilar artery and anterior brainstem can be approached. Glassock's triangle is exposed. Boundaries of this triangle– laterally is the line extending from foramen spinosum to the arcuate eminence, medial is the GSPN and at the base the 3rd division of the trigeminal nerve. Miller advocates drilling bone along an imaginary line extending from the tip of the vertical crest to the junction of the petrous carotid artery and cranial nerve V_3 until the cochlea is identified. Main advantage of this approach is hearing preservation. Drawback is limited exposure of the posterior fossa.

Middle Fossa Transtentorial Approach (Kawase)

Indications are aneurysms of the midbasilar artery, petroclival meningioma that extend into the parasellar region (spheno-petroclival meningioma). It can be accomplished with an anterior or posterior petrosectomy or a combined petrosal approach. Hearing is preserved.

Technique

The dura is opened above and below the superior petrosal sinus (SPS). Cranial nerves 4th and 5th are identified. Superior petrosal sinus is clipped between cranial nerves 5th and 7th with care not to sacrifice petrosal vein. Tentorium is cut until tentorial notch is seen. Tentorium can be tented up with retention sutures exposing the petroclival region from cranial nerves 3rd and 7th Mobilization of 5th nerve can be accomplished in Meckels cave. Dorello's canal is seen through this exposure.

Complications

Injury to 4th cranial nerve as a result of tentorial incision. The risk of temporal lobe retraction is higher than in the former procedures.

Retrolabyrinthine presigmoid – It was first described by Hitselberg in 1972. The concept of this procedure is based on its allowing entry into the cerebellopontine angle (CPA) anterior to the sigmoid sinus, thus lessening the need for cerebellar retraction. Originally described for partial sectioning of the fibers of the sensory roots of cranial nerve 5th for trigeminal neuralgia. Used for selective sectioning of the vestibular division of cranial nerve 8th for vertigo and for endolymphatic duct surgery. Can be used to remove small acoustic tumors.

Disadvantages

Limited exposure, which can be compromised even further by a large dominant SS or when the mastoid air space is contracted (crowded mastoid).

Trans-sigmoid Approach

Can be used as a part of any posterior transpetrosal approach. Exposure is increased by ligating SS usually between superior and inferior petrous sinus or between vein of Labbe and superior petrosal sinus. A preoperative angiogram is essential to document the patency of the torcula. Temporary clipping across sigmoid sinus for assessing temporal lobe swelling or cerebellar swelling can be done.

Retrosigmoid (Suboccipital) Approach

Suboccipital craniectomy is completed between the transverse sinus above and the sigmoid sinus laterally. Maximal approach for posterior fossa lesions is achieved. Dura is opened based superiorly and laterally.

Complications

In 9% of cases a high jugular bulb may make drilling of the meatus impossible and is hence fraught with increased bleeding and air embolism.

Translabyrinthine Approach

Indications: Done in patients with non-serviceable hearing and for vestibular neurectomy in intractable vertigo when hearing is lost.

Surgical technique: Sinodural-angle is exposed. The angle between the sigmoid sinus [SS], the middle fossa dura above and posterior fossa dura below is called sinodural angle. The roughly triangular area of bone bounded by sigmoid sinus, superior petrosal sinus and bony labyrinth (solid angle) is known as Trautmann's triangle. This bone is drilled to expose the presigmoid posterior fossa dura.

Advantages: After drilling the labyrinth, the tumor is encountered together with superior and inferior vestibular nerve and facial nerve is protected. It is in contrast to middle fossa approach where facial nerve is immediately beneath the dura.

Disadvantages: Time consuming and sacrifice of hearing. Inadequate exposure of tentorium, foramen magnum and petroclival area. It may be difficult to control vascular structures, e.g. anterior inferior cerebellar artery (AICA) if inadvertent injury occurs.

Transotic Approach

It allows more extensive approach. Dissection can be done anteriorly to visualize CPA and petrous apex.

Indications

Same as translabyrinthine approach. Schwannoma, meningioma, hemangioma, arachnoid cysts and mucosal cysts involving IAC can be dealt. Transotic approach circumvents the problem of high jugular bulb. This approach can be used for large vestibular schwannomas because it provides an additional corridor inferior to 7th nerve. Other advantage is that there is less chance of CSF leak because of closure of eustachian tube.

Transcochlear

Developed by House and Hitselberg. Cochlea is removed. Facial nerve is transposed

Indications: Large tumor of CPA anterior to internal acoustic meatus and approximately 2/3rd of clivus and for aneurysms of middle and lower basilar artery.

Complications: Loss of hearing, sometimes GSPN is injured which results in dry eye, facial nerve palsy because of traction via GSPN, CSF leak, meningitis.

Infralabyrinthine Approach

Indications: Cholesterol granuloma of petrous apex. Can be used in conjunction with suboccipital approach for resection of meningioma of petrous ridge with extension into temporal bone but without involvement of labyrinth. Hearing is preserved. Difficulties:

A high jugular bulb will give small corridor. Preoperative coronal CT scan will depict the gap between jugular bulb and labyrinth, a height <1 cm is a contraindication for the procedure. Complications like injury to 7th nerve, jugular bulb, CSF leak, etc.

Esthesioneuroblastoma

This tumor arises from olfactory epithelium of the nasal cavity. It has a bimodal distribution, males and females are equally involved. Epistaxis and nasal obstruction are common complaints. Nasal inspection reveals a fleshy mass in the nose. The tumor may extend into the anterior cranial fossa and orbits. MRI clearly delineates the extent of the tumor. CT may show the amount of bony destruction. Cervical nodes are a favorite site for metastasis. Tumor is staged by modified Kadish staging which has been seen to correlate with the outcome. In stage A and B, there is no intracranial extension; intracranial extension is seen in stage C and metastasis in stage D. Histological grading has not been seen to consistently predict the outcome. Treatment is surgery and radiochemotherapy. Recurrence is usual. Survival in stage D is short.

Choroid Plexus Papillomas

These benign tumors arise from neuroepithelial lining of choroid plexus. These tumors usually are seen in children. Lateral ventricles are the commonest sites. This tumor is in contra-distinction to other pediatric tumors which are commonly seen in infratentorial compartment. Common symptoms are features of raised ICP. This tumor is notorious for production of excessive amounts of CSF. The etiology of hydrocephalus is excessive CSF production and mechanical obstruction. These tumors calcify and intensely enhance on contrast. These tumors can get complicated by carcinoma. Brain invasion is usually a feature of choroids plexus carcinoma. Surgical excision is usually through transcortical route. Survival rates are high if the excision of the tumor is complete or near complete.

Cranial Ependymomas

These tumors are common in children. These tumors arise from the floor of the 4th ventricle near area postrema. Vomiting is a salient complaint. Hydrocephalus is common. Other features of midline posterior fossa syndrome may exist. MRI is the investigation of choice. Calcification and hemorrhage are common. Incidence of calcification in ependymomas is higher than in medulloblastomas, but the overall incidence of medulloblastomas is much higher than in ependymomas; hence the commonest posterior fossa midline tumor in children with calcifications is medulloblastoma. CSF dissemination is known. In adults, ependymomas are common in supratentorial compartment. Surgery followed by chemoradiotherapy is the treatment option. Overall prognosis is poor. Histopathology reveals perivascular pseudorosettes and ependymal rosettes. Immunohistochemistry reveals positivity for S-100 protein and vimentin. Aberrations in chromosome 22 is the commonest anomaly.

Medulloblastomas

Medulloblastoma is considered to be one among the primitive neuroectodermal tumors (PNET's). These tumors are common in children and constitute about 1/4th of all pediatric brain tumors. Clinical presentation is of posterior fossa syndrome. Calcification is seen in about 1/3rd of tumors, less than in ependymomas. Imaging reveals an iso to hypodense lesion with or without calcifications. CSF rim is usually seen anterior to the tumor at the level of 4th ventricle, while as in ependymomas, since these arise from the 4th ventricular floor, this CSF cleft is not seen. Treatment is surgery followed by radiochemotherapy. Staging of the tumor is done by TNM stage (Changs staging). These are WHO grade IV tumors. Histopathology reveals true rosettes. Synaptophysin stains positive in these tumors. Medulloblastomas have been reported in patients with P53 mutations.

Colloid Cysts

These are located in the roof of the third ventricle near foramen of Monro. These arise from the remnants of post velar arch. These are benign lesions and because of their strategic location these may cause acute hydrocephalus and sudden death. Headache is the commonest symptom and headache classically gets relieved by change in the head posture. Classical drop attacks are because of acute hydrocephalus causing compression on the leg fibers of the corticospinal tract. CT shows non-enhancing hyperdense or isodense lesion depending on the viscosity of the contents of the colloid cyst. Stereotactic aspirations of the cyst have been tried in the past but the cyst recollects again. Other options in the past have been bilateral VP shunts to decompress both the lateral ventricles. Endoscopic excision usually is never complete. Open surgery and complete excision of the cyst is the gold standard. In absence of hydrocephalus, transcallosal approach is preferred and in presence of hydrocephalus, a transventricular-subchoroidal route is the corridor of choice. Transcortical-transventricular approach has the disadvantage of inducing seizures while as transcallosal interforniceal approach runs the risk of injury to fornix.

Dysembryoplastic Neuroepithelial Tumor [DNET]

These are benign tumors usually involving the temporal lobe. Most of the tumors have cysts within. Tumors may be calcified. The tumor mimics gangliogliomas on imaging. Seizure is the commonest symptom. These are WHO I tumors. Surgery is the treatment of choice.

Low Grade Gliomas

These are glial tumors of the CNS for which the expected survival is usually 5–10 years. Mostly young adults are involved. Seizure is a common symptom. Other symptoms are of raised ICP. Neurodeficit depends on the location of the tumor. The tumor usually shows no or minimal enhancement. Calcifications may be seen in up to 20% of tumors. MRI usually reveals a hypo to iso-intense lesion on T_1-weighted sequence and hyperintense on T_2-weighted. Good prognostic factors in low grade gliomas are young age, absence of neurologic deficits, seizures as presenting symptom, no raised ICP features. Low grade gliomas can be managed conservatively till the period when either enhancement increases or neurodeficits set in. De-differentiation into higher grade tumors is a drawback of conservative management. Oligodendrogliomas with 1p 19q mutations are chemosensitive. Treatment is surgical debulking. Tumors involving the eloquent cortex or tumors with no mass effect can be managed conservatively.

Brainstem Gliomas

These are common in children and account for 20% of CNS tumors. According to Epstein classification, these tumors are classified into focal diffuse, cervicomedullary and dorsally exophytic. Diffuse variety is the commonest. Usual presentation is of multiple cranial nerve deficits. Hydrocephalus sets in late in the disease process. Ataxia is another common symptom. MRI is the investigation of choice. Tumors as most of the other tumors are hypointense on T_1-weighted and hyperintense on T_2-weighted. In case of focal or dorsally exophytic subtypes, surgery has a role. However in diffuse brainstem gliomas which usually involve the pons, surgery is attended with high morbidity and mortality rates. Hence radiotherapy is considered primary modality of treatment in such cases.

VON HIPPEL-LINDAU DISEASE (VHL)

Criteria

Type 1: Without pheochromocytoma

Type 2A: With pheochromocytoma and Renal cell carcinoma (RCC)

Type 2B: With pheochromocytoma but without RCC

Genetic defect in short arm of chromosome-3.

75% of hemangioblastomas involve – cerebellum. 23% – spinal cord. 2% – brainstem, etc.

20% of cerebellar hemangioblastoma have VHL. All VHL have cerebellar hemangioblastoma.

50% of VHL have retinal hemangioma but only 20% are symptomatic. 40% have RCC, 30% have pancreatic cysts. 5% have pheochromocytoma. 10% have increased erythropoietin. 3/4th have nodule with cyst, nodule is hypodense on CT, enhancing briskly on contrast. Tumor is composed of vascular spaces lined with proliferating endothelial tissue. RCC has to be differentiated from hemangioma on histopathology. In RCC – EMA positive cells contain glycogen and cells display mitotic figures, in hemangioma - tumor cells are EMA negative, cells contain fat and mitosis is absent. Death is due to RCC, pheochromocytoma, pancreatic carcinoma.

Hemangioblastoma

It is a benign vascular tumor. Male predominance, Age–40 years. In familial – age is less. About 1/4th tumors are associated with Von Hippel-Lindau disease. VHL gene is a tumor suppressor gene. In sporadic cases – loss of both copies of the alleles. In familial – where one copy is already absent, loss of only one copy of the allele. Embryology – arises from the primitive choroid plexus which gets trapped into the developing cerebellum at 12th week of life. The clinical diagnosis of VHL is based on the presence of capillary hemangioblastoma in the central nervous system or retina associated with VHL associated tumors, or a family history. There are Type 1, Type 2A and Type 2B variants of VHL. Only type 1 is without pheochromocytoma. VHL is an autosomal-dominant disease which is transmitted through VHL gene. Cerebellum is the commonest site of involvement by hemangioblastomas. Other sites are spinal cord, optic nerve, brainstem and filum terminale. The commonest symptoms are of raised ICP. Optic nerve hemangioblastoma presents with severe visual loss. Spinal hemangioblastomas may cause SAH. The commonest segment of spinal cord involved is the dorsal cord. About half of the spinal cord hemangioblastomas have tumor syrinx. 24-hour urinary vanillylmandelic acid levels of >8 mg are suggestive of pheochromocytoma. Contrast CT abdomen can help in diagnosing these lesions. Renal cell carcinoma: 25% patients VHL get it Special features of RCC in VHL – bilateral, multicentricity – early age – male predominance.

10% of VHL develop pheochromocytoma. Pheochromocytoma in VHL is bilateral. Other condition whether B/L pheochromocytoma is seen is MEN-1a, NF-I and familial pheochromocytoma. Polycythemia is seen in 15% of hemangioblastoma, it is not seen in spinal hemangioblastoma. Polycythemia may act as a marker for recurrence after treatment Polycythemia is seen in 1/4th of patients with hemangioblastoma. This is secondary to increased levels of erythropoietin secreted by the tumor cells. Contrast craniospinal MRI is the investigation of choice for hemangioblastoma. The tumor reveals intense enhancement. T_2-weighted images best display flow voids suggestive of increased vascularity.

Contrast craniospinal MRI is the investigation of choice for hemangioblastoma. The tumor reveals intense enhancement. T_2-weighted images best display flow voids suggestive of increased vascularity. Angiography: four patterns:

1. Vascular mural nodule within an avascular cyst
2. Doughnut ring of abnormal vessels surrounding an avascular space representing an avascular cyst
3. Large solid vascular mass
4. Multiple small widely separated vascular nodules

HPE: endothelial cells, pericytes

USG abdomen: Renal cysts

Ophthalmological examination–retinal angiomas and optic nerve hemangioblastoma.

60% spinal hemangioblastomas are intramedullary, 40% are EM-ID.

Syrinx is common – because of transudation of fluid and dissection of gray matter.

Treatment is surgical. Tumor shall be excised in toto. Postoperative radiotherapy has a role in incompletely resected tumors in a setting of VHL. Histopathology reveals stromal cells with rich capillary network. The tumor qualifies for a WHO grade I tumor. Operative mortality for cystic lesion – 2%. Operative mortality of solid lesion – 15%. Recurrence rate is 3–10% after total excision.

Chondrosarcoma

Three histologic types:

Classic, Mesenchymal and dedifferentiated.

Skull base – Classic variety is the commonest. Age – 2nd to 3rd decade, extradural in location.

Tumor origin may involve clivus, sphenoethmoid junction, cavernous sinus, foramen magnum, petrous apex. Chordoma is midline, chondroma is – median. CT-isodense, MRI T_1-Isointense, T_2-hyperintense Bone destruction, Calcification – 40%. Heterogenous contrast enhancement.

Untreated chordomas – 1 year survival, after surgery – 1.5 years, Surgery + Radiotherapy – 5 years

5 year survival – 33%, 10 year survival – 20%

Surgical Approaches

Anterior—Transoral, transphenoid, transethmoid, maxillary, subfrontal

Lateral—Pterional, subtemporal transpetrous, subtemporal – infratemporal,

Lateral and posterolateral – presigmoid, retrolabyrinthine, translabyrinthine

Heavy particle radiation is effective.

Radiosurgery for small lesions.

Trigeminal Neuromas

These are benign tumors of 5th cranial nerve. These usually arise from roots or ganglion. Clinical symptoms include trigeminal neuropathy, weakness of muscles of mastication, deafness, cerebello-pontine angle syndrome. Deafness may be conductive or sensorineural. Tumors arising from the ganglion are more painful. If the tumor extends into post-fossa – symptom of 7th and 8th nerves. 10% of trigeminal neuromas have no 5th nerve, symptoms, 6% of 5th nerve tumors have 8th nerve dysfunction. *[10% of 8th nerve schwannomas have 5th nerve symptoms*]. Trigeminal pain is common if tumor arises from ganglion (50%) than from root (30%).

Tumors are located in inter-dural plane. Jefferson has classified trigeminal schwannomas into A, B, C, depending upon whether the tumor is located in middle fossa, posterior fossa or both respectively. These tumors cause a classical truncated appearance of the petrous margin. Small tumors (≤3 cm) are amenable to radiosurgery. The common surgical corridors are orbitozygomatic and subtemporal. Tumors located in the posterior fossa need sub-occipital craniotomy.

X-ray – middle fossa erosion, erosion of pterygoid plates, erosion of petrous tip (truncation). MRI – hypo on T_1W, hypo on T_2W, homogenous enhancement. DSA – medial displacement of precavernous segment, shift of basilar artery, 20% have tumor blush from branches of precavernous segment and ECA.

Surgical approaches - Orbito-zygomatic approach, Subtemporal intradural/extradural, Subtemporal transtentorial.

Facial nerve schwannoma

It is the 3rd cranial nerve in order of frequency which gives rise to schwannoma. Arises from sensory fibers, commonest segment involved is tympanic segment. Presentation is of hearing loss, facial palsy (50%). 20% have acute facial nerve palsy and 30% have insidious onset. Treatment – Non-serviceable ear – translabyrinthine approach, serviceable ear – middle fossa approach.

Paraganglioma of Carotid Body and Temporal Bone

Carotid body – more common – 12% are malignant, equal M:F ratio

Temporal bone – 3% – malignant, common in females

Shamblin classification for carotid body tumor

Grade I-can be dissected from carotid artery

Grade II-Partial encasement of carotid artery

Grade III-Total encasement of carotid artery

Glasscock-Jackson Classification for Temporal Bone Paraganglioma

i. Small tumors involving jugular bulb, mastoid, middle ear
ii. Tumor extending under internal auditory canal, might have intracranial extension
iii. Tumor extending into petrous apex, might have intracranial tumor
iv. Tumor extending beyond petrous apex into clivus or infratemporal fossa, might have intracranial extension.

Primary CNS Lymphoma

Associated with AIDS, immune-suppression. In transplant patients risk is 100-fold

Age – 4th–6th decade

Signs and Aymptoms

Raised ICP (60%), stroke, e.g. hemianopsia (7%), demyelination – meningioencephalitis (25%).

About 5% of patients of primary CNS lymphoma have systemic disease at the time of diagnosis. Nearly all PCNSL are associated with EBV in HIV related cases while as only 50% of systemic lymphomas in HIV population is EBV related.

Imaging

Periventricular, usually single, multiple in immune suppressed, subependymal spread, meningeal involvement also seen, reactive gliosis + meningeal involvement and skull involvement – usually in secondary CNS lymphoma.

CT – Hyperdense, enhances on contrast.

MRI – Isointense on T_1 and T_2.

Histopathology-B-cell, angiocentricity, central necrosis if HIV associated, bleed and calcification – unusual, sometimes ring enhancement (+), edema is less as compared to GBM/metastasis

D/D – Toxoplasmosis, abscess, metastasis, GBM, Dural based lymphoma can mimic a meningioma.

Treatment – Steroid effect lasts only for 6 months, effect stops – 1 week later after stopping, before biopsy steroids should be stopped.

Surgery – If impending herniation, or mass effect, no response to steroids, or if recurrence after radiochemotherapy

RT – to tumor (60cGy) to tumor and whole brain (40cGy)

Chemotherapy – CHOP regime, based on breakdown of blood-brain barrier (bbb) since the bbb gets restored after initial response, so concerns about further chemotherapy. So people have started intra-arterial mannitol to break bbb then give iv cyclophosphamide + high dose methotrexate (MXT)

Sandwich treatment: High dose-MXT + steroids – radiotherapy – High dose cytosine arabinoside.

PCV regime has also been used as adjuvant therapy after RT.

In presence of meningeal lymphoma – Ommaya reservoir – instill MXT – 15 mg, Hydrocortisone 15 mg, Cytoarabinoside – 75 mg twice weekly – till CSF is clear, then weekly for 1 month, then monthly for 1–2 years.

Intracranial Sarcoma

Presentation is raised ICP, seizures and neurodeficit. Arises from brain, meninges, cranial nerves, skull, secondaries from extracranial sarcomas

Common in children, M:F = equal

Origin:

i. Denovo
ii. Arising within a glioma (gliosarcoma)
iii. Meningosarcoma
iv. Postradiation

Histopathological subtypes – Fibrosarcoma, spindle cell sarcoma, polymorphic sarcoma

Gliosarcoma – hard, well delineated, attached to dura, may mimic a meningioma at surgery and even on DSA. Gliosarcoma common in temporal lobe, center of gliosarcoma is necrotic, median survival after surgery is 4 months. Post-radiation sarcoma - mean latent period – 10 years, Histopathology-usually a fibrosarcoma. Treatment is surgery.

Meningeal Hemangiopericytoma

Arises from perivascular pericytes (mesenchymal component) of meninges. Common in males, 35–45 years. Highly vascular, from pial and dural vessels. Sites – parasagittal, tentorial, sphenoid ridge. Does not induce hyperostosis. CT/MRI– same as meningioma. Positive for vimentin, negative for epithelial membrane antigen (EMA). Treatment – surgical excision, preoperative embolization. High chances of local recurrence and metastasis (50%). RT has a role – 4000–6000 cGy. Adriamycin has a role.

Choroid Plexus Papilloma (CPP)

Benign tumor, ependymal origin. In children from trigone of lateral ventricle, in adults common in 4th ventricle. Hydrocephalus, papilledema, increased ICP without localization. CSF production increases, obstruction of CSF path, recurrent bleeding, subarachnoid scarring – all contribute to hydrocephalus. CSF analysis reveals – increased pressure, increased protein xanthochromia. Radiology- tumor calcification (20%). CT-isodense and intense enhancement. DSA tumor blush fed by choroidal artery, early venous shunting is seen in choroid plexus carcinoma and ependymoma, this feature can differentiate them from CPP. Treatment – surgery

Intracranial Lipomas

Arises from abnormal persistence and maldifferentiation of menix primitive. Clinical – 1/3rd are asymptomatic and 2/3rd are symptomatic. Symptoms depend upon the site. Associated anomalies are also common. Imaging–lipomas are hypodense on CT scan, calcification sometimes may be present, no enhancement, MRI – hyper on T_1 and T_2, no edema, no enhancement. DSA – in corpus callosal lipomas there may be single pericallosal artery, or pericallosal artery aneurysm

Pericallosal lipomas: constitute 50% of intracranial lipomas, seizures-common, headache – next common

Cerebellopontine lipomas – more in males, 8th nerve dysfunction, no intervening capsule between it and the 8th nerve. Surgery is not indicated for 2 reasons – it is not known that symptoms are caused by it, and preservation of nerve is very difficult.

Sylvian lipoma – MCA travels through it, symptoms – seizures, no surgery is needed.

Ambient and Quadrigeminal cistern lipomas – 4th cranial nerve travels through it, it may be duplicated or even absent, hydrocephalus is secondary to aqueductal malformation and rarely because of compression, other signs and symptoms are of upward gaze paresis, ataxia, VP shunt needed.

Medullary cistern lipoma – encloses lower cranial nerves however never causes lower cranial nerve palsy, causes truncal and appendicular ataxia.

Gliomas

30% of grade I – progress to glioblastoma multiforme (GBM). 50% of grade II – progress to GBM at recurrence. 50% of recurrent oligodendroglioma are malignant and 20% recur as GBM

Good prognosis factors for low grade gliomas

Young age, no preoperative neurologic deficit, long history of symptoms, seizure as the presenting symptom, gross total surgical removal.

Outcome for low grade gliomas:

Median survival – 7 years, 5 years survival – 65%, 10 years survival – 40%.

Tuberous Sclerosis (TS)

Definite criteria for TS

One primary feature OR

Two secondary features OR

One secondary + two tertiary features

Probable TS

One secondary + one tertiary OR

Three tertiary

Probable

One secondary OR

Two tertiary

Vogt's triad – seizures, mental retardation, adenoma sebacum, 6% have subependymal giant cell astrocytoma (SEGA). Subependymal nodules – look like candle drippings, are calcified, may become malignant.

Ataxia Telengectasia

Autososmal dominant, degeneration of purkinje cells of cerebellum. Signs and symptoms- ataxia, cutaneous telangiectasia of face, degeneration of myelinated fibers of peripheral nerves and posterior columns, degenerative changes in posterior roots and sympathetic ganglia. Patients are prone to develop leukemia/lymphomas. Death occurs by 2nd decade.

Sturge-Weber Syndrome

Angiomas in V_1 or V_2 distribution of trigeminal nerve and leptomeningeal venous angiomatosis.

The underlying brain shows cortical atrophy and calcification of 2nd, and 3rd cortical layers. Presentation is seizures. Klippel-Trenaunay-Weber syndrome is a spinal variant of Sturge-Weber syndrome.

Hereditary Hemorrhagic Telangiectasia (HHT)

Autosomal dominant disorder. Systemic fibrovascular dysplasia. Patients have telangiectasia, AVM, aneurysm. Any patient with SAH, epistaxis and cutaneous telangiectasia,, should be suspected of having HHT.

Ganglioglioma

Mean age of onset is 12-years, temporal lobe is the commonest lobe involved, commonest symptom is seizure, raised ICP is rare. Radiologically – 10% lesions are calcified. CT scan – Iso/hypo/hyper dense, enhancement in 50% cases. MRI – Hypo on T_1, hyper on T_2, swollen gyri on T_2. For seizures AEDs. Treatment – surgical. If recurrence occurs – re-exploration. Radiotherapy is indicated if HPE reveals malignant features.

HPE – multipolar displaced neurons with neoplastic glial element, reticular fibers also seen, electron microscopy – reveals dense core granules in cells, immunohistochemistry – positive for synaptophysin.

Metastatic Brain Tumors

18% cancers in body seed to brain. 5% are solitary, common in supratentorial compartment. Cancer lung is the commonest cause of brain metastasis. In lung cancers, adenocarcinoma and undifferentiated cancers spread more than squamous cell carcinoma. After cancer lung, breast cancer is the second source of metastasis. Of all tumors, melanoma has the highest tendency to seed to brain, and causes hemorrhagic metastasis. Presentation depends upon the site, 10% stroke like secondary to bleed, 10% have papilledema, focal weakness is seen in 40%. Seizures are more common in multiple metastasis.

Patients with metastasis to pituitary gland are mostly asymptomatic however in some patients.

Symptomatic triad of headache, visual symptoms, diabetes insipidus is seen. Predilection of posterior pituitary lobe to metastasis is because of abundant blood supply through inferior hypophyseal artery. Metastasis can seed a meningioma—because of abundant blood supply. Treatment: Surgery, surgery is indicated if the primary is well controllable.

Other indications for surgery in metastases – tumor bleed, metastasis with mass effect, posterior fossa metastasis with hydrocephalus.

Radiosurgery is indicated if size <3 cm, no mass effect

Chemotherapy for germ cell tumor, breast carcinoma

Radiotherapy is the primary treatment for leukemia, lymphoma, germ cell tumor

About 15% of patients with systemic cancer have primary brain tumors rather than metastasis so tissue sampling is necessary.

Meningiomas

Increased incidence with age. Meningiomas – 15% of brain tumors, 25% of spine tumors.

Intraventricular meningioma – 10% in children, 4% in adults. In children, male predominance, childhood meningiomas are more malignant. In adults F:M = 2:1. High association with breast cancer. Chromosome 22, deletion of tumor suppressor gene. Tumors possess D_1 (not D_2), estrogen, androgen, progesterone, glucocorticoids and somatostatin receptors. Highest recurrence with sphenoid wing meningiomas. Aneuploidy is associated with malignant tumors, more peritumoral edema, large size, multiple tumors tending to recur.

Imaging: Calcification 20% enlargement of foramen spinosum. Hyperostosis (20%).

Angiogram- mother-in-law appearance, sunburst appearance, tortuous arteries and veins, tumor blush, corkscrew appearance of vessels. CT-hyperdense on plain and enhancement on contrast, bone hyperostosis, and on MRI most of them are isointense on T_1 and T_2-weighted sequences, however depending on the histopathology each meningioma has a different intensity signal. Besides, MRI shows flow voids on T_2-weighted sequence and dural tail on contrast.

Epidermoids, Dermoids

Ectodermal inclusion tumors, benign, slow growing. Dermoids present at 20-years and epidermoids at 20–40 years. Dermoids are midline in location. Dermoid contain a cystic lining and contains stratified squamous epithelium, teeth, bones and sebaceous glands and hair. Midline dermoid cysts are usually associated with spina bifida, cleft lip/palate. In bones dermoids cause lytic lesions with sclerotic margins.

Vestibular Schwannoma [VS]

10% have 7th nerve palsy. 10% have 5th nerve symptoms usually sensory because motor fibers are resistant and located inside. Hemifacial spasm can also be seen. 10% have no hearing loss.

Two Stages of Growth

Intracanalicular

Extracanalicular

Grades-T_1 – intracranalicular, T_2 intra + extracanalicular, T_{3a} – filling the cerebellopontine cistern, T_{3b} – reaching up to the brainstem, T_4 – distorting the brainstem.

Size – 2.5 cm will cause audiovestibular symptoms, 2.5–3.5 cm will cause audiovestibular and trigeminal symptoms, >3.5 cm will lead to any other additional symptom.

Usual gap between audiovestibular and trigeminal symptom is 1.5–2 years. There is no coordination between size and degree of hearing loss. Stapedial reflex- Highly sensitive (95%) but poor specificity. Speech discrimination score of <90% is abnormal, up to 75% of auditory fibers should be damaged before it produces a pure tone loss. This test has a very low sensitivity. Brainstem evoked response audiometry cannot be done if hearing loss is >70 dB. Interaurel latency is more specific, up to 0.2 millisec is normal. Sensitivity and specificity of BERA is 90%. Contrast MRI is more sensitive to pick-up small tumors than BERA. 10% of [VS] have NF-2. Purely intracanalicular – 15%. Purely extracanalicular – 10%. Both – 75%. Peritumoral cysts are seen with tumors >25 mm in size.

Cerebellar Astrocytoma

These constitute10% of pediatric CNS tumors, peak age–8 year, M:F = equal, 10% malignant. Presentation is of raised ICP, ataxia, nystagmus which is in the direction of the lesion. Vermian astrocytoma (85%)- usually solid. Hemispheric tumor is cystic. Bleed into the tumor is one of the causes of rapid deterioration. Imaging- nodules – enhance, but cyst wall does not. Prognosis is good.

Medulloblastoma

20% CNS tumors in children M:F – 4:3. Children with medulloblastoma are older than children with ependymoma. Peak age– 7 years. Symptoms and signs- raised ICP.

Treatment – shunt, 19% chances of metastasis

Prognostic factors – Age <2 years and neurological deficit-bad prognosis, age >7 years – good prognosis. Stage of tumor dictates the prognosis. Staging has been proposed by Chang.

Histopathological Subtypes

Desmoplastic – good prognosis

Medulloblastoma with extreme nodularity-good prognosis

Medullomyoblastoma – bad prognosis

Treatment – surgery

Radiotherapy: 5000 – 5500 cGy tumor bed
4000 – 4500 cGy whole brain
3000 – 3500 cGy Spine

Chemotherapy – (PCV) prednisolone, CCNU, Vincristine.

Brainstem Gliomas

15% of CNS tumors in children

Epstein classification

a. Diffuse infiltrating
b. Exophytic
c. Focal
d. Cervicomedullary

Age – usually <20 year, can occur in adolescence also. Vomiting is a common feature since tumors arise from the floor of 4th ventricle. Initially tumors do not enhance, but as the time goes, tumor starts attaining malignant characteristics and starts enhancing. Diffuse tumor – bad prognosis. Median survival – 18 months. 50% are malignant tumors.

Treatment – surgery for exophytic and focal solid or cystic tumors.

If after surgery for a focal solid lesion, there is 50% or less residual tumor and patient is neurologically preserved – no need for radiochemotherapy. Patient can be followed up, any deterioration or increase in size will warrant radio-chemotherapy. In case after surgery, patient has not improved – radio-chemotherapy. For diffuse tumors – radio-chemotherapy.

Ependymomas

5% of pediatric tumors. Mean age – 5 years. Male predominance. 1/2 supratentorial, 1/2 infratentorial. In adults – 1/3rd supratentorial and 2/3rd infratentorial. Infratentorial – solid, Supratentorial – cystic

Treatment – surgery, radiotherapy – 4500 rads, chemotherapy has a role in delaying recurrence.

Operative mortality – 10%, 5 year survival – 60%, 10 year survival – 50%.

Prognostic Factors

a. Tumor grade
b. Post-op residual tumor

Median survival 50-months in supratentorial and 30-months in infratentorial.

Pituitary Tumors

MEN-I – 20% patients have pituitary tumors. Only 3% pituitary tumors have MEN-I. Sparsely granulated tumors are more aggressive, common in females, rapidly growing. 99% of acromegaly is caused by pituitary tumors. There is correlation between tumor size and PRL levels. Therapy for prolactinomas with Bromocriptine induces fibrosis, calcification and amyloid deposition in tumor

ACTH-producing Adenomas

These secrete ACTH and endorphins. In Cushing's disease: 80% are microadenomas and 20% are macroadenomas, 10% of microadenomas are invasive and 60% of macroadenomas are invasive.

Diencephalic Syndrome

Cause – tumors of diencephalon, i.e. hypothalamus, optic nerve glioma, suprasellar arachnoid cysts, epidermoids, craniopharyngioma, suprasellar germinoma. Children are emaciated but appear muscular because of loss of subcutaneous fat. Emaciation is disproportionate to the amount of vomiting and anorexia. Rotatory nystagmus in 50%. Growth hormone (GH) levels will be higher, these levels would not improve after adequate caloric intake, a feature which differentiates it from anorexia nervosa. Lipolysis is secondary to GH, though in acromegaly and gigantism there is no lipolysis. Treatment – directed to cause.

Craniopharyngioma

Presents as raised ICP, visual loss, short stature, diabetes insipidus, 5–30% of craniopharyngiomas have hydrocephalus.

Endocrine deficiency is as –

60% have GH deficiency, 50% have FSH and LH deficiency, 30% have ACTH deficiency, 30% have TSH deficiency.

Blood supply of craniopharyngioma: Acom artery, Pcom artery, meningohypophyseal trunk, never from posterior circulation unless it invades the floor of 3rd ventricle. Postoperative diabetes insipidus occurs in 70%. Recurrence – after total resection is seen in 19%, after subtotal resection in – 60% whereas after subtotal resection + radiotherapy – 29% patients have recurrence. 10% survival is 92% after total resection and 90% after subtotal + radiotherapy. Postoperative neuropsychological dysfunction occurs in 40%. Vision improves in 90% after surgery.

Low Grade Gliomas (LGGs)

Advantages of surgery

Debulk it, 2 log cell kill and make it amenable to radiotherapy.

Reduce the chances of dedifferentiation.

Achieve biopsy.

Reduce the proliferating pool.

Decrease the number of inherently resistant cell pool to radiotherapy.

Points against surgery

Chance of neurological deficit.

Length of survival does not depend on amount of debulking

Amount of cells which can be tackled by bodies immune system – 10^5

After Radiotherapy - Tumor can grow in 3 ways

Early - because of edema, Delayed – because of demyelination, Late – Necrosis (6 m–2 years)

Hypothalamic Glioma

Classification by Begard et al:

i. Extends from chiasm anteriorly
ii. Chiasm and extends superiorly into 3rd ventricle
iii. Extends into 3rd ventricle to varying extent
iv. Extends posteriorly into the optic tracts

Indications for Considering Observation in Vestibular Schwannoma

Long h/o auditory symptoms in a patient of any age and size of tumor.

Elderly patients with mild symptoms.

Incidental with no symptoms.

Intrameatal tumor with non-serviceable hearing loss.

Sites of Glomus

Glomus jugulare. Glomus intravagale. Carotid body tumor. Glomus tympanicum (tympanic branch of 9th cranial nerve). Spine, orbit, adrenal, organ of zuckerkandl, bladder wall.

Temporal bone paraganglioma: *These arise from:*

1. Tympanic branch of 9th nerve
2. Adventitia of jugular bulb

3. Tympanic canaliculus
4. Promontory
5. Lesser petrosal nerve
6. Auricular branch of vagus

Branches from ascending pharyngeal artery supply the paraganglia of the temporal bone

In patients with positive family history of paragangliomas 1/3rd will have a second paraganglioma

Histiocytosis X

Diagnosis

Presumptive – Light microscopy

Probable – Positive staining for S_{100} + CD_4

Definitive – Birbeck granule + CD_1

Types

i. Eosinophilic granuloma
ii. Hand-Schiller-Christian disease -Bony lesions, exophthalmos, diabetes insipidus
iii. Letter-Sewer disease – Acute fever, pancytopenia, hepatomegaly, skin eruptions and pulmonary infiltrates

Meningiomas

75% homogenously hyperdense. 25% isodense. Calcification – 20%. Peripheral edema – 60%

CECT – uniform intense enhancement (90%). Iso to slightly hypo on T_1W, variable on T_2W.

T_2 signal may correlate with histopathological features.

90% of fibroblastic tumors are hypointense on T_2W and 2/3rd of meningothelial/angioblastic are hyperintense on T_2W. Mushrooming (inhomogeneous enhancement indistinct tumor brain interface) seen in 10% benign and 20% malignant tumors.

Arachnoid Cyst

D/D of arachnoid cysts

Epidermoid and dermoid cysts, ependymal cyst, lipoma, cystic gliomas, Porencephalic cyst

Overall cysts will be isointense to CSF except inflammatory, hemorrhagic and malignant

Cystic glioma – Edema will be seen

Epidermoid – Frond like appearance insinuates, does not displace the structures

A suprasellar arachnoid cyst can give rise to Bunny-Head appearance, should be distinguished from aqueductal stenosis with dilated lateral ventricles.

Cysticercal Cyst

	T_1	T_2
Vesicular	Hypo	Hyper, no enhancement, no edema
Colloidal	-	Edema + enhancement
Calcifying	Iso/hypo	Hypo
Calcified	Iso	Hyper

Paraganglioma of Cauda Equina

Common in males, 5th decade. 5 cm distal to conus tip, opposite to L_{2-3} space. Commonest roots L_3 or L_4. Intradural, intra-arachnoid tumor, sometimes associated with NF-1. Familial tumors may be multicentric. Paraganglioma of cauda equina do not produce hormones. Signs and symptoms– LBA, radiculopathy. Cauda-equina syndrome, conus-cauda syndrome.

Imaging: Hyperintense on T_1W, enhances on contrast

I_{123}-MIBG (meta-iodo-benzyl-guanidine) – differentiation from ependymoma/neurofibroma.

Pathology: Zell ballen pattern, argyrophil granules, positive stain for synaptophysin.

Electron microscopy – dense core vesicles, GFAP – negative.

Malignancy is governed by lymph node or distant metastasis. If tumor recurs – re-exploration +radiotherapy

Vertebral Hemangiomas

Seen in elderly females, 5th decade, commonest benign tumor of spine

Thoracolumbar – 2/3rd one level is involved, 1/3rd multiple levels are involved

Usually vertebral body is involved, sometimes posterior elements are also involved

Two histologic types: *(1) Cavernous (2) Capillary*

Cavernous – dilated vascular spaces with single layer endothelial covering

Capillary – smaller vascular spaces

Mostly asymptomatic. Symptoms – pain, paraparesis, scoliosis. X-ray – vertebral striations

MRI –Hyper on T_1 and T_2, hyperintensity is secondary to fat content. More hyperintense-less aggressive. X-ray may show reduced vertebral body height.

Treatment: Pain – radiotherapy

Neurologic deficit: Surgical decompression.

If lesion is predominantly involving the posterior elements laminectomy followed by embolization. If lesion is predominantly involving the body-enbolization followed by corpectomy and spinal instrumentation.

EVOKED POTENTIALS

In patients in whom language sites are identified, the resection margin is taken within 1–2 cm of cortical areas important for speech function. In patients in whom the primary motor and sensory cortices are mapped, the resection margin is taken closer to the cortical margins (up to 0.5 cm). The resection is stopped if speech function deteriorates but is resumed if full recovery occurs within 5 minutes. During cortical stimulation, simultaneous recording with electrocorticography is not performed because of the tailored craniotomy openings in these patients. Significant changes include amplitude decrease greater than 50% or increases in latency of more than 10% from baseline; these changes should be communicated to the surgeon. SSEP changes lag behind MEP changes by an average of 16 minutes. Thus, a major concern of SSEP monitoring is that by the time monitoring changes become apparent, irreversible neurological injury may have already occurred. Additionally, SSEPs have a low sensitivity for detection of nerve root injury and thus may miss damage caused by aberrant pedicle screw placement or nerve root traction. These deficiencies limit the overall efficacy of SSEPs as a standalone monitoring tool; thus, SSEPs should be used primarily as an adjunct to other forms of monitoring.

Cerebellar Astrocytomas

Some tumors recur early but some quite late — well beyond the time one would have predicted according to Collins' Law. This proposition states that a patient can be considered cured of his neoplasm if he has survived treatment without evidence of disease for a follow-up period of 9 months plus his age at diagnosis. The assumptions underlying this Law are: l) that the tumor grows by simple exponential doubling at a constant rate; 2) that the recurrent tumor should attain approximately the same size as the original to produce similar clinical signs; and 3) that the recurrent tumor should not have taken longer to reach that size than did the original, the longest possible time for which would be if the onset had been at conception. The exceptional biological behavior of cerebellar astrocytomas resembles that of optic gliomas but contrasts with that of other intracranial neoplasms, such as medulloblastomas and ependymomas or other tumors. *J. Neurosurg 1988;68*

CURRENT STANDARD OF CARE AND TREATMENT OF GBM

The current standard of care for patients with GBM includes maximal safe resection, followed by concurrent radiation therapy (RT) to the resection cavity and chemotherapy (with temozolomide (TMZ), followed by adjuvant TMZ). Surgical resection alone results in a median survival of approximately 6-months. Combined, surgical resection and RT extend median survival to 12.1 months. Addition of TMZ further extends the median survival to 14.6 months.

Surgical Resection

Surgery remains an important component in the treatment of GBM. It allows for a histologic confirmation of the diagnosis as well as cytoreduction. Surgery may also serve a therapeutic role by reducing the intracranial pressure, and depending on the location of the tumor, occasionally leads to recovery of some neurological function. The principal contraindications to resective surgery are poor performance status (Karnofsky performance scale [KPS] <70), advanced age, eloquent location or extensive bihemispheric involvement. The goal of surgery is to achieve gross total resection of the contrast enhancing component of the tumor, without compromising neurological function. Gross total resection may not be possible based on anatomic structures invaded by the tumor. Advances in surgical imaging techniques, such as intraoperative magnetic resonance imaging (MRI), diffusion tensor imaging, awake craniotomy, cortical mapping, stereotactic guidance, and fluorescent-guided resection, have facilitated delineation of tumor borders and can help optimize maximal safe surgical resection.

Fluorescent-guided Resection

Fluorescent-guided resection utilizes 5-amino-levulinic-acid that localizes to tumor but not the surrounding normal brain and fluoresces when exposed to light of a specific wavelength. This fluorescence can be used to guide tumor resection by identifying tumor tissue that may otherwise appear normal. Studies comparing fluorescence-guided resection with standard white light resection have shown that patients undergoing fluorescence-guided resection were more likely to have a gross total resection and were more likely to be progression free at 6-months. Although maximal surgical resection remains important, ultimately GBM does not have a surgical "answer".

Chemo-radiotherapy

The combination of RT plus TMZ is the most efficacious adjuvant therapy to prolong survival after primary resection. Treatment following surgery usually consists of 6 weeks of RT to the surgical cavity and TMZ, followed by 6 adjuvant cycles of TMZ.

The current standard of care for RT in GBM is focal, fractionated external beam radiation therapy (EBRT) to the surgical resection cavity and to a 2 cm margin of surrounding brain tissue. Usually, 60 Gy of RT is delivered in fractions of 2 Gy over 6-weeks. Ionizing radiation induces single-strand and double-strand breaks in the DNA of proliferating cells. Other modes of delivering RT have being investigated, including brachytherapy, but none have been proven more effective than the current standard approach. TMZ, an oral alkylating chemotherapeutic agent, causes DNA damage and triggers a cascade of events leading to tumor cell apoptosis. Recently, TMZ was added to the standard of care for GBM treatment. Previously, chemotherapy had no demonstrable clinical benefit, and RT alone remained the standard of care after surgical resection. In 2005, a clinical trial demonstrated that concurrent RT and TMZ followed by adjuvant TMZ significantly prolonged the median survival more than that of radiation alone (14.6 months versus 12.1 months; $p < 0.001$). At the 5-year analysis of this study, more patients treated with TMZ were alive. These findings established the therapeutic benefit of TMZ in combination with RT, establishing the so-called "Stupp regimen" standard of care for GBM treatment. Despite these advances, the median progression-free survival time is only 7 months. When given in combination with RT, patients receive 75 mg/m^2/day of TMZ for 6 weeks. For adjuvant therapy following completion of RT, patients receive 150 mg/m^2/day of TMZ for 5 days every 28 days for at least 6 cycles. As mentioned earlier, TMZ derives its therapeutic benefit from adding a methyl group to purine bases of DNA, which leads to DNA damage and triggers a cascade of events that leads to tumor cell apoptosis. The primary cytotoxic target of TMZ is O6-methylguanine. The methyl group added to O6-methylguanine can be removed by O6-methylguanine methyltransferase (MGMT), which is a DNA repair protein that functions to remove methyl groups from the O6 position of guanine. Removal of this methyl group confers resistance of tumor cells to TMZ and other alkylating chemotherapeutic agents by protecting cells from their DNA-damaging effects.

Carmustine Wafers

Implantation of carmustine wafers into the resection cavity is another Food and Drug Administration (FDA) approved treatment of GBM. Similar to TMZ, carmustine is a DNA alkylating agent. Biodegradable wafers impregnated with carmustine line the tumor resection cavity, allowing for delivery of chemotherapy. Carmustine is released into the surrounding brain tissue immediately after tumor resection and its effects last for several weeks. In clinical trials, carmustine wafers used in combination with radiation and TMZ have been shown to modestly prolong survival in subsets of patients. However, because there are complications associated with the use of wafers, including infection, swelling, need for removal, and impairment of wound healing, they are not used routinely at most centers.

MOLECULARLY TARGETED THERAPIES

Genetically, GBM is a highly heterogeneous tumor harboring multiple recurrent and non-recurrent genetic alterations. Within the same tumor, cytogenetically related and unrelated clones coexist. Due to recent progress in genomics, several aberrantly activated pathways and mutated genes have been implicated in the pathogenesis and malignant progression of GBM. These findings have inspired the investigation of molecularly targeted therapies designed to target tumor-specific recurrent genetic alterations as a novel approach to treating GBM. Many mutations occur in receptor tyrosine kinases (RTKs) or components of their downstream signaling pathways, making them potential targets for drug development and evaluation in clinical trials. The majority of growth factor receptors are transmembrane glycoprotein RTKs with extracellular ligand-binding domains and intracellular kinase domains. Activation of these RTKs triggers a cascade of downstream signaling events, and inappropriate activation of these signaling pathways is thought to drive tumor growth, survival, invasion into normal brain, and secretion of angiogenic factors. Thus, inhibition of these pathways and their downstream intracellular signaling components is the goal of molecularly targeted approaches to treatment of GBM.

Molecularly targeted therapies can broadly be divided into small molecule inhibitors and monoclonal antibodies. Small molecule inhibitors are non-polymeric, organic compounds able to cross cell membranes and target specific intracellular constituents. Many small molecule inhibitors are tyrosine kinase inhibitors (TKIs), which function by selectively targeting the intracellular kinase domain of RTKs, blocking receptor activation of downstream signaling pathways. Single kinase inhibitors have activity against only one RTK, whereas as multikinase inhibitors have activity against several different RTKs. Conversely, monoclonal antibodies, too large to cross cell membranes, are used to target cell surface proteins and other extracellular peptides. In clinical trials, targeted agents are generally studied as single agent therapies in recurrent GBM or used in combination with RT and TMZ for treatment of newly diagnosed GBM. Overall, the results of multiple clinical trials with various molecularly targeted agents have demonstrated only modest therapeutic benefit.

Inhibition of Growth Factor Receptor Pathways

Amplification of EGFR signaling is one of the most common genetic alterations seen in GBM. Over 60% of GBM overexpress EGFR, and in about half of these, over-expression is the result of a mutant form of the receptor, EGFR VIII, which has a constitutively active kinase domain. EGFR over-expression promotes tumor growth, survival, angiogenesis, and invasion. EGFR is also over-expressed in other cancers, and a variety of small molecule tyrosine kinase inhibitors and some monoclonal antibodies have been investigated for their potential to block aberrant EGFR signaling.

Gefitinib and Erlotinib are oral small molecule which bind to intracellular kinase domain of EGFR, they inhibit the activation of its downstream signaling pathways. In preclinical models of GBM, gefitinib and erlotinib have demonstrated antiproliferative and antiinvasive effects, potent inhibition of EGFR, and prolonged survival. Unfortunately, in clinical trials, they have shown limited therapeutic efficacy. Both gefitinib and erlotinib have been studied as monotherapy in recurrent GBM and in combination with RT and TMZ for newly diagnosed GBM, but neither agent provided any clinical benefit. Several additional clinical trials using erlotinib in combination with radiation and TMZ have shown that erlotinib enhances tumor cell sensitivity to radiation. Other studies, however, have not shown the same results. Overall, small molecule EGFR TKIs have provided minimal to no benefit in clinical outcomes.

Cetuximab is a chimeric murine-human monoclonal antibody that blocks activation of EGFR by its ligands. Cetuximab binding also leads to internalization and down regulation of EGFR, and it has been suggested that cetuximab may have antibody dependent cytotoxic effects on the GBM cells it binds. In preclinical models of GBM, cetuximab decreased growth and prolonged survival. Unfortunately, in clinical trials, cetuximab has shown limited therapeutic benefit and has not improved patient outcomes. Over-expression of PDGFR signaling is another frequent alteration found in GBM. PDGF stimulates tumor growth through autocrine signaling, promoting angiogenesis through paracrine effects on adjacent endothelial cells.

Imatinib is a small molecule multikinase inhibitor that binds PDGFR as well as several other RTKs. Imatinib blocks the PDGFR kinase domain to prevent activation of its downstream signaling pathways. Unfortunately, similar to EGFR inhibitors, clinical trials with imatinib demonstrated a lack of therapeutic efficacy and minimal clinical benefit. Initially, these results were attributed to the presence of drug efflux pumps at the blood-brain barrier actively removing imatinib from the brain. Thus, subsequent clinical trials administering hydroxyurea with imatinib were conducted. Results of these trials, however, showed that addition of hydroxyurea did not improve outcomes.

Inhibition of Angiogenic Pathways

GBM is a highly vascularized tumor characterized by extensive angiogenesis. Vascular endothelial growth factor (VEGF), a critical mediator of angiogenesis, is highly over-expressed in GBM. VEGF has been correlated with clinical outcomes, including time to recurrence and survival. Several small molecule inhibitors and monoclonal antibodies have been developed to block this signaling. Antiangiogenic therapies are currently the most advanced group of targeted therapies for GBM, and there have been multiple clinical trials demonstrating their therapeutic efficacy.

Bevacizumab is a humanized monoclonal antibody that binds and neutralizes the VEGF ligand, preventing activation of its receptors. In clinical trials of recurrent GBM, bevacizumab demonstrated clinical benefit and improved progression-free survival. Bevacizumab is thought to improve outcomes by reducing angiogenesis, decreasing growth of tumor cells expressing VEGF, disrupting the microvasculature of the tumor leading to increased tumor hypoxia, and increasing tumor cell sensitivity to RT. It is currently undergoing clinical trials for use in combination with radiation and TMZ for treatment of newly diagnosed GBM. To date, the results of these clinical trials have shown some promising results, but additional trials are also currently underway to confirm clinical benefit. Despite encouraging results in preclinical trials, clinical trials with these agents have demonstrated limited therapeutic benefit, and in some trials, were associated with high toxicity rates. Cilengitide is another novel antiangiogenic therapy being studied in GBM. It is a cyclized pentapeptide small molecule inhibitor that selectively blocks activation of the αvβ3 and αvβ5 integrins. The integrins are a family of cell adhesion molecule transmembrane glycoprotein receptors that mediate cell-matrix and cell-cell interactions. In GBM, the αvβ3 and αvβ5 integrins are widely overexpressed in GBM cells and tumor vasculature, and in addition to VEGF, they are key mediators of angiogenesis, tumor growth, and metastasis. Several clinical trials have shown that cilengitide is well tolerated with minimal toxicity, and ongoing clinical trials are investigating its therapeutic efficacy and clinical benefit.

INHIBITION OF INTRACELLULAR SIGNALING PATHWAYS

Immunotherapy

Immunotherapy attempts to harness the immune system to selectively destroy tumor cells. It includes both passive and active strategies. Passive immunotherapy uses antibodies, immune cells, or other components of the immune

Brain Tumors (Important Theory)

system to target the tumor cells. This approach does not require activation of the patient's native immune response; rather, immune cells are activated *ex vivo* and then reinjected. Passive immunotherapy involves use of monoclonal antibodies, cytokine-mediated therapies, and adoptive cell transfer approaches. Active immunotherapy attempts to stimulate the patient's native immune response against the tumor. Active immunotherapy includes peptide-based and cell-based approaches. These therapies are often referred to as cancer vaccines. Currently, most immunologic therapies available are antibody-based therapies, some of which were discussed earlier. There are, however, several cancer vaccines being evaluated as treatment for GBM in clinical trial.

Passive Immunotherapy: Adoptive Cell Transfer

Adoptive cell transfer uses stimulated immune effector cells to generate cell-based cytotoxic responses to attack GBM cells. In this approach, autologous immune cells are activated *ex vivo* and re-administered. The cells can be given systemically or intratumorally. The two main immune cells used in adoptive cell transfer are lymphocyte-activated killer (LAK) cells and cytotoxic T lymphocytes (CTLs)

Active Immunotherapy: Cancer Vaccines

Active immunotherapy is similar in concept to vaccination. It boosts the patient's native immune response against the tumor cells by priming it with antigen exposure. Several sources of GBM-related antigen may be used in active immunotherapy, which include intact tumor cells, tumor cell lysate, tumor-derived peptides and mRNA, and synthetic peptides. Active immunotherapy approaches include peptide-based therapies and cell-based therapies. In peptide-based therapies, GBM-related antigens are administered to the patient as a vaccine to stimulate an immune response. The antigens used for cancer vaccines are usually small peptides, around nine amino acids in length, which are capable of activating cytotoxic T-lymphocytes.

Rindopepimut is an injectable peptide vaccine designed to stimulate an immune response against a specific EGFRvIII antigen. EGFRvIII variant is a constitutively active, mutant form of EGFR expressed in GBM. A segment of this mutant peptide has been used as a vaccine to generate EGFRvIII-specific antibodies. In clinical trials of patients with GBM expressing EGFRvIII, rindopepimut has shown some promising results, but clinical trials have not been completed. In cell-based therapies, APCs are activated with GBM-related antigens, rather than the antigen itself, to prime the immune system and then injected into the patients to generate an immune response. As DCs (dendritic cells) are professional APCs, they are typically used. The DCs are typically collected from the patient's autologous peripheral blood mononuclear cells, cultured in the presence of growth factors and matured, activated *ex vivo* with tumor-related peptides, and then readministered to generate an antitumor response.

GENE THERAPY

Gene therapy for the treatment of cancer involves the delivery of genetic material, which includes transgenes, toxins, and viruses, into tumor cells for therapeutic purposes. The genetic material is typically packaged within a vector for delivery into cells. There are a variety of different vectors, which include both viral and nonviral vectors. Some gene therapies have shown promising results in preclinical trials, Lack of clinical benefit is, at least in part, likely due to the low transfection efficiency of most viral vectors. Retroviruses and adenoviruses are among the earliest and most widely studied viral vectors for use in gene therapy. Retroviruses are a large family of enveloped RNA viruses. They contain a reverse transcriptase that, following transduction, allows them to integrate their genetic material in the host DNA. Retroviruses selectively infect actively dividing cells, which allows them to target rapidly dividing GBM cells while sparing normal brain cells. A major drawback is that they may be unable to target the relatively quiescent GSCs that may be responsible for tumor resistance to treatment and recurrence. Another drawback of retroviruses is that they are unstable and difficult to produce at high titers.

Conditionally Cytotoxic Gene Therapy

Conditionally cytotoxic gene therapy, also referred to as enzyme-prodrug activating therapy or suicide gene therapy, is the most commonly used gene therapy approach in GBM. In conditionally cytotoxic approaches, the transgene for a noncytotoxic enzyme is delivered into tumor cells, and this enzyme remains noncytotoxic until the administration of a noncytotoxic prodrug. Upon prodrug administration, the enzyme converts the noncytotoxic prodrug into a toxic metabolite that induces tumor cell death. For enzyme-prodrug activating therapy to be successful, the enzyme transgene must be delivered exclusively into tumor cells, and its enzymatic activity must be high enough to kill tumor cells without causing toxicity to surrounding normal cells or inducing a systemic immune response. In most enzyme-prodrug therapies, there is a significant bystander effect. This occurs when the cytotoxic metabolite is transmitted, via gap junctions or by diffusing through extracellular space, to cells that were not originally transduced with the enzyme. Since expression of the enzyme gene will not occur in all tumor cells, this bystander effect is important in amplifying the cytotoxicity of the enzyme-prodrug therapy.

Directly Cytotoxic Gene Therapy

Directly cytotoxic gene therapy, otherwise known as targeted toxin therapy, utilizes surface molecules overexpressed in GBM to target toxins directly into tumor cells to cause tumor cell death. This can be accomplished through viral vector-mediated delivery of transgenes for highly toxic proteins or with recombinant molecules: **Immunotoxins**. Immunotoxins consist of a tumor-specific monoclonal antibody or ligand conjugated to a toxin. The antibody or ligand component binds selectively to surface molecules overexpressed in GBM and induces internalization of the immunotoxin. Upon internalization, the toxin triggers a cascade of intracellular events that lead to tumor cell apoptosis. Commonly used toxins are **Pseudomonas** exotoxin (PE) and **Diphtheria** exotoxin.

Immunostimulatory Gene Therapy

Immunomodulatory gene therapy uses the genetic material of cytokines, lymphocytes, or other immune modulators to enhance the host immune response to the tumor. Immunomodulatory approaches are based on the expectation that antitumor immune responses, activated by tumor-specific antigen expression, would effectively eliminate tumor cells. Unfortunately, often tumors develop mechanisms to evade these immune responses, creating an immune suppressive tumor microenvironment. Thus, the goal of immunostimulatory gene therapy is to improve the immune response against the tumor.

Oncolytic Virotherapy

In oncolytic virotherapy, unlike in other approaches, viral toxicity is directly responsible for tumor cell death. Oncolytic viral vectors are engineered as conditionally replicating viruses that specifically infect and replicate within tumor cells, while sparing the surrounding normal brain. Oncolytic virotherapy takes advantage of the innate ability of lytic viruses to lyse and kill their host cells following infection. Upon lysis, virions spread to infect the surrounding tumor cells, propagating their toxicity. In order to be safe and effective, oncolytic viral vector replication and lytic destruction must be limited to tumor cells only, while being relatively avirulent in normal brain cells. This can be accomplished by attenuating the virus to allow restriction of its replication to rapidly dividing cells, permitting them to infect and lyse tumor cells but not normal, non-replicating brain cells. Additional molecular strategies used to accomplish this include deletion of components of the viral genome necessary for viral replication that are not expressed in normal cells but aberrantly expressed in cancer cells, Insertion of promoter sequences into the viral genome that drive the expression of replication genes under the control of unique transcription factors overexpressed in cancer cells, and engineering viral capsid proteins that use unique molecular targeting to selectively transduce cancer cells.

OTHER NOVEL THERAPIES

A variety of other novel approaches for the treatment of GBM are currently being investigated. The NovoTTF-100A is a device that uses alternating electric fields to disrupt cell division, and it is currently being studied as a treatment option for GBM. The use of thermal lasers to denature tumor tissues is another area being investigated. Laser interstitial thermal therapy (LITT) is a minimally invasive thermoablative procedure that uses a laser to create low-powered thermal energy that heats and destroys tumor cells. LITT has been used for several decades for the treatment of GBM and other tumors; however, its use has been limited due to several technical limitations, mainly difficulty in regulating the dose of LITT delivered to individual patients. In order to overcome these technical limitations, the NeuroBlate

System (Monteris Medical, Inc.) was developed with technical advances, such as real-time MRI-guided thermography to facilitate detection of thermal damage to tissue, that allow for safer and more precise delivery of LITT for treatment of GBM. Results of trials have demonstrated that the NeuroBlate System LITT has a favorable safety profile in patients with GBM; however, additional studies assessing clinical efficacy and outcomes still need to be conducted.

Chemotherapy for GBM

Under normal physiological conditions, the BBB exclude large hydrophilic agents from the brain parenchyma. The BBB within tumors is known to be leaky. Unfortunately, agents that are active against gliomas in vitro but do not cross an intact BBB and have shown little efficacy in clinical trials. Therefore, the chemotherapeutic agents that have been used successfully for treating pts with HGGs are relatively lipophilic and can readily cross an intact BBB.

Nitrosoureas: Nitrosoureas were the first drugs to be widely used in the treatment because they readily cross BBB. The nitrosoureas that have been most commonly used are. BCNU, ACNU, CCNU. In meta-analysis of 12 randomized controlled trials, which compared RT alone with RT plus nitrosourea therapy for high grade gliomas, a 6% increase in 1-year survival as well as 2-month increase in median survival was found. Since TMZ has come into wide spread use, nitrosoureas have been used less and less, often except for the local delivery of BCNU via gliadel wafers.

Procarbazine: It is an alkylating agent causing DNA alkylation interferes with protein synthesis. It was studied in a large randomized trial that began in 1976 and was reported in 1983 by Green et al. In this study, single agent procarbazine was almost as beneficial as BCNU. Procarbazine found wide spread use in the PCV combination. As a single agent it is generally administered once daily for 28–30 days with a month break between cycles.

Temozolomide: Temozolomide is an oral 2nd generation methylating agent. It has nearly 100% bioavailability after oral administration and readily crosses BBB. CSF concentration may reach 40% that of serum concentration. Temozolomide modifies DNA at several sites most notably O-6 position of guanine. TMZ induces DNA methylation of guanine at O6 position (O6-MG; as well as 7-methylguanine (N7-MG; and 3 methyladenine (N3-MA). O6-MG incorrectly pairs with thymine and triggers the mismatch repair (MMR) system leading to double strand break of the genome that result in the arrest of cell cycle and induction of apoptosis. MGMT – a key molecule for TMZ resistance. MGMT specifically removes the methyl/alkyl group from the O6-position of guanine and restore the guanine to its normal form escaping from DNA strand breaks. Thus, the expression of MGMT in tumors has a protective effect against alkylating agents-dependent cell death correlating between MGMT activity and TMZ resistance. MGMT expressing tumor cells exhibit 4- to 10-folds increase of resistance to TMZ, BCNU, and their related compounds. MGMT is an important drug resistance factor and an ideal target for suppression of drug resistance. TMZ is generally well tolerated. Common adverse effects are; nausea, vomiting, constipation, myelosuppression and fatigue. Since there is far less cumulative myelosuppression with TMZ than with nitrosoureas, it can be taken safely for a much longer time. A unique side effect of TMZ is pseudoprogression. The transient enhancement of diseased area on MRI that gives the impression of progression despite the overall benefit of chemotherapy and RT. Pseudoprogression often precedes recovery and is believed to be inflammation or necrosis. TMZ cycle should be continued even if pseudoprogression continues and only after 3-cycles should treatment be evaluated. Studies reported that up to 50% of progression cases are pseudoprogression which can be alleviated with continued TMZ administration. As TMZ degrades within hours and its effects are dose dependent, patient adherence to dosing schedules is integral to treatment. In newly diagnosed cases 75 mg/m^2 per day for 6 weeks f/b As an adjuvant for 5 days each 28 day cycle. Dose for 1st adjuvant cycle 150 mg/m^2 per day for 5 days, Dose for subsequent cycles (max_6 cycles) 200 mg/m^2 for 5 days. For recurrent GBM, 150 mg /m^2 for 5 days, each 28 days cycle. Alternate schedule exist and should be modified if hematological toxicity becomes severe. The clinical study looked at the effects of concurrent EBRT and daily TMZ for six weeks followed by adjuvant five day cycles of TMZ for six months compared to EBRT alone. This trial showed that EBRT plus TMZ significantly improved survival of patients with newly diagnosed GBM without reducing quality of life.

Chemotherapy for Recurrent High Grade Glioma

Treatment of patients with recurrent HGG is generally disappointing. The progression-free-survival (PFS) is about 2-months for GBM and 3-months for anaplastic glioma. In multi-centric trials with TMZ the PFS at 6-months was 46%.

Bevacizumab was recently approved by FDA for treatment of GBM, which has failed treatment with TMZ. A variety of TMZ regimens have been investigated for recurrent GBM. It is not clear which of these is most effective. Once such strategy is low dose continuous daily TMZ.

Carboplatin 560 mg/m^2 IV at 4-week intervals; continued until disease progression, unacceptable toxicity, or for 12-additional courses after achieving maximal response. The PCV regimes have been used for many years for initial therapy and recurrent disease. Due to toxicity its use has diminished considerably since the availability of TMZ and Bevacizumab. Single agent Irinotecan has been used for treatment of recurrent HGGs with limited success.

Side effects include nausea, vomiting, diarrhea, constipation, secondary malignancy, mucositis or stomatitis, hypersensitivity and serum sickness, pneumonitis / pulmonary fibrosis, nephrotoxicity, myelosuppression (cumulative), hemolytic anemia CNS depression, nightmares, insomnia, hallucinations, thromboembolism, rash, pigmentation, photosensitivity, myocardial infarction and anorexia.

IRINOTECAN

It is a topoisomerase inhibitor-1, in chemical terms, it is a semisynthetic analogue of the natural alkaloid camptothecin. Irinotecan prevents DNA from unwinding by inhibition of topoisomerase 1. Irinotecan is activated by hydrolysis to SN-38, an inhibitor of topoisomerase I. This is then inactivated by glucuronidation by uridine diphosphate glucuronosyltransferase. The inhibition of topoisomerase I by the active metabolite SN-38 eventually leads to inhibition of both DNA replication and transcription. The most significant adverse effects of irinotecan are severe diarrhea and extreme suppression of the immune system. Irinotecan-associated diarrhea is severe and clinically significant, sometimes leading to severe dehydration requiring hospitalization or intensive care unit admission. This side-effect is managed with the aggressive use of antidiarrheals such as loperamide or co-phenotrope with the first loose bowel movement. The recommended dosage for its use as a single agent is 125 mg/m^2 i.v. every 4 weeks followed by a 2-week rest, or 350 mg/m^2 i.v. every 3 weeks. When used in combination with leucovorin and 5-FU, the recommended regimens are irinotecan 125 mg/m^2 i.v., LV 200 mg/m^2 bolus, and 5-FU 500 mg/m^2 bolus weekly for 4 weeks. The combination of irinotecan plus temozolomide for chemotherapy of recurrent malignant glioma has produced consistently high response rates and encouraging 6-month PFS, despite the majority of patients having progressed following RT. In another phase II trial, a combination of irinotecan with BCNU had activity against recurrent or newly diagnosed malignant glioma comparable to irinotecan alone but with apparent increased toxicity. The combination of irinotecan and thalidomide demonstrated promising activity in patients with recurrent GB. Thirty-two patients were treated in 6-week cycles with irinotecan (125 mg/m^2 weekly for 4 weeks with 2 weeks off) and thalidomide (100 mg daily, initial dose, increased as tolerated to a maximum of 400 mg daily). The study was designed to detect an improvement in 6-month PFS compared with historical controls. Results demonstrated a median PFS of 13 weeks, with eight patients (25%) achieving PFS at 6 months. Finally, the intriguing data for irinotecan and bevacizumab combination therapy suggest that there is a synergy between topoisomerase I inhibitors and anti-VEGF therapies, with acceptable toxicity. The inclusion of irinotecan and bevacizumab in the treatment of patients with newly diagnosed malignant glioma may significantly improve their survival.

ETOPOSIDE

It is a topoisomerase II inhibitor. Etoposide was first synthesized in 1966 and U.S. Food and Drug Administration approval was granted in 1983. Its chemical make-up derives from podophyllotoxin, a toxin found in the American Mayapple. Penetration of etoposide into the cerebrospinal fluid, brain tumor, and brain tissue after intravenous administration was investigated in patients presenting with malignant brain tumors. A relatively low dose (55-65 mg/m^2) was used to compare intravenous with oral administration. A relatively low dose of etoposide injected intravenously penetrates the brain tumor at an efficacious concentration. Plasma and cerebrospinal fluid levels of etoposide after oral administration (50-150 mg/day) were also studied so as to determine the adequate oral dose for the treatment of malignant brain tumors. The peak plasma concentration after intravenous administration ranged from 7.01 to 10.47 micrograms/ml, varying in proportion to the injected dose, whereas that after oral administration was lower, namely, 1.44–4.99 micrograms/ml. Common adverse effects are; hypotension, alopecia, pain and or burning at the IV site, constipation or diarrhea, metallic food taste, bone marrow suppression.

BRAIN METASTASIS IMAGING, CLINICAL FEATURES AND MANAGEMENT

Dissemination of Brain Metastasis

Commonly located beneath the gray-white matter junction and superficial distal arterial fields. CNS metastases most often involved the brain parenchyma, leptomeninges, and spinal epidural space. Distribution of lesions reflects the blood flow with approximately 80% in cerebrum, 15% in cerebellum, and 5% in brainstem. Clinical features depends on the area of metastasis.

NEUROIMAGING OF METASTATIC BRAIN DISEASE

Contrast CT scans are often the initial imaging modality for symptomatic patients with unknown brain metastases. On MRI, most show mild T_1-hypointensity with T_2-hyperintensity and FLAIR hyperintensity. Metastases tend to be most commonly located in the supratentorial compartment with the exception of those from renal cell carcinoma that tend to be infratentorial. On MRI, mild hypointensity with T_2-hyperintensity and FLAIR hyperintensity. Hemorrhagic metastases demonstrate hyperdensity on NCCT and T_1-hyperintensity on non-contrast MRI. Metastases from malignant melanoma may demonstrate T_1-hyperintensity because of hemorrhage or melanin components.

LEPTOMENINGEAL METASTASIS

The leptomeninges may be the site of metastases from

1. Primary CNS malignancies (34%)
2. Extra-cranial hematological (11%)
3. Solid (46%) malignancies.

Solid tumors include adenocarcinomas from breast, lung (small cell type), stomach, and malignant melanoma. Observed as curvilinear o nodular pial enhancement along the basal cisterns or sulci in 35%.

Hydrocephalus In 13%.

Cranial nerve deposits in 11%.

DURAL METASTASES

Commonly caused by systemic breast carcinoma, pulmonary adenocarcinoma, squamous cell carcinoma, and renal cell carcinomas. More prone to recurrent disease (>41%). Overall survival is similar to that of patients with parenchymal disease.

SPECT

Provides physiological imaging with a variety of radiopharmaceuticals. 99mTc-HMPAO, 123I-IMP, and thallium-201 (201TI). Metastases often show decreased uptake with the exception of hypervascular metastases, such as malignant melanoma. 99mTc-MIBI demonstrates only a 50% sensitivity for brain metastases.

PET

Measures metabolic activity charged positrons. Preferred over SPECT because of higher intrinsic resolution. 18F-fluorodeoxyglucose positron-emission tomography (FDG-PET). commonly done. Methionine -, tyrosine-, and choline-labeled PET scanning are newer technologies that are based on amino acid membrane transport, protein synthesis, and phospholipid uptake. Absolute quantification of cerebral blood flow and uses functional imaging to define eloquent cortex. Advantages of PET are:

Evaluation of suspected metastatic lesions.

Whole-body staging in a convenient single examination.

Possible detection of the primary systemic tumor.

Perfusion MRI

Provides visual maps of the regional variations in cerebral microvasculature caused by intrinsic differences between tumoral and nontumoral capillary systems. Exploits the T_2 signal changes occurring during passage of contrast through the cerebrovascular system to attain cerebral blood flow and cerebral blood volume (CBV) information. Lack of angiogenesis suggests tumor-mimicking lesions i.e., radiation necrosis cerebral abscess, and tumefactive demyelination. Perfusion MRI evaluation of the peritumoral T_2-hyperintensity reliably differentiate the metastatic from high-grade gliomas. Isolated dural-based metastasis, differentiation from meningioma can be done. Intratumoral rCBV measures are elevated in meningiomas because of increased vascularity and lack of BBB but are only mildly elevated in a number of metastatic tumors.

Hypervascular metastases from malignant melanoma, renal cell carcinoma, or Merkel carcinoma, however, may present with an elevated rCBV.

Spectroscopic MRI

Provides semiquantitative evaluation of metabolite levels to characterize brain tumors. Commonly measured metabolites include choline (Cho), lactate (Lac), lipids (Lip), **N**- acetylaspartate (NAA), and creatine and creatine phosphate (Cr). Metastases show elevated Cho levels, Lac and Lip resonances, and decreased NAA and Cr levels, with subsequently increased Cho /Cr and Cho/Cho (normal) and decreased NAA/Cr ratios. Peritumoral MRS can be used to differentiate metastasis from high grade glioma.

Functional Imaging: Relationship of tumor margins with eloquent cortex and may change the operative approach. Performed with PET, magnetoencephalography (MEG), and functional MRI (fMRI).

FUNCTIONAL IMAGING

MEG has the best temporal resolution, because it directly measures neuronal activity. MRI has the advantage of concurrent acquisition of anatomic and functional images. PET and MEG require separate acquisition and fusion of the anatomic images. fMRI also has better spatial resolution than PET and MEG, but decreased precision.

Intraoperative Imaging

Neuronavigation systems improve lesion targeting and resection of tumor tissue. Frame-based and frame-less stereotactic systems suffer from diminished accuracy as the duration of surgery increases. Intraoperative ultrasound has unprecedented real time scanning, but suffers from suboptimal definition of small lesions and tumor margins. Intraoperative MRI has emerged as an important imaging guidance tool because of its superior spatial resolution and sensitivity.

Post-therapeutic Imaging

MRI is routinely performed after surgical resection to evaluate for residual tumor and assess for potential complications (within 24 hours).

Radiation necrosis cannot be distinguished from residual or recurrent tumor by conventional imaging methods. Nuclear medicine imaging detects the typical hypometabolism within areas of radiation necrosis.

IMAGING STRATEGY

CT retains a limited but important role as an initial diagnostic tool to exclude neurosurgical emergencies. A contrast-enhanced MRI study with volumetric 3D sequences and diffusion data should be performed. Spectroscopic and Perfusion MRI should be performed to help differentiate metastases from other tumor and tumor-mimicking lesions. Both MRS and pMRI can also be used to guide stereotactic biopsy to the most proliferative area of the tumor.

CSF ANALYSIS

On single or multiple CSF sampling, 75 to 80% sensitivity and 95 to 100% specificity. Analysis of CSF is superior to MRI for detection of hematological malignancies (sensitivity, 89–95% versus 39–48%). For solid tumors (sensitivity, 46% versus 100%). Neuroimaging and CSF analysis should be considered complementary tools.

MANAGEMENT OPTIONS

Surgery

Radiotherapy

Radiosurgery

Palliative treatment

National Comprehensive Cancer Network recommendations.

TREATMENT GUIDELINES

For patients with a resectable new solitary metastasis or a symptomatic metastasis with mass effect, surgery followed by WBRT is recommended, WBRT for patients with active systemic disease and poor prognosis. RPA Class 3; palliative care. RS can be used for palliative care also. RS should be considered when surgery is contraindicated. Generally, metastases 3 cm or less in diameter, without abundant surrounding edema can be treated with RS. For tumors less than 3 cm in diameter, surgical resection and WBRT should be considered.

Surgery in Recurrent Metastases

Shown to improve survival and quality of life in patients with recurrent disease. (Arbit E, et al. **Cancer** 76:1995, Bindal RK, et al. **J Neurosurg** 83:1995.). Remove necrotic tissue use localized adjunctive therapies, including brachytherapy and local chemotherapy adjunct. Surgical debulking and intraoperative histological confirmation.

Whole-Brain Radiation Therapy (WBRT): Treatment of choice for metastases that impinge on eloquent areas, or are too large, numerous, or disseminated for surgery or RS. Response rates after WBRT vary, (complete or partial responses 60%).

Acute toxicities, after treatment, may include nausea or vomiting, alopecia, hearing loss, acute or subacute skin reactions, and somnolence.

Long term complications; necrosis, personality and memory changes (both short- and long term memory), and neurocognitive deficits.

The object of RS in treating brain metastases is to deliver a high dose of radiation to a target volume, destroying all cells within the target boundaries. RS systems are the Gamma Knife and the linear accelerator. Brain metastases are well suited for RS.

They are often small, radiographically well-circumscribed, pseudospherical tumors that are noninvasive, and they are often located at the gray-white junction, where toxicity to critical structures is low. Maximum tolerated RS dose for brain tumors is directly related to the tumor size. Maximum tolerable doses are 24 Gy (<20 mm; 18Gy (21 to 30 mm) and 15 Gy (31 to 40 mm).

CHEMOTHERAPY

For patients with metastases from chemosensitive tumors, such as germ cell tumors or lymphoma, chemotherapy should be administered first, with radiotherapy reserved for relapse.

Surgery or Radiosurgery

The tumor location and size and the presence of edema are important considerations. Tumors that are large, in a favorable location for resection, and are associated with mass effect should be surgically resected. Surgery should also be considered for patients with an unknown primary lesion or at the time of a possible first metastasis from a known primary lesion because of the need for tissue diagnosis. Small tumors (3 cm) should be treated with RS if they are unresectable. Small tumors that are resectable and are associated with minimal edema can treated with either surgery or RS.

Seizures

Seizures are a presenting symptom in approximately 20% of patients with brain metastases. Phenytoin, carbamazepine, and valproic acid are frequently used as first-line agents, along with newer agents in selected circumstances. American Academy of Neurology now recommends that anticonvulsants should be administered only to those patients at risk for seizure, and their use should be minimized to single therapy at the lowest effective dose.

ROLE OF ANTICONVULSANTS

Meta-analysis of the available data showed that prophylactic anticonvulsants do not seems to significantly reduce the risk of a first seizure.

Anticonvulsant-related side effects were especially common in brain tumor patients (20–40%). A combination of multiple anticonvulsants is needed to control seizures adequately.

EMBRYOLOGY OF INTRAVENTRICULAR MENINGIOMAS

The presence of arachnoid cell nests in the normal choroid plexus stroma has been illustrated in the literature, and a thorough examination of the choroid plexus usually reveals small or sometimes larger collections of these cells. The presence of these cells in the choroid plexus has been explained by various investigators. The choroid plexus develops initially from an invagination of a mesenchyme in the thin, roof area of the myelencephalon during the 6th week of gestation. In the 7th to 9th weeks, the telencephalic choroid plexus has started to develop a loose mesenchymal stroma, which is covered by a layer of cells derived from the ependyma. Arachnoid tissue is transported together with the choroid plexus as the ventricular system invaginates, and by 20 to 40 weeks, the central stroma of the choroid plexus contains meningocytes, connective tissue, and blood vessels. Meningiomas arise from arachnoid cap cells, which are specialized cells in arachnoid granulations. In a similar fashion, intraventricular meningiomas arise from arachnoid cells contained with- in the choroid plexus. Meningothelial inclusion bodies are normally found in the arachnoid and choroidal tela, and meningiomas arise from this mesenchymal stroma of the choroid plexus. Third ventricle tumors may arise from the tela of the velum interpositum, which is the space between the two layers of tela in the roof of the third ventricle that contains the posterior medial choroidal arteries and internal cerebral veins. Fourth ventricle meningiomas characteristically arise from choroids or interior tela choroidea. Ventricles of the brain provide space for tumor expansion, and until the cerebrospinal fluid pathways are mechanically occluded, manifestations are mild and nonspecific. Cushing and Eisenhard described five clinical features of lateral ventricle tumors: 1) pressure symptoms with ipsilateral headache; 2) contralateral macula splitting homonymous hemianopia; 3) contralateral sensorimotor paresis, more marked sensory involvement, and numbness over trigeminal distribution; 4) cerebellar involvement in more than half of patients; and 5) paralexia, worsened by surgical intervention in left-sided tumors.

Regardless of their locations, most of the clinical symptoms are due to increased IP. Lesions grow into the ventricular cavity until they produce obstructive hydrocephalus. Visual field deficits may be seen in 25% of patients and seizures are rare. Cerebellar signs may be seen in fourth ventricle tumors, and hypothalamic features with or without endocrinopathy may be seen in third ventricle tumors. Manifestations of NF2 may be evident on clinical and neurological evaluation. Fibroblastic meningiomas, the most common type in the lateral ventricles,

Lateral ventricle tumors are fed by lateral–posterior choroidal vessels, whereas those in the temporal horn receive their blood supply from the anterior choroidal artery. Tumors in the atrium are supplied by both anterior and posterior choroidal arteries. Third ventricle tumors are supplied by medial posterior choroidal vessels, whereas fourth ventricle tumors derive their blood supply from choroidal branches of the PICA.

MULTIPLE CHOICE QUESTIONS

1. **The triad in McCune-Albright's syndrome is:**
   a. Endocrinopathy, fibrous dysplasia, cafe au lait spots
   b. Endocrinopathy, vestibular schwannoma, Café au lait spots
   c. Craniopharyngioma, fibrous dysplasia, Café au lait spots
   d. None of the above
   Ref. Youmans, 5th/e, p3590

2. **Optic pathway gliomas are:**
   a. Oligodendrogliomas
   b. Pilocytic astrocytomas
   c. Gangliogliomas
   d. Tanycytic ependymomas
   Ref. Youmans, 5th/e, p3595-9

3. **Optic pathway gliomas can present with the following features, except:**
   a. Macrocephaly b. Visual failure
   c. Precocious puberty d. Gigantism
   Ref. Youmans, 5th/e, p3595-9

4. **The treatment of choice for diffuse chiasmatic glioma is:**
   a. Surgery
   b. Biopsy only
   c. Biopsy and radiotherapy
   d. None of the above
   Ref. Youmans, 5th/e, p3595-9

5. **All the following are long term sequel of cranial irradiation in children, except:**
   a. Aneurysm formation
   b. Secondary malignancies
   c. Moya Moya syndrome
   d. Visual failure
   Ref. Youmans, 5th/e, p1715, p3681-3

6. **Which of the following tumors is radio-curable?**
   a. Medulloblastoma b. Germinoma
   c. Ependymoma
   d. Metastatic renal cell carcinoma
   Ref. Youmans, 5th/e, p4023-4

7. **The maximum incidence of calcification is in:**
   a. Medulloblastoma b. Craniopharyngioma
   c. Ependymoma
   d. Choroid plexus papilloma
   Ref. Youmans, 5th/e, p1207-19

8. **Which of the following tumors is staged with TNM grading?**
   a. Ependymoma
   b. Dysembryoplastic neuroepithelial tumor
   c. Medulloblastoma
   d. Pituitary adenoma
   Ref. Youmans, 5th/e, p1031-40

9. **Which of the following tumors has a mural nodule?**
   a. Pilocytic astrocytoma
   b. Hemangioblastoma
   c. Medulloblastoma with extreme nodularity
   d. 'a' + 'b'
   Ref. Youmans, 5th/e, p986-988, 1053-60

10. **The commonest division of 8th cranial nerve from which tumor arises is:**
    a. Cochlear division
    b. Superior vestibular division
    c. Inferior vestibular division
    d. Equally from all the divisions
    Ref. Youmans, 5th/e, p1147-74

11. **The most sensitive diagnostic tool for detecting early 8th nerve schwannoma is:**
    a. Brainstem evoked response audiometry
    b. Contrast MRI
    c. Air meatography
    d. High resolution CT scan
    Ref. Youmans, 5th/e, p1147-64

ANSWERS

1. a. **2.** b. **3.** d. **4.** c. **5.** a. **6.** b. **7.** b. **8.** c. **9.** d. **10.** b.
11. b.

12. All the following about cystic 8th nerve schwannoma are true, except:
   a. They present with dysgeusia
   b. Internal auditory meatus is not dilated
   c. Facial nerve preservation during surgery is difficult
   d. They arise from cochlear division

   Ref. Youmans, 5th/e, p1147-64

13. The treatment of choice for small vestibular schwannomas with brainstem compression is:
   a. Radiosurgery
   b. Suboccipital craniotomy and tumor decompression
   c. Suboccipital craniotomy, cerebellar hemispherectomy and tumor decompression
   d. Wait and watch

   Ref. Youmans, 5th/e, p1147-64

14. Which of the following tumors in pediatric age group is less common?
   a. Cerebellar astrocytoma
   b. Brainstem glioma
   c. Optic pathway glioma
   d. Tentorial meningioma

   Ref. Youmans, 5th/e, p3655-70

15. Which of the following tumors arises from remnants of postvelar arch?
   a. Germinoma of posterior third ventricle
   b. Choroid plexus tumors
   c. Colloid cyst
   d. Intraventricular meningioma

   Ref. Grenberg, 4th/e, p289

16. All the following about colloid cyst are true, except:
   a. Radiosurgery is the treatment of choice
   b. Headache is the commonest symptom
   c. It is a neuroepithelial tumor
   d. It can cause sudden death

   Ref. Greenberg, 4th/e, p289

17. All the following lesions cause chronic temporal lobe epilepsy, except:
   a. Gangliogliomas
   b. DNET's
   c. Pleomorphic xanthoastrocytoma
   d. Glioblastoma multiforme

   Ref. Kleihues, p 96

18. Following is/are the types of cortical sulci:
   a. Axial
   b. Limiting
   c. Collateral
   d. All the above

   Ref. Schmidek and Sweet 4th/e, p781

19. All the following about occipital transtentorial approach are true, except:
   a. The approach may damage the occipital lobe
   b. May damage the splenium of the corpus callosum
   c. Provides an excellent view above and below the tentorial notch
   d. It is contraindicated in those tumors that straddle the tentorial notch

   Ref. Youmans, 5th/e, p1022

20. In which of the following diseases dysplastic gangliocytoma of the cerebellum is found:
   a. von Hippel Landau syndrome
   b. Lhermitte-Duclos disease
   c. Gorlins syndrome
   d. MEN-IIb

   Ref. Turkish Journal of Neurosurgery 2011; 21(4):651-54

21. The most common location for posterior fossa meningioma is:
   a. Tentorium
   b. Torcula
   c. CP angle
   d. Jugular fossa

   Ref. Youmans, 5th/e, p1119-22

ANSWERS

12. d.	**13.** b.	**14.** d.	**15.** c.	**16.** a.	**17.** d.	**18.** d.	**19.** d.	**20.** b.	**21.** c.

22. All the following lesions are amenable to radiosurgery, except:

a. Pituitary adenoma
b. Craniopharyngioma
c. Colloid cyst
d. AVM

Ref. Youmans 5th/e, p4053-68

23. Which of the following meningiomas causes skull bone thickening?

a. Falcine meningioma
b. Parasagittal meningioma
c. Intraventricular meningioma
d. Tentorial meningioma

Ref. Youmans, 5th/e, p1111-2

24. The commonest meningioma involving the brain is:

a. Posterior fossa meningioma
b. Tentorial meningioma
c. Convexity meningioma
d. Parasagittal meningioma

Ref. Youmans, 5th/e, p1111

25. All the following tumors are supplied by external carotid artery branches, except:

a. Falcine meningioma
b. Convexity meningioma
c. Parasagittal meningioma
d. None of the above

Ref. Schmidek and Sweet, 4th/e, p735

26. Which of the following modalities is helpful in avoiding injury to the eloquent cortex?

a. Functional MRI
b. Wada test
c. Fiber tracking
d. All the above

Ref. Youmans, 5th/e, p448-9, 2503-8

27. All the statements regarding 7th cranial nerve are true, except:

a. It originates in pontomedullary sulcus
b. Its origin is 2 mm posterior to the 9th nerve
c. A tuft of choroid plexus extends just inferior to its origin
d. None of the above

Ref. Greenberg, 4th/e, p267

28. Which of the following tumor does not undergo malignant change?

a. Psammomatous meningioma
b. Craniopharyngioma
c. Pilocytic astrocytoma
d. Sub-ependymal giant cell astrocytoma

Ref. Youmans, 5th/e, p986-8, 1099-127, 1207-19

29. All the following statements about epidermoid and dermoid cysts are true, except:

a. Epidermoids are commonly found laterally and dermoids inc the midline
b. Epidermoids tend to be isolated, while as dermoids are associated with other congenital lesions
c. Epidermoids cause bacterial meningitis and dermoids cause aseptic meningitis
d. Epidermoids contain keratin, dermoids contain keratin and hair

Ref. Youmans, 5th/e, p1226-44, 4259

30. Which of the following tumors has highest incidence of hemorrhagic metastasis?

a. Melanoma
b. Choriocarcinoma
c. Small cell carcinoma
d. Lymphoma

Ref. Youmans, 5th/e, p1078

31. All the following statements about surgical procedure for vestibular schwannomas are true, except:

a. Translabyrinthine route is the most direct route
b. Retrosigmoid approach is the best for large tumors
c. Temporal lobe retraction is a definite risk in middle fossa approaches
d. Disadvantage of translabyrinthine route is that there is maximum cerebellar retraction

Ref. Youmans, 5th/e, p1149-52

ANSWERS

22. c. **23.** b. **24.** c. **25.** a. **26.** d. **27.** b. **28.** a. **29.** c. **30.** b. **31.** d.

32. All the following about trigeminal schwannomas are true, except:

a. 10% have no 5th nerve symptoms
b. If the tumor extends into the posterior fossa 7th and 8th nerve symptoms will be seen
c. Truncation of petrous apex is found
d. Facial pain is more common if tumor arises from root than if it arises from ganglion

Ref. Neurosurgery Review 2010;34(2):159-71

33. All the following statements about facial nerve schwannoma are true, except:

a. It arises from sensory fibers
b. Tympanic segment is mostly involved
c. 50% have facial palsy
d. It never causes hearing loss

Ref. Skull base 1991; vol 1:51-6

34. All the following statements about hemangiopericytoma are true, except:

a. Arises from perivascular pericytes
b. Commoner in males
c. It is highly vascular
d. Radiotherapy has no role

Ref. Youmans, p1133-8

35. All the following about choroid plexus papilloma are true, except:

a. It is a benign tumor
b. In children it arises from trigone and in adults from 4th ventricle
c. It causes increased CSF production
d. It rarely displays calcification

Ref. Youmans, 5th/e, p3612

36. All the following statements about intracranial lipomas are true, except:

a. Arises from abnormal persistence and maldifferentiation of menix primitive
b. Curvilinear calcifications are noted
c. It produces lot of perilesional edema
d. It does not enhance on contrast

Ref. Youmans, 5th/e, p3948-9

37. All the following are good prognostic factors in low grade gliomas, except:

a. Young age
b. No preoperative neurologic deficit
c. Long history of symptoms
d. Raised ICP as the presenting symptom

Ref. Youmans, 5th/e, p981-94

38. All the following statements about von-Hippel-Landau (VHL) disease and hemangioblastomas are true, except:

a. Most often cerebellum is involved
b. There is mutation of short arm of chromosome-7
c. 50% of VHL have retinal hemangioblastomas
d. 20% of cerebellar hemangioblastomas have VHL complex

Ref. Youmans, 5th/e, p1053-4

39. In which of the following phakomatosis, there is mutation of chromosome-9?

a. Tuberous sclerosis
b. VHL
c. NF-2
d. Rendu-Osler-Weber disease

Ref. Youmans, 5th/e, p811-2

40. Vogt's triad is seen in which of the following conditions?

a. Tuberous sclerosis
b. NF-1
c. Ataxia telangiectasia
d. VHL

Ref. Youmans, 5th/e, p811-2

41. All the following statements about Sturge-Weber syndrome are true, except:

a. There are cutaneous angiomas along 1st or 2nd division of 5th cranial nerve
b. There is leptomeningeal venous angiomatosis
c. The underlying brain shows calcifications in 4th and 5th cortical layer
d. Seizure is one of the presentations

Ref. Youmans, 5th/e, p813

ANSWERS

32. d. **33.** d. **34.** d. **35.** d. **36.** c. **37.** d. **38.** b. **39.** a. **40.** a. **41.** c.

42. All the following statements about ganglio-gliomas are true, except:
- a. Frontal lobe is the commonest site
- b. Seizure is usual presentation
- c. 10% lesions are calcified
- d. 50% lesions are contrast enhancing

Ref. Youmans, 5th/e, p981-4

43. All the following statements about brain metastasis are true, except:
- a. Carcinoma lung is the commonest cause
- b. Half of the metastasis to brain are solitary
- c. Choriocarcinoma causes hemorrhagic metastasis to brain
- d. Most of the solitary metastasis are from thyroid

Ref. Youmans, 5th/e, p316-20

44. All the conditions cause hyperostosis of sphenoid ridge, except:
- a. Fibrous dysplasia
- b. Sphenoid wing meningioma
- c. Paget's disease
- d. Trigeminal schwannoma

Ref. Youmans, p1115, 3590-1

45. What percentage of vestibular schwannomas causes 5th nerve symptoms?
- a. 5%
- b. 10%
- c. 20%
- d. 40%

Ref. Greenberg, 4th/e, p261-2

46. All the following statements about differentiating vestibular schwannomas and CP angle meningiomas are true, except:
- a. In the former internal acoustic meatus is dilated, and in latter it is normal
- b. In the former incidence of micro-hemorrhages is less than in latter
- c. In the former, the angle between the tumor and the petrous is acute and in latter it is obtuse
- d. In the former the epicenter of the tumor is on internal acoustic meatus and in latter it is away

Ref. Osborn, Section 3, p29-31, 108-9

47. All the following tumors have bimodal peaks in age distribution, except:
- a. Esthesioneuroblastoma
- b. Craniopharyngioma
- c. Medulloblastoma
- d. Vestibular Schwannoma

Ref. Youmans, 5th/e, p1207-19, 1333-41

48. Which of the following criteria fits into the diagnosis of von-Hippel Landau disease?
- a. Two or more hemangioblastomas in neuraxis
- b. One hemangioblastoma and one visceral manifestation
- c. Both 'a' and 'b'
- d. None of the above

Ref. Greenberg, 4th/e, p292

49. All the following statements about null cell adenomas are true, except:
- a. These are negative for all hormones
- b. These are chromophilic adenomas
- c. These cause stalk effect
- d. Cell of origin is unknown

Ref. Youmans, 5th/e, p1172-5

50. All the following statements about diencephalic syndrome are true, except
- a. Described first by Russell
- b. Rotatory nystagmus is seen in 50% patients
- c. Children appear muscular
- d. Growth hormone levels are decreased

Ref. Greenberg, 4th/e, p254

51. Which of the following factors causes growth in tumors after radiotherapy?
- a. Edema
- b. Necrosis
- c. Demyelination
- d. All the above

Ref. Youmans, 5th/e, p659-700, 4015-24

52. All the following about pseudotumor orbit are true, except:
- a. It is an inflammatory condition of orbit
- b. Etiology is unknown
- c. Bilateral pseudotumor can occur in polyarteritis nodosa, Wegner's granulomatosis, sarcoidosis
- d. Lateral orbitotomy is the treatment of choice

Ref. Youmans, 5th/e, p1376

ANSWERS

42. a. **43.** d. **44.** d. **45.** b. **46.** b. **47.** d. **48.** c. **49.** b. **50.** d. **51.** d. **52.** d.

53. All the following statements about Histiocytosis-X are true, except:
- a. Definitive diagnosis is by looking for Birbeck granule
- b. Eosinophilic granuloma, Hand-Schiller-Christian disease and Letter-Sewer disease are three forms of it
- c. Commonest extra-skeletal unifocal site is liver
- d. Prognosis is calculated by Lahey's score

***Ref.* Youmans, 5th/e, p1400-1**

54. Method of Oon is used to check the position of:
- a. Pineal gland
- b. Pituitary gland
- c. Manmillary bodies
- d. Tectal plate

***Ref.* Greenberg, 4th/e, p548**

55. Hematocrit is elevated in one of the following tumors:
- a. Astroblastoma
- b. Ependymoma
- c. Hemangioblastoma
- d. Medulloblastoma

***Ref.* Youmans, 5th/e, p1053-4**

56. In which of the underlying conditions hyperostosis of skull is not usually seen?
- a. Neurofibromatosis
- b. Meningioma
- c. Sinus pericranii
- d. Fibrous dysplasia

***Ref.* Youmans, 5th/e, p1403-4**

57. All the following are features of sinus pericranii, except:
- a. These usually occur in the midline
- b. These may communicate with superior sagittal sinus
- c. These may be congenital or traumatic
- d. These cannot be differentiated from vascular malformations of the scalp

***Ref.* Youmans, 5th/e, p1403-4**

58. The most common cranial nerve involved in sarcoidosis is:
- a. Olfactory nerve
- b. Optic nerve
- c. Facial nerve
- d. Vestibulocochlear nerve

***Ref.* Youmans, 5th/e, p1435-9**

59. All the following elements constitute the components of the middle column as per Denis's three-column theory, except:
- a. Posterior longitudinal ligament
- b. Posterior half of the vertebral body
- c. Posterior annulus fibrosus
- d. Posterior neural arch

***Ref.* Youmans, 5th/e, p4962**

60. One of the indications of operating upon a spinal fracture is when:
- a. Vertebral body height is reduced by 10%
- b. Fracture fragments are displaced in the spinal canal for >1 cm
- c. Vertebral body height is reduced by 20%
- d. When the fracture is a stable fracture

***Ref.* Youmans, 5th/e, p4999**

61. Sacral chordomas arise from:
- a. Embryonic remnants of nucleus pulposus
- b. Embryonic remnants of annulus fibrosus
- c. Ecchordosis physaliphora
- d. None of the above

***Ref.* Pediatric Neurosurgery, 2011;47:22-30**

62. The cut-off size that distinguishes a spinal osteoma from an osteoblastoma is:
- a. 0.5 cm
- b. 1.0 cm
- c. 1.5 cm
- d. 2.0 cm

***Ref.* Pediatric Neurosurgery, 2011;47:22-30**

63. Which of the following statements is true about Mafucci's syndrome?
- a. Multiple osteochondromas are seen
- b. Subcutaneous hemangiomas are associated
- c. There is a risk that chondromas may become malignant
- d. All the above

***Ref.* Youmans, 5th/e, p1387**

ANSWERS

53. c. **54.** a. **55.** c. **56.** c. **57.** d. **58.** c. **59.** d. **60.** b. **61.** c. **62.** c. **63.** d.

64. All the following features are true about epidermoids and dermoids, except:
a. Both arise from ectoderm
b. Both grow from desquamation of epithelium and glandular secretion
c. Both are hypodense on CT scan
d. None of the above
Ref. Youmans, 5th/e, p1224-6, 3691-2, 4259-60

65. The most common primary malignant tumor of orbit in pediatric age group is:
a. Malignant nerve tumor
b. Rhabdomyosarcoma
c. Neuroblastoma
d. None of the above
Ref. Youmans, 5th/e, p 1375

66. The following statements about pseudotumor of orbit are true, except:
a. It occurs mostly in females
b. Third to sixth decade is commonly involved
c. It is an autoimmune process
d. Infection of the orbit can mimic it clinically
Ref. Youmans, 5th/e, p1376-7

67. All the following statements about hemangioma of skull are true, except:
a. The commonest variety is a cavernous hemangioma
b. MRI shows the lesion to have significant flow voids
c. Lesion may cause headache because of distension of the inner and outer bone tables
d. Curettage of the lesion is the commonest procedure of choice
Ref. Youmans, 5th/e, p1384

68. All the following factors induce or increase brain edema, except:
a. Atrial natriuretic peptide
b. Serotonin
c. Bradykinin
d. Vasopressin
Ref. Youmans, 5th/e, p801

69. All the following statements about steroids are true, except:
a. Steroids are effective irrespective of the integrity of the blood brain barrier
b. Steroids reduce vasogenic edema
c. Steroids have no or minimal effect on cytotoxic and interstitial edema
d. None of the above
Ref. Youmans, 5th/e, p801-2

70. All the following conditions are associated with increased risk of brain tumors, except:
a. Ionizing radiation
b. Exposure to pesticides
c. History of allergic disorders
d. Viral infections
Ref. Youmans, 5th/e, p673-5

71. Which of the following pituitary tumors do not usually cause mass effect?
a. Corticotrophic adenomas
b. Somatotrophic adenomas
c. Prolactinomas
d. None of the above
Ref. Youmans, 5th/e, p1170-4

72. Which of the following conditions is not a predisposing factor for pituitary apoplexy?
a. Bromocriptine therapy
b. Head injury
c. Petrous sinus sampling
d. Cranial radiotherapy
Ref. Youmans, 5th/e, p1175-6, 1202-3

73. In which of the following brain tumors, a viral infection of brain has a dominant role in its etiopathogenesis?
a. Pleomorphic xanthoastrocytoma
b. Lymphoma
c. Ganglioglioma
d. Ependymoma
Ref. Youmans, 5th/e, p1067-74

ANSWERS

64. b. **65.** b. **66.** a. **67.** b. **68.** a. **69.** a. **70.** c. **71.** a. **72.** c. **73.** b.

74. All the following tumors are seen in close relation with ventricle of the brain, except:
a. Ganglioglioma
b. Central neurocytoma
c. Lymphoma
d. Ependymoma
Ref. Youmans, 5th/e, p981-4

75. All the following statements about brain metastasis are true, except:
a. The common metastatic tumors are from lung and breast in adults
b. In children, the commonest tumors to metastasize are neuroblastoma and rhabdomyosarcoma
c. Metastasis are more common at gray-white junction
d. Metastasis are more common along the MCA territory
Ref. Youmans, 5th/e, p1077-3

76. In which of the following conditions, a synergistic effect of Epstein-Barr-virus and plasmodium falciparum on the etiopathogenesis is well known?
a. Metastasis from carcinoma cervix
b. Burkitt's lymphoma
c. Ganglioglioma
d. Pleomorphic xanthoastrocytoma
Ref. Seminars in cancer biology 2009;19(6): 411-20

77. All the following statements which differentiate high grade gliomas from low grade gliomas (LGG's) are true, except:
a. The incidence of seizures in high grade gliomas (HGG) is more than in low grade gliomas (LGG's)
b. Enhancement on contrast administration is heterogenous in HGG's than in LGG's
c. HGG's usually involve elderly population and LGG's involve the young adults
d. Rosenthal fibers on histopathology are seen in LGG's while as high mitotic index is seen in HGG's
Ref. Youmans, 5th/e, p981-94

78. All the following tumors are subtypes of low grade gliomas, except:
a. Ganglioglioma
b. Pleomorphic xanthoastrocytoma
c. Primitive neuroectodermal tumor
d. Subependymal giant cell astrocytoma
Ref. Youmans, 5th/e, p997-1007

79. A 5-year-child presents with history suggestive of lower cranial nerve palsy and also has gait difficulty. The commonest lesion MRI shows among the following brainstem lesions is:
a. Cervicomedullary glioma
b. Diffuse pontine glioma
c. Focal brainstem glioma
d. Dorsally exophytic glioma
Ref. Youmans, 5th/e, p984-6

80. A 7-year-old boy from Uganda presents with headache, proptosis of two weeks' durations. His imaging reveals a skull base lesion with extension into the orbits. The most likely diagnosis is a:
a. Plasmacytoma b. Histiocytoma
c. Burkitt's lymphoma d. Neuroblastoma
Ref. AJNR, case of the week 2009;March 30: 444-52

81. All the following tumors are small round cell tumors, except:
a. Lymphoma b. Neuroblastoma
c. Medulloblastoma d. Glioblastoma
Ref. Kleihues

82. All the following conditions are associated with a high-risk of medulloblastoma, except:
a. Ataxia-telangiectasia b. Tuberous sclerosis
c. Gorlin's syndrome d. Cowden's disease
Ref. Youmans, 5th/e, p811-2

83. In which of the following tumors ultrastructure reveals a typical 9+1 pattern of cilia?
a. Ependymoma b. Glomus jugulare
c. Schwannoma d. None of the above
Ref. Youmans, 5th/e, p1046

ANSWERS

74. a. **75.** b. **76.** b. **77.** a. **78.** c. **79.** b. **80.** c. **81.** d. **82.** b. **83.** a.

84. All the following statements about hemangioblastomas of the brain are true, except:
a. These are seen in von-Hippel-Landau disease
b. This tumor is common in men than in women
c. It is more commonly seen in infratentorial compartment than supratentorial
d. This tumor is a grade II WHO tumor
Ref. Youmans, 5th/e, p1053-4

85. Which of the following conditions gives rise to precocious pseudopuberty?
a. Pituitary adenoma b. Pineal tumors
c. Opticochiasmatic glioma
d. Thalamic glioma
Ref. Youmans, 5th/e, p1013

86. Which of the following markers is present in the serum of Pineal endodermal sinus tumor?
a. Alpha-fetoprotein
b. Beta-human chorionic gonadotropin
c. Carcinoembryonic antigen
d. None of the above
Ref. Youmans, 5th/e, p1014

87. According to the modified Chang classification for medulloblastoma, stage T_2 tumor means:
a. Tumor ≥ 3 cm in size invading one adjacent structure or filling the 4th ventricle partially
b. Tumor ≤ 3 cm in size involving the vermis and filling the 4th ventricle fully
c. Tumor ≤ 3 cm in size, limited to vermis, roof of 4th ventricle or cerebellar hemisphere
d. Tumor ≥ 3 cm exiting through the aqueduct and involving the 3rd ventricle or midbrain or down past the foramen of Magendie
Ref. Youmans, 5th/e, p1034-6

88. All the following are complications of radiotherapy to brain tumors, except:
a. Radionecrosis
b. Peritumoral edema
c. Moya-Moya syndrome
d. Subdural hematomas
Ref. Youmans, 5th/e, p1715-21, 2195-6

89. All the following features differentiate dermoids from epidermoids, except:
a. Dermoids present in late adulthood while as epidermoids present in teen age population
b. Dermoids are usually located in the midline while as epidermoids are usually not restricted to midline
c. Dermoids are easy to excise than epidermoids
d. Posterior fossa dermoids are associated with Klippel-Feil anomaly, but such association is not seen in epidermoids
Ref. Youmans, 5th/e, p1224-6, 3691-2, 4259-60

90. Which is the commonest clinical finding in a patient with corpus callosum glioma involving the frontal lobes?
a. Urinating in public
b. Disinterest in surroundings
c. Making silly jokes
d. None of the above
Ref. Youmans. 5th/e, p830

91. All the following are the features of paraneoplastic cerebellar degeneration, except:
a. Presence of pleocytosis in CSF
b. Presence of anti-40 antibodies in serum
c. Cross reaction of anti-Yo antibodies with mossy fibers
d. Usually seen in patients with ovarian or breast cancer
Ref. Youmans, 5th/e, p832

92. Match the serum antibodies with each of the following disease process:
a. Limbic encephalitis, (1) anti-yo 1, *anti-Yo*
b. Paraneoplastic cerebellar degeneration, (2) anti-Ri
c. Opsoclonus, (3) anti-Hu 3, anti-Hu
Ref. Youmans, 5th/e, p830-3

93. All the following are usual sites for extraneural metastasis for intracranial meningiomas, except:
a. Lungs b. Liver
c. Spinal cord d. Lymph nodes
Ref. Journal of Clinical Oncology 2010; 20(29):e214-5

ANSWERS

84. d. **85.** b. **86.** a. **87.** a. **88.** d. **89.** a. **90.** b. **91.** b. **92.** a. **93.** c.

94. In which of the following intracranial lesion serum CA19-9 is elevated?

a. Metastatic melanoma
b. Metastasis from lung carcinoma
c. Epidermoid
d. Teratoma

Ref. Youmans, 5th/e, p4259-60

95. Which malignancy can complicate an intracranial epidermoid?

a. Adenocarcinoma
b. Squamous cell carcinoma
c. Transitional cell carcinoma
d. None of the above

Ref. Youmans, 5th/e, p4259-60

96. Which of the following spinal lesions can present with hydrocephalus?

a. Dermoid
b. Meningioma
c. Neurofibroma
d. a and c

Ref. Youmans, 5th/e, p4826-7

97. Giant spinal schwannomas are defined as:

a. When the tumor extends over 2 or more vertebral levels
b. When the tumor extends over 3 or more vertebral levels
c. When the tumor size is 5 cm or more in size
d. None of the above

Ref. Journal of Korean Neurosurgical Society 2010;47(6):454-7

98. All the following statements are true, except:

a. NF-2 codes for merlin
b. Merlin is also known as schwannomin
c. Merlin is a cytoskeletal sphingolipid
d. Loss of merlin leads to the development of meningioma

Ref. Youmans, 5th/e, p1105-8

99. The following statements about astrocytomas are true, except:

a. Fibroblastic growth factor expression is elevated in the astrocytes
b. Both fibroblast growth factor receptors; FGFR1 and FGFR2 are elevated
c. Low grade astrocytomas exhibit the alpha subunit of the FGFR1
d. None of the above

Ref. Youmans, 5th/e, p727

100. The role of platelet derived growth factor has been best established in which of the following brain tumors?

a. Ependymomas
b. Meningiomas
c. Astrocytomas
d. Medulloblastomas

Ref. Youmans, 5th/e, p729

101. Which of the following molecules is involved in invasion in malignant gliomas?

a. Fibronectin
b. Laminin
c. Tenascin
d. All the above

Ref. Youmans, 5th/e, p761

102. Which of the following characteristics describes squalamine?

a. It is derived from dogfish stark
b. It is a steroid
c. It has anti-angiogenic properties
d. All the above

Ref. Youmans, 5th/e, p779

103. All the following mediators are responsible for brain edema, except:

a. Atrial natriuretic peptide
b. Histamine
c. Serotonin
d. None of the above

Ref. Youmans, 5th/e, p801

104. The most sensitive test to diagnose carcinomatous meningitis is:

a. Contrast MRI
b. CSF examination
c. PET scanning
d. Double-dose contrast CT scan

Ref. Greenberg, 4th/e, p322-3

ANSWERS

94. c. **95.** b. **96.** d. **97.** a. **98.** c. **99.** b. **100.** c. **101.** d. **102.** d. **103.** a. **104.** b.

105. All the following are features of carcinomatous meningitis, except:

a. Intraventricular and subarachnoid enhancing nodules
b. Widening of spinal canal
c. Enhancing cisterns
d. Maintenance of normal CSF protein levels

Ref. Greenberg, 4th/e, p322-3

106. All the following statements regarding aneurysmal bone cysts of spine are true, except:

a. These are common in females
b. These are benign cysts and never undergo malignant transformation
c. Curettage and bone grafting is the usual treatment
d. Radiotherapy, embolization are other alternatives to surgery

Ref. Pediatric Neurosurgery 2011;47:22-30

107. All the following statements about chordoma are true, except:

a. Chordoma have a low grade malignant potential
b. Females are affected more than males
c. Chordomas have a tendency for recurrence
d. Heavy particle irradiation has advantage over conventional radiotherapy

Ref. Pediatric Neurosurgery 2011;47:22-30

108. Hyperthyroidism caused by pituitary tumor is:

a. Primary hyperthyroidism
b. Secondary hyperthyroidism
c. Mixed hyperthyroidism
d. None of the above

Ref. Youmans, 5th/e, p1172-74

109. Which of the following features does not characterize pituitary tumors?

a. Headache is a feature
b. Inferior temporal quadrantnopia is the initial field defect on perimetry
c. Diabetes insipidus is a common finding
d. b and c

Ref. Youmans, 5th/e, p1174

110. The commonest metastatic tumor to brain in children is:

a. Ewing's sarcoma
b. Germ cell tumor
c. Leukemia
d. Wilm's tumor

Ref. Pediatric Neurosurgery 2011;47:31-7

111. All the following characteristics differentiate meningiomas from hemangiopericytomas, except:

a. Meningiomas have broader dural tail than hemangiopericytomas
b. Hemangiopericytomas are more vascular than meningiomas
c. Meningiomas cause hyperostosis of bone while as hemangiopericytomas cause bone erosion
d. All meningiomas are histopathologically benign while as all hemangiopericytomas are histopathologically malignant

Ref. Youmans, 5th/e, p1133-38

112. Which of the following pituitary tumors has no fixed site of origin within the pituitary gland?

a. PRL secreting
b. GH secreting
c. Gonadotrope secreting
d. Glucocorticoid secreting

Ref. Youmans, 5th/e, p1171

113. Aneurysmal bone cysts of spine usually include the posterior elements of:

a. Cervical spine
b. Dorsal spine
c. Lumbar spine
d. Sacral spine

Ref. Pediatric Neurosurgery 2011;47:22-30

114. The commonest sarcoma involving a pediatric spine is:

a. Osteosarcoma
b. Ewing's sarcoma
c. Chondrosarcoma
d. None of the above

Ref. Pediatric Neurosurgery 2011;47:22-30

ANSWERS

105. d. **106.** b. **107.** b. **108.** b. **109.** d. **110.** c. **111.** d. **112.** c. **113.** b. **114.** b.

115. The most common brain metastasis in males is from:
a. Lung b. Skin
c. Kidney d. Thyroid
Ref. Youmans, 5th/e, p1077-93

116. Following are the radioresistant metastasis to brain, except:
a. Melanoma b. Renal cell carcinoma
c. Osteosarcoma d. Germ cell tumors
Ref. Youmans, 5th/e, p1024-5

117. The most probable diagnosis for a pineal region tumor with moderately elevated levels of HCG and its high radiosensitivity and diabetes insipidus at presentation is:
a. Pineocytoma
b. Germinoma
c. Endodermal sinus tumor
d. None of the above
Ref. Youmans, 5th/e, p1014

118. Collier's sign is seen in lesions around the:
a. Dorsal midbrain
b. Frontal lobe
c. Craniovertebral junction
d. None of the above
Ref. Youmans, 5th/e, p1013

119. In which of the following lesions, the apparent diffusion coefficient is the lowest?
a. Brain abscess
b. Cerebral lymphoma
c. Cystic astrocytoma
d. Metastasis
Ref. AJNR 2010;31:60-6

120. The best investigation to differentiate a cerebral lymphoma from toxoplasmosis of brain is:
a. Functional MRI
b. Diffusion tensor imaging
c. Thalium-201 scan
d. Magnetic resonance spectroscopy
Ref. Youmans, 5th/e, p1069

121. In which subtype of brainstem gliomas is surgery a good option?
a. Diffuse b. Dorsally exophytic
c. Cervicomedullary d. None of the above
Ref. Youmans, 5th/e, p984-5

122. Which of the following lesions has the following characteristics - these lesions are common in females; erode the petrous apex, can cause conductive hearing loss, patient has weakness in chewing and patient may get a corneal ulcer?
a. Trigeminal schwannoma
b. Chordoma of clivus
c. CP angle epidermoid
d. Vestibular schwannoma
Ref. Youmans, 5th/e, p1344-8

123. All the following statements are true except:
a. Epidermoids and dermoids have female preponderance
b. Epidermoids occur in slightly older age group as compared to dermoids
c. Hair follicles being among the contents of dermis, transformation into squamous cell carcinoma is seen more often than in epidermoids
d. Both the lesions cause lytic lesions of skull
Ref. Youmans, 5th/e, p1224-6, 3691-2, 4259-60

124. Following are the differential diagnosis of intraventricular tumors:
a. Ependymoma
b. Choroid plexus carcinoma
c. Meningioma
d. All the above
Ref. Youmans, 5th/e, p1240-1

125. A 4-year-old boy complaints of repeated vomitings without headache. His neurological examination reveals features of midline posterior fossa syndrome, his most probable diagnosis is:
a. Ependymoma
b. Germinoma
c. Cerebellar astrocytoma
d. Meduloblastoma
Ref. Youmans, 5th/e, p1043-8

ANSWERS

115. a. **116.** d. **117.** b. **118.** a. **119.** b. **120.** c. **121.** b. **122.** a. **123.** c. **124.** d.
125. a.

126. The following tumors are arranged in decreasing order of their incidence of calcification:

a. Craniopharyngioma – medulloblastoma – ependymoma - cerebellar astrocytoma
b. Craniopharyngioma – ependymoma – medulloblastoma – cerebellar astrocytoma
c. Ependymoma – craniopharyngioma – cerebellar astrocytoma – medulloblastoma
d. Medulloblastoma – cerebellar astrocytoma – craniopharyngioma -ependymoma

Ref. Youmans, 5th/e, p1031-40, 1207-19, 1043-8

127. Following tumors have bimodal distribution for age:

a. Medulloblastoma
b. Craniopharyngioma
c. Cerebellar astrocytoma
d. All the above

Ref. Youmans, 5th/e, p1031-40, 1207-19

128. All the following effects of steroids on brain tumors are true, except:

a. It reduces the capillary permeability
b. It reduces the tumor blood volume
c. It has apoptotic effect on lymphomas
d. The maximum dose in adults is 50 mg/day

Ref. Youmans, 5th/e, p801

129. Commonest sites of extraneural metastasis of meningiomas are:

a. Lungs
b. Liver
c. Orbit
d. Mediastinum

Ref. Greenberg, 4th/e, p259

130. The commonest site of extracranial site of meningiomas is:

a. Lung
b. Orbit
c. Ovary
d. None of the above

Ref. Youmans, 5th/e, p1118-9

131. All the following statements about meningiomas are true, except:

a. Meningiomas mostly are benign tumors
b. These constitute about 20–25% of brain tumors
c. All meningiomas have a dural tail
d. Most of the meningiomas are vascular tumors

Ref. Youmans, 5th/e, p1099-127

132. Which of the following statements about meningiomas is/are true?

a. Meningiomas express estrogen and progesterone receptors
b. Meningiomas express estrogen, progesterone and androgen receptors
c. Meningiomahs express estrogen and dopaminergic receptors
d. All the above

Ref. Youmans, 5th/e, p1108

133. All the following statements about meningiomas are true, except:

a. Meningiomas produce hyperostosis of bone
b. Meningiomas contain calcium
c. Enplaque meningiomas are highly vascular
d. Angiography reveals mother-in-law appearance

Ref. Greenberg, 4th/e, p258

134. The classical chiasmal syndrome is seen in:

a. Olfactory groove meningiomas
b. Tuberculum sellae meningiomas
c. Diaphragm sellae meningiomas
d. None of the above

Ref. Al Mefty p 397

135. The commonest site of intracranial schwannoma is:

a. Oculomotor schwannoma
b. Vestibular schwannoma
c. Trigeminal schwannoma
d. Trochlear schwannoma

Ref. Greenberg, 4th/e, p262

136. Which of the following brain tumors is least likely to bleed?

a. Pituitary adenomas
b. Pilocytic astrocytomas
c. Oligodendrogliomas
d. Glioblastoma multiforme

Ref. Youmans, 5th/e, p986-8

ANSWERS

126. b. **127.** d. **128.** d. **129.** b. **130.** b. **131.** c. **132.** d. **133.** c. **134.** b. **135.** b. **136.** b.

137. Histopathological examination of a metastatic 'calvarial' tumor is most likely to reveal origin from:

a. Kidney b. Breast
c. Thyroid d. Lung

Ref. Greenberg, 4th/e, p313

138. Which chromosome deletion is seen in oligodendrogliomas ?

a. 1p, 19q b. 13p, 3q
c. 18p, 6q d. None of the above

Ref. Kleihues p 60

139. All the following statements are true, except:

a. In primary optic atrophy, the whole disk is chalky white
b. In secondary optic atrophy, the whole disk is pale white
c. In Foster-Kennedy syndrome, there is bilateral secondary optic atrophy
d. Myopic disc are very pale and have a crescent of pallor around

Ref. Greenberg, 4th/e, p32

140. In which of the following conditions, sella is 'J' shaped?

a. Pituitary adenoma
b. Optic nerve glioma
c. Rathke cleft cyst
d. Diaphragm sella meningioma

Ref. Greenberg, 4th/e, p548

141. In which of the following conditions, the phenomenon of T-2 shine through effect is commonly displayed on MRI scan:

a. Hemangioblastoma
b. Metastasis
c. Dysplastic gangliocytoma of cerebellum
d. Pineoblastoma

Ref. Turkish Journal of Neurosurgery

142. A 50-year-old male reported with history of sudden onset of headache and hemiparesis. Imaging revealed a frontotemporal hematoma with perilesional edema and upon contrast administration, the lesion shows enhancement. The crush biopsy reveals small rounded cells. The most possible diagnosis on Hematoxylin-eosin staining expected is:

a. Neurocytoma b. Tuberculoma
c. Astrocytoma II d. Oligodendroglioma

Ref. Greenberg, 4th/e, p256-7

143. A 40-year-old male reports with 3 months history of headache and 1 month history of vomiting. CT reveals a hyperdense lesion in the left parietal lobe. There is homogenous enhancement of the lesion, and there is no dural tail sign. Patient was put on steroids and planned for an MRI brain. While on steroids, plain CT was repeated which revealed central hypodensity in the brain. The most possible diagnosis is a:

a. Meningioma b. Lymphoma
c. Astrocytoma II d. Metastasis

Ref. Youmans, 5th/e, p1067-74

144. Patients with a partially resected intracranial epidermoid if asked for regular follow-up to rule out the rare chance of complication viz. development of a squamous cell carcinoma shall be followed by screening the serum for:

a. Prolactin levels
b. Interleukin-1
c. Carcinoembryogenic antigen levels
d. None of the above

Ref. Youmans, 5th/e, p1224

145. One of the causes of precocious puberty is a:

a. Pituitary adenoma
b. Hypothalamic hamartoma
c. Optic-chiasmatic glioma
d. None of the above

Ref. Youmans, 5th/e, p2578

146. A 7-year-old boy reports with headache of 6 months' duration and vomiting of 1-month duration. His MRI brain showed an intra-ven-tricular lesion, iso-intense on T1W and hyperintense on T2W. Histopathology revealed a cellular tumor with cells having scant cytoplasm and round nuclei with finely

Brain Tumors (MCQs)

ANSWERS

137. b. **138.** a. **139.** c. **140.** b. **141.** c. **142.** d. **143.** b. **144.** c. **145.** b.

speckled chromatin. Immunostain for GFAP was negative and synaptophysin was positive. The most probable diagnosis is:

a. Neurocytoma
b. Oligodendroglioma
c. Subependymal giant cell astrocytoma
d. None of the above

Ref. Kleihues, p108

147. Which of the following surgical approaches is not done for resection of: Trigeminal schwannomas of middle fossa?

a. Subtemporal approach
b. Orbitozygomatic approach
c. Postauricular approach
d. Extradural temporopolar approach

Ref. Youmans, 5th/e, p1349

148. Stage IB in juvenile angiofibroma means:

a. Tumor extension into one or more paranasal sinuses
b. Tumor extension into pterygopalatine fossa
c. Tumor extending into the cheek
d. None of the above

Ref. Youmans, 5th/e, p1353

149. All the following are features of eosinophilic granuloma, except:

a. It is a local manifestation of Langerhan cell histiocytosis
b. It may present as a local scalp swelling
c. X-ray skull reveals a punched-out lesion
d. After surgical excision, recurrence never occurs

Ref. Greenberg, 4th/e, p314

150. Which of the following description correlates with class-B of glomus jugulare?

a. Tumor confined to the middle ear
b. Involvement of intralabyrinthine or apical spaces of the temporal bone
c. Tumor involving the middle ear or mastoid bone, without infralabyrinthine space involvement
d. Intracranial extension

Ref. Youmans, 5th/e, p1298

151. In modified Kadish staging of esthesio-neuroblastoma, stage C tumor means:

a. Tumor beyond nasal cavity and paranasal sinuses
b. Tumor with metastasis
c. Tumor confined to the nasal cavity
d. Tumor extension to the paranasal sinuses

Ref. Youmans, 5th/e, p1335

152. Which of the following is not a feature of McCune-Albright syndrome?

a. Polyostotic fibrous dysplasia
b. Endocrine dysfunction
c. Champagne cork appearance of bone on imaging
d. Cafe's au lait spots

Ref. Youmans, 5th/e, p1401

153. All the following brain tumors are resistant to radiotherapy, except:

a. Melanoma
b. Medulloblastoma
c. Sarcoma
d. Renal cell carcinoma

Ref. Youmans, 5th/e, p1038

154. A middle aged woman reports with visual disturbances. She also has elevated prolactin levels. MRI brain shows a lesion between the anterior and the posterior pituitary lobes. The lesion is hyperintense on T_1-weighted sequence and does not enhance on contrast administration. The most likely diagnosis is a:

a. Prolactinoma
b. Ectopic germinoma
c. Craniopharyngioma
d. Rathke cleft cyst

Ref. Greenberg, 4th/e, p289

155. Which of the following lesions can produce diencephalic syndrome/gelastic seizure/ diabetes insipidus/precocious puberty?

a. Optic nerve glioma
b. Hypothalamic hamartoma
c. Pineal region germinoma
d. Brainstem glioma

Ref. Youmans, 5th/e, p3596

ANSWERS

146. a. **147.** c. **148.** a. **149.** d. **150.** c. **151.** a. **152.** c. **153.** b. **154.** d. **155.** b.

156. The arcuate defect in the visual fields is caused by:

a. Pituitary tumor b. Craniopharyngioma
c. Optic nerve gliomas d. Hydrocephalus

Ref. Bickerstaff, 6th/e, p45

157. Which of the following is associated with bilateral sylvian fissure arachnoid cysts?

a. Glutariaciduria type-I
b. Tay-Sach's disease
c. Neiman-pick's disease
d. None of the above

Ref. Youman p3290

158. All the following are true for pineal region tumors, except:

a. Germinomas are radioresistant
b. Pineocytomas do not require radiotherapy
c. Germinomas associated with elevated β-hcg levels may have a less favorable prognosis
d. Prophylactic spinal radiation is given currently only once there is evidence of spinal metastasis

Ref. Youman p1024-25

159. All the following statements about radiotherapy in pituitary adenomas are true, except:

a. Residual pituitary adenomas with major parasellar extensions are best treated by radiotherapy
b. Fractionated radiotherapy has a larger mean time to remission than stereotactic radiosurgery
c. New hormone deficiencies are more common in radiosurgery group than in patients receiving fractionated radiotherapy
d. Patients who have previously received radiotherapy to sella, have high incidence of CSF leaks at 2nd surgery

Ref. World Neurosurg. 2015;83(6):1173-9

160. Which feature is not seen in intra-axial lesion:

a. Containment of all the margins of the lesions within the brain parenchyma
b. Thickening of the cortex rather than buckling
c. Enhancement of the overlying leptomeninges
d. Extensive vasogenic edema

Ref. Youman's p835

161. All the following statements about temozolamide are true, except:

a. It is an oral drug active against low grade gliomas
b. Its active metabolite is 3-methyl-imidazole-4-carbox-gamide
c. It causes alkylation of DNA
d. Alkylation of O^6 position of guanine is the target lesion it produces

Ref. Youman's p882

162. Malignant gliomas can have local and distant recurrence. The distal recurrence is arbitrarily defined as:

a. More than 1 cm from the original tumor site
b. More than 2 cm from the original tumor site
c. More than 3.5 cm from the original tumor site
d. More than 5 cm from the original tumor site

Ref. Youman p757

163. Which of the following is not a paraneoplastic syndrome?

a. Cerebellar degeneration
b. Limbic encephalitis
c. Myoclonus
d. Dyskinesias

Ref. Youman p832

164. The radiological feature of extra-axial lesion include:

a. An obtuse margin with brain parenchyma
b. Buckling of the cortex
c. Dural tail
d. All the above

Ref. Youman p835

165. Which of the following drugs is used as a medical treatment for the medulloblastoma?

a. Temozolomide b. Cisplatin
c. Mebendazole d. Doxorubicin

Ref. Neuro Oncol. 2015;17(4):545-54

166. Which are of the following is not an agent for tumor embolization?

a. NBCA b. Onyx
c. Gelatinized foam d. Lipiodol

Ref. Interv Neuroradiol. 2015 Oct;21(5): 624-30

ANSWERS

156. c. **157.** a. **158.** a. **159.** c. **160.** c. **161.** a. **162.** b. **163.** d. **164.** d. **165.** c. **166.** d.

167. In which of the following conditions patient gets bobble-head doll movements?

a. Sylvian fissure arachnoid cyst
b. Craniopharyngioma
c. Suprasellar arachnoid cyst
d. None of the above

Ref. J Pediatr Neurosci 2015;10(1):18-21

168. Which of the following secondary changes can explain progression of lesion in operated case of brain glioma who has received radiotherapy?

a. Radiation necrosis
b. Tumor recurrence
c. Radiation induced neoplasm
d. All the above

Ref. JNS 1995, 82, 436-44

169. Among the below mentioned tumors which brain tumor violates the Collin's law?

a. Medulloblastoma b. Ependymoma
c. Brainstem glioma d. Cerebellar astrocytoma

Ref. JNS 1988, 68, 41-7

170. Calcification is usually seen in following brain tumors, except:

a. Pleomorphic xanthomatous astrocytoma
b. Ganglioglioma
c. Pilocytic astrocytoma
d. Hemangioblastoma

Ref. AJNR, Apr. 2015

171. All the following statements about pituitary adenomas are correct, except:

a. Adenomas bigger than 1 cm are macroadenomas
b. Adenomas bigger than 5 cm are giant adenomas
c. A figure-of-8 appearance is seen in imaging
d. Adenomas are usually isointense to the grey matter

Ref. AJNR, Feb. 17, 2014

172. All the following statements about granular cell tumor of pituitary are true, except:

a. These are purely intrasellar lesions
b. These present with usual disturbances and headaches
c. These are iso-intense on T_1W
d. These are hyperdense in CT

Ref. AJNR, Jan 2, 2014

173. Which of the following statements about cystic meningiomas are true?

a. There are 4 types of cystic meningiomas based on the location of the cyst
b. Cyst occurs because of degeneration necrosis, direct secretion or reactive changes
c. Microcystic meningioma and schwannoma with cystic change are the differential diagnosis
d. All the above are true

Ref. AJNR, Oct 21, 2013

174. All the following symptoms can be caused by intraventricular mass lesions, except:

a. Headache
b. Visual field defects
c. Hemiparesis
d. Seizures

Ref. Neurosurgery Focus, 20(3);E9, 2006

175. Which of the following statements regarding paraneoplastic syndrome is correct?

a. Eaton-Lambert syndrome is the commonest paraneoplastic syndrome
b. Retinopathy is also a feature of PNPS and is usually associated with small cell cancer of lung
c. Stiff women's syndrome is associated with breast cancer
d. All the above

Ref. Adams, p728

ANSWERS

167. c. **168.** d. **169.** d. **170.** d. **171.** b. **172.** a. **173.** d. **174.** d. **175.** d.

EXPLANATION

1. There are three types of fibrous dysplasia: monostotic (MC-70%), polyostotic. McCune Albright syndrome is characterized by polyostotic fibrosis dysplasia, endocrine hyper-function, café-a-lait pigmentation of the skin and other extra-skeletal abnormalities.
2. Optic pathway gliomas (OPG's) are included as one of the representatives of childhood supratentorial tumors. They represent 1% of all CNS tumors, 3–5% of all pediatric brain tumors, 65% of the patients are less than 5-years of age. They occur with equal frequency in males and females. The majority of the pediatric low grade astrocytomas in the hypothalamic / chiasmatic region are pediatric low grade gliomas. There may be other gliomas such as fibrillary astrocytomas and ganglioglioma but anaplastic astrocytoma and PNET are rare. Pilocytic astrocytomas have typical Rosenthal's fibers and eosinophillic granular bodies.
3. The signs and symptoms are dependent on the location and direction of tumor growth and the structures involved. The predominant clinical manifestations are visual disturbances, hydrocephalus and endocrine dysfunction. Children may exhibit a decrease in visual field deficits. If the tumor is located in the intra-orbital space, proptosis with deviation of the affected eye can occur. Suprasellar gliomas extending into the third ventricle often causes obstructive hydrocephalus. Hydrocephalus is manifested as macrocephaly and failure to thrive in infancy. Older children may present with endocrine dysfunction and failure to thrive
4. Surgical resection is not feasible for gliomas diffusely involving the optic pathway including optic chiasma, tracts, optic radiations and brain stem. These structures are treated non-surgically with chemotherapy or radiotherapy or both.
5. Radiation therapy to cranium is associated with radiation induced neoplasia. Criteria for radiation induced neoplasia include (1) tumor must occur in the irradiation field (2) it cannot be present before radiotherapy (3) tumor must differ from histologically from irradiated tumor and (4) there must be no genetic predisposition.
6. Brain germinomas are extremely responsive to both radiation therapy and chemotherapy with long term recurrence rate of 90%. Radiotherapy has historically been the treatment of choice and presently the standard treatment is multimodal i.e. surgery + chemotherapy + radiotherapy.
7. CT scan shows calcification which occurs in 50–90% of pediatric craniopharyngiomas. CT is also superior in demonstrating the anatomy and size of sphenoid sinus when transsphenoidal route is anticipated. The calcifications have craggy popcorn like appearance with egg-shell lines. About 40–50% ependymomas show calcification and about 20% medulloblastomas are also calcified, however the overall incidence of medulloblastomas is much higher than that of ependymomas such that the commonest cause of calcification in posterior fossa is a medulloblastoma. About 10% of choroid plexus papillomas are calcified.
8. Chang and colleagues classified medulloblastoma patients on the basis of two parameters. Tumor stage (T) and metastasis (M). M-stage is particularly important in estimating prognosis and directing adjuvant therapy.

   M_0: No evidence of gross, cerebrospinal or hematogenous metastasis.

   M_1: Positive microscopy of CSF cytology.

   M_2: Gross nodular seeding involving the cerebellar subarachnoid space or ¾ ventricle

   M_3: Gross nodular seeding of the spinal subarachnoid space

   M_4: Extra neural metastasis.

10. Arises from the vestibular component of the vestibule-cochlear nerve. In recent surgical studies, the most common origin has been from the superior vestibular nerve followed by inferior V. nerve. The extent of cerebellopontine spread is variable but it is the meatal origin that gives acoustic neuromas their 'ice-cream-cone' shape. The growth rate is about 0.4–2.4 mm/year. In NF-2 the tumor occurs at young age and has more unpredictable growth (1.3mm/year). These patients have bilateral tumors. Microscopic appearance – Antoni A and Antoni B pattern.
11. MRI with paramagnetic contrast have greatly increased the sensitivity of imaging in the detection of vestibular schwannomas and in the distinction between other CPA pathology. Vestibular schwannomas are the most common tumor seen within CP angle (70 to 80%) followed by meningiomas and the epidermoids. Vestibular schwannomas should be distinguished from meningiomas by various imaging features which include acute angle

with the petrous bone, ice-cream cone appearance, evidence of microbleeds, epicenter of the tumor on the meatus, absence of calcification, etc. in favor of the vestibular schwannomas.

12. Cystic tumors are believed to have more aggressive surgical course. There is higher risk of facial nerve injury too. The facial nerve preservation drops from 93 to 88% in patients with cystic tumors. Intra-op dissection is tedious.

13. Tumor size and extension along with preoperative hearing level are important predictors of likelihood of hearing preservation. The sub-occipital approach has good results of hearing preservation. The middle fossa approach is best used for small laterally placed tumors. One of the key points which dictates the feasibility of radiosurgery is associated brainstem compression, since edema can be a difficult complication after radiosurgery any evidence of brainstem compression on imaging is a contraindication for radiosurgery for fear of worsening of symptoms.

14. As a whole gliomas (astrocytomas) are most common (50%). In this group, the pilocytic are most common (about 25%). The second group medulloblastoma which occurs in the fourth ventricle from neural stem cells in 15-20%. Craniopharyngiomas also form a huge bulk, infact in some series of pediatric brain tumors these constitute The others are of neuroepithelial origin which includes ependymomas (10%), PNET (1.9%), ganglioglioma (2.5%).

15. Colloid cyst arises from remnants of postvelar arch. Benign cyst, incidence 0.5% to 1%; most commonly located in the roof of the third ventricle. It can lead to acute hydrocephalus, due to blockage of foramen Monro. Treatment options include microsurgical or endoscopic excision or conservative management.

16. Most common symptom is headache of varying intensity. Acute hydrocephalus which leads to sudden death due to blockage of foramen of Monro. It is neuroepithelial in origin. Treatment of choice is microsurgical / endoscopic excision. Radiosurgery has no role.

17. Gangliocytoma (WHO-I) and ganglioglioma (WHO-I or III) are well differentiated tumors. They frequently occur in temporal lobe. Ganglioglioma is most common tumor associated with temporal lobe epilepsy (40%). DNET (WHO-Grade I) is a low grade tumor that occurs in children and young patients with history of long standing resistant seizures. Resection is curative even partial resection usually stops seizure activity. Pleomorphic xanthoastrocytoma (WHO grade-II), typically arises in superficial cerebral location in children and young adults with history of seizures. Temporal lobe is favored site. Glioblastoma multiforme (WHO-IV) can cause seizures but is not responsible for chronic seizures as the life span is short after the diagnosis.

20. Dysplastic gangliocytoma of the cerebellum (Lhermitte Duclos disease) – WHO grade-I. It is characterized by: Cerebellar location. Gross enlargement of folia on MRI. Disorganized cerebellar cortical histology (large ganglion cells predominate). A layer of molecular axons in outer molecular layer. Association with Cowden's syndrome (50%) cases. Treatment primarily surgical. MRI shows a typical tigroid pattern on coronal T_2-sections, also T_2-shine-through–phenomenon is seen in this lesion. Malignant transformation is very rare.

21. 10% of all intracranial meningomiomas arises in posterior fossa. Almost half (50%) in CP angle, 40% are tentorial or cerebellar convexity. 10% - clival and foramen magnum.

Incidence of brain tumors (data with postmortem examination included):

i. Meningiomas (40%)
ii. Gliomas (35%)
iii. Pituitary adenoma (13%).

Incidence of brain tumors (postmortem examination excluded):

i. Gliomas (43%)
ii. Meningiomas (21%)
iii. Pituitary adenoma (17%).

Meningiomas constitute 1–4% of all brain tumors in children (<18 years of age).

23. Hyperostosis is characteristic feature of meningiomas especially enplaque meningioma. Parasagittal meningioma is one that fills parasagatil angle with no brain tissue between the tumor and SSS. Also associated with hyperostotic bone is present. Falcine meningioma arises from falx and is completely concealed by overlying cortex. So hyperostosis is absent. Intraventricular meningiomas arise from arachnoid cells of choroid plexus and tela choroidae (1% all intracranial meningiomas). 90% are located in trigone of lateral ventricle.

24. Distribution of intracranial meningiomas:

Convexity – 35%. Parasagittal – 20%. Sphenoid ridge – 20%. Intraventricular – 5%. Tuberculum sellae – 3%. Infratentorial – 13%. Others – 4%.

WHO grading of meningiomas

Grade I	**Grade II**
(FMT-PALMM)	
Fibrous meningioma	Atypical meningioma
Meningothelial meningioma	Clear cell meningioma
Transitional meningioma	Chordoid meningioma
Psammomatous meningioma	
Angiomatous meningioma	
Lymphoplasmacyte – rich meningioma	
Metaplastic meningioma	
Microcystic meningioma	

Grade I

Rhabdoid meningioma

Papillary meningioma

Anaplastic (malignant) meningioma

25. Most meningiomas are supplied by meningeal artery which is a branch of ECA, however at few sites branches from ICA supply these tumors viz. falcine and orbital meningiomas via branches of ophthalmic artery, tentorial meningiomas via tentorial branch of ICA (Cassinari and Bernasconi).

26. Following modalities can be useful to avoid injury to eloquent area of brain. Functional MRI and PET are used mostly in preoperative period. Functional MRI – depends on local oxygen demand of cerebral tissue, PET depends on difference of regional blood flow. Wada test (amobarbital), developed by Wada in 1949. Anatomic localization of motor strip. This technique is based on Taylor-Haughton lines. The motor strip is typically located 4–5 cm post to coronal suture in mid-sagittal plane.

27. The motor nucleus of seventh nerve is located at the pontomedullary junction. Motor fibers ascend within pons and forms sharp bend (internal genu) around the sixth nerve nucleus, forming visible bump in the floor of 4th ventricle wall facial colliculus. Cranial nerves caudal to it also exit the brainstem posterior to it.

28. Psammomatous meningioma – is included WHO grade-I meningioma, so does not under go malignant transformation. Remember WHO grade-I meningioma are (FMT-PALMS). Recurrence of the meningioma depends on the grade of tumor (WHO) and Simpson-class of excision. Simpson grade-I, II, III and IV have 10-yr recurrence rate of 9%, 19%, 29%, 40% respectively.

29. Epidermoid may be cranial or spinal. Average age at diagnosis in 40 years. The tumor grows similar to normal skin. Epidermoid is composed of stratified, keratinized squamous epithelium. The cyst contains accumulation of desquamated epithelial elements, keratin and cholesterol whereas dermoid cyst contains both dermal and epidermal elements. Epidermoids can get complicated by squamous cell carcinoma which can be corroborated by increased CEA levels in the serum. Carbohydrate antigen $CA_{19\text{-}9}$–level can be used for follow-up case, after excision of epidermoids.

30. Incidence of brain metastasis differs when age is taken into consideration. More common in adults than children. Adult metastasis are from lung, breast, renal, skin and colon cancers. In children leukemia followed by lymphomas. Hemorrhagic brain metastasis are from choriocarcinoma followed by melanoma.

31. The three main surgical approaches for vestibular schwannoma are:

i. The standard option is retrosigmoid approach, with this approach large tumors can be handled. There is an excellent view of cranial nerves and smaller tumors allow the surgeon to attempt hearing preservation.

ii. *Middle fossa approach:*
   a. For small medially placed tumors.
   b. Not ideal for tumor with significant extra-canalicular extension. With this approach, there is risk of temporal lobe injury due to retraction.

iii. *Trans-labyrinthine:* It has advantage of identification of facial nerve at IAC and offers good approach for patient with large tumors and no hearing. It is the most direct route. However tumors reaching medially are a relative contraindication to this approach as access is difficult.

32. Overall facial hypoesthesia is much more common symptoms as compared to pain. Tumors arising from ganglion usually produce more pain in contrast to tumors from root. Abducent nerve palsy is next common symptom closely followed by VII-VIII nerve. Less than 10% of patients have lower cranial nerve involvement. Conventional X-ray demonstrates erosion of the petrous apex.

34. Stereotactic and conventional external beam radiotherapy have been investigated as potential therapeutic options. Small tumors not associated with peritumoral cyst, are likely to respond best to treatment. Local control rates are 85–95% at 2-years and 65–86% at 5-years

35. Choroid plexus papillomas comprise about 0.5–0.6% brain neoplasm in adults and 2–5% of intracranial neoplastic lesions in children. In about 20% pediatric case, these tumors show malignant transformation and approximately half arise within atrium. These are WHO – classified grade-I tumors. Imaging shows tumors frequently contain calcifications, and hemorrhagic cysts. Surgical removal is the treatment of choice.

36. Intracranial lipomas represent post-neurulation abnormality occurring from an abnormality in meninx primitiva. Meninx primitivia, the anlagen of the pia and arachnoid from neurocrest. Mostly found at cisterns of lamina-terminalis, pericallosal cistern, velum interpositum and suprasellar, quadrigeminal and CP angle. They mostly present raised ICP. Do not enhance on contrast. Perilesional edema is not a feature.

37. Good prognostic factor for LGG are:

Age younger than 40-years at diagnosis, Seizure as presentation, absence of neurodeficit. KPS more than 70. MMSE score greater than 26/30. Tumor diameter less than 5cm. Absence of contrast enhancement. Histopathological factors associated with better prognosis are MIB-1, labeling index less than 8%. Histologic diagnosis of either low grade oligodendroglioma or oligoastrocytoma. Gemistocytic astrocytomas have a relatively poor prognosis.

38. VHL – is an autosomal dominant neoplasia syndrome. The word phakomatosis is misnomer for it as there is no cutaneous marker for this entity. There is germinal mutation of VHL-gene, (CNS manifestation include hemangioblastoma and endolymphatic sac tumors (10%). VHL syndrome (25–40%). The incidence of retinal haemingioblastoma in VHL patients is 25–60%.

39.

Tumor syndrome	Common gene involvement	Common chromosome Involvement	Associated CNS lesion
NF-1	NF-1	22, 17	Pilocytic astrocytoma including optic nerve, gliomas GBM.
NF-2	NF-2	22	Vestibular schwannomas, meningioma, ependymomas.
Tuberous sclerosis	TS	9q, 12q, 15q	Subependymal giant cell astrocytoma
Von-Hippel-Lindau	VHL	3p 26	Haemingioblastoma
Turcot	APC	5q, 21	Gliomas, medulloblastoma, pituitary adenomas
Gorlin	Parched homolog (PTCH, $PTCH_2$)	9q 22, IP 32	Medulloblastomas
Cowden	Phosphatase and tumor homolog (PTEN)	10q22-23.	Dysplastic gangliocytoma

40. Tuberous sclerosis is autosomal dominant, sporadic outnumber familial cases. The defect is in genetic loci 16 P13 which encode protein products hamartin and tuberin. The classical clinical findings include seizures, mental retardation and skin lesions, although this triad is found only in 29% of patients. Skin lesion include ash leaf spots, shagreen patches, subungal fibroma and faint angiofibroma (adenoma seabaeam). CNS lesions include cortical tubers, subependymal nodules (SEN's), white matter linear migration lines, trans-mantle cortical dysplasia and subependymal giant cell tumors.

41. SWS or encephalotrigeminal angiomatosis is included among neurocutaneous syndromes. The characteristic finding include leptomeningeal angiomatosis with tropism for occipital and parietal lobes. Ipsilateral vascular malformations in V_1 and V_2 division of trigeminal nerve. Epilepsy affects 75–90% of patients. MRI is gold standard for diagnosis. CT and plain films can also demonstrate calcification and cerebral "tram-tracking". Patients with large unilateral intracranial lesions may improve after functional hemispherotomy.

42. Well differentiated neuroepithelial tumor WHO grade-I, can occur anywhere in brain but most common location is temporal lobe (85%). Enhancement after gadolinium has been found to vary from no enhancement to heterogenous enhancement. The most common clinical presentation is seizures, followed by headache, dizziness, ataxia (posterior fossa). Lesions are typically cystic with solid component and calcifications are common.

43. Lung: 50–60%, Breast: 15–20%, Skin (melanoma): 5–10%, Gastrointestinal: 4–6%, Genitourinary: 3–5%. Others: 3–5%, Unknown: 4–8%. Most common cause of solitary metastasis is lung.

44. Fibrous dysplasia characterized by abnormal fibro-osseous proliferation, can affect any bone, monostotic – single bone, polyostotic – with multiple bone involvement, part of McCune – Albright syndrome, imaging – sunburst appearance. Paget's disease: may be lytic (osteoclastic) scelerotic (osteoblastic) – hyperostotic and mixed, imaging – cotton wool appearance. Meningiomas usually cause hyperostosis, Trigeminal schwannomas are known to cause truncation of petrous apex.

45.

Symptoms and signs			
Symptoms	**% age**	**Signs**	**% age**
Hearing loss	98%	Abnormal corneal reflex	33%
Tinnitus	70%	Nystagmus	26%
Dysequilibrium	67%	Facial hypoesthesia	26%
Headache	32%	Facial weakness	10%
Facial numbness	10%	Abnormal eye movement	11%
Diplopia	10%	Papilledema	10

47. Vestibular schwannomas is typically seen in 4th and 5th decades. In NF_2, the younger age group is involved, have more unpredictable growth rate and usually aggressive. If VS occurs before the age of 40 years, then patient should be evaluated for NF_2. Craniopharyngioma, medulloblastoma and esthesioneuroblastoma have 2-peaks in pediatric and adult group. Infact for craniopharyngiomas, histopathologic type also varies in the 2-groups viz, papillary and adamantinomatous.

49. They present only after they obtain sufficient size to produce mass effect. On careful history, symptoms of hypopituitarism are present. Moderate hyperprolactinemia due to stalk compression may also present. Many pituitary adenomas previously thought to be null cell adenomas were later found to be FSH- and LH- secreting tumors. Surgery is the treatment of choice.

50. Diencephalic syndrome originally described by Russell is characterized by suprasellar glioma in infancy that is manifested as lack of weight gain and emaciation. Paradoxically these children because of loss of subcutaneous fat appear muscular. Their growth hormone levels are increased. They may have nystagmus or head bobbling. Optic pathway hypothalamic gliomas should be considered in differential diagnosis of failure to thrive in children.

51. Radiation reaction may be:

i. **Acute:** acute skin reaction inform of desquamation and erythema, fatigue, temporary alopecia, acute visual complications, serous otitis, nausea.

ii. **Subacute (several weeks or month of RT):**

a. Demyelination resulting in nausea, vomiting, ataxia, dysphasia and cerebellar ataxia.

b. Radiation necrosis in absence of tumor progression, is seen typically and manifested in this period. Magnetic resonance spectroscopy may show lactate peaks in necrosis and choline peaks in tumor progression. Conformation may need either a stereotactic or excision biopsy.

c. Late – after several month to years –angiopathy – decline in cognitive function, dementia, ataxia and confusion.

53. LCH (Langerhan cell histiocytosis) is characterized by uncontrolled histiocyte proliferation and includes:-

Eosinophilic granuloma, Hand-Schiller-Christian disease. Letter-Sewer disease.

Predominantly occurs in children and adolescents with mean age at incidence being 12- years. Bone is involved in 80–90%, lung is most common non-osseous site followed by liver and other organs viz, skin, hypothalamus, posterior pituitary and lymphatic system. The most common and simplest form is solitary lytic lesion-designated as eosinophilic granuloma which accounts for 60–80% of cases. Histologically marked by clonal proliferation of S-100 positive histiocyte cells in clusters mixed with eosinophils. Electron microscopy reveals Birbeck's granules.

57. Sinus pericranii is an abnormal collection of veins adherent to outer table of skull in communication with the intracranial venous sinuses via dilated diploic and emissary veins of the skull. The lesion is most commonly located in midline draining into SSS. Skin over the lesion may be hairless and tinged blue. It may be associated with blue nevus syndrome, vascular malformations, cavernous hemangioma, capillary telangectasia and aneurysm of internal cerebral vein. The etiology may be spontaneous, congenital and traumatic. Slow progression of the lesion is the norm, although spontaneous regression has been reported. When disease is progressive, surgical excision may be carried.

58. Sarcoidosis is a chronic, multisystem granulomatous disease of unknown cause. Only 5% of the sarcoidosis patients have neurological manifestations. Any site of the central or PNS can be affected by sarcoidosis. Cranial neuropathy is the most frequently encountered neurological manifestations, 50% have multiple cranial nerve involvement. Dysfunction of facial nerve is the commonest cranial neuropathy seen in (>50%). It may be unilateral or bilateral.

59. Denis 3-column model of the spine attempts to identify CT criteria of instability of the thoracolumbar spine fractures.

a. Anterior column – anterior of half of disc and vertebral body (VB) includes anterior annulus fibrous (AF) and anterior longitudinal ligament.

b. Middle column – posterior half disc and VB, posterior annulus fibrosis and posterior longitudinal ligament.

c. Posterior column – posterior arch with interposed posterior ligament column and ligamentum flavum.

60. Indications of surgery in spinal fracture are:

Loss of >50% height, kyphotic angulation – 20° of one segment, residual spinal canal ≤50% of normal, three or more contiguous fractures, middle column fracture.

61. Chordomas are tumors which arise from the remnants of the notochord. Though the nucleus pulposus represents the remnant of the notochord, these tumors do not arise from it but from the non-neoplastic remnants of the notochord, called ecchordosis physaliphora, which are thought to exist in the vertebral body. These tumors are locally aggressive and are notorious for their recurrence. About 10% of sacral chordomas are malignant. Treatment of sacral chordoma is surgery followed by radiotherapy. Heavy particle irradiation has shown good results for chordomas.

62. Osteomas are benign tumors. Their size is 1.5 cm, and if the size is 1.5 cm or more, these qualify for osteoblastomas which are again benign lesions. Usually the posterior column of the spine is involved. These tumors usually do not recur after total removal unlike aneurysmal bone cysts. The common spinal segments involved by osteomas are lumbar followed by cervical.

63. Maffucci's syndrome is associated with multiple osteochondroma which do have malignant potential. On CT osteochondromas shown popcorn appearance.

64. Epidermoids are more common. Dermoids occur in midline and epidermoids laterally. Dermoids are often associated with congenital malformations. When there is intracranial extension, the cyst may rupture and result in meningeal irritation known as Mollaret's meningitis. Cholesterol within the cyst gives hypodense appearance on

Self Assessment & Review of Neurosciences

CT. Dermoids occur commonly at anterior fontanalle and occipital squama. Dermoid grow by both desquamation and glandular secretion. Dermoids on CT and MRI have similar appearance as of fat.

65. Tumors of the orbit can be primary or other tumors which extend into orbit. The most frequent orbital tumors in adults are lymphoid tumors, cavernous hemangiomas and meningiomas where as rhabdomyosarcoma and capillary hemangioma predominate in children.

67. Rare tumors of calvaria, F:M – 3:1 and more common in frontal and parietal bone, 15% patients have multiple lesions. On X-ray 'Sunburst or honeycomb" pattern, Local tenderness and swelling are clinical manifestations, headache may also occur, On contrast imaging enhancement is typical, flow voids are not seen, enblock resection is treatment of choice. Simple curettage has chances of recurrence.

68. Types of brain edema:Vasogenic edema, Cytotoxic, Interstitial, Osmotic

Mediators involved in vasogenic brain edema are: Vascular endothelial growth factor (VEGF), Angiopoietin-1, Aginopoeitin-2, FGF (fibroblast), HGF (hepatocyte), IL-3, IL-4, IL-8, Vascular permeability factor.

Cytotoxic edema – nitric oxide (vasodilator)

Bradykinin, substance P, leukotrienes, serotonin and histamine, vasopressin induce or mediate edema at various levels. For cytotoxic, osmotic and interstitial edema, the main therapeutic option is to reverse the cause. For vasogenic edema, steroids and decongestants have profound role.

69. Steroids have profound role in vasogenic edema (of tumor). Steroids reduce brain edema by decreasing the vascular permeability. They stabilize the blood brain barrier. They have transient effect in hydrostatic edema but no role in cytotoxic edema.

71. Most patients with corticotroph adenomas come to medical management because of clinical problems of steroid excess. Because these tumors are typically small and confined to sella, symptoms referable due to mass effect are seldom presenting complaints.

72. Pituitary apoplexy – abrupt and acute hemorrhagic manifestation of pituitary adenoma. The clinical syndrome is easily recognized consisting of acute headache, meningismus, visual impairment, ophthalmoplegia and altered sensorium. Without intervention, patient may die of SAH, increased ICP or succumbs to life threatening hypopituitarism. It may be the first presentation of pituitary adenoma. Most commonly occurs in hormonally active tumor (acromegalic and Cushing). Predisposing factors include bromocriptine therapy, anticoagulant usage, diabetic ketoacidosis, head trauma, estrogen therapy and pituitary irradiation.

73. About 2–13% of AIDS patients develop primary central nervous system lymphoma. HIV related primary CNS lymphoma is typically a large cell lymphoma with immunoblastic and more aggressive features. Infection by Epstein-Barr virus (EBV), a ubiquitous pathogen normally suppressed by intact immune system likely has a role in the pathogens of PCNSL. CSF analysis may reveal markers of the virus.

74. Ganglioglioma is an infrequent tumor of CNS. Most commonly is present in temporal lobe (85%). It is the most common tumor found in temporal lobe epilepsy. These tumors are classified WHO grade-I. Another tumor frequently found in the temporal lobe which induces epilepsy is DNET (dysembryoplastic-neuroepithelial-tumor). This also qualifies for a WHO grade-I. The commonest cause of temporal lobe epilepsy is medial temporal lobe sclerosis. MRI will show hyperintensity in the medial temporal lobe and volumetry shows temporal lobe volume loss with dilatation of the temporal horn of the lateral ventricle.

79. Most children with diffuse pontine glioma have evidence of cerebellar dysfunction (87%), multiple lower cranial nerve palsies (77%) and motor paresis and sensory changes secondary to lung tract involvement. Involvement of cerebellar peduncles result in ataxia which can be truncal or appendicular.

82. Familial cancer syndromes associated with medulloblastoma include.

Gorlin's syndrome (multiple nevoid basal cell carcinoma). Rubinstein-Taybi syndrome. Ataxia-telangectasia. Turcot's syndrome (polyposis-glioma). Li-fraumani syndrome (germline TP_{53}). Neurofibromatosis. Tuberous sclerosis

84. WHO grade-I tumor, 25–40% - associated with VHL-syndrome, more frequently in males 1.5–2 times. Brainstem, spinal cord and cerebellum (90%). 30% supratentorial, 2% of all intracranial neoplasms but 7–12% of posterior fossa tumors.

85. Clinical manifestation of pineal tumors.

Symptoms of increased ICP pressure from obstructive HCP. Brainstem and cerebellar compression. Endocrine dysfunction – rarely encountered. Such symptoms may develop early in disease process even before the tumor is radiographically apparent. Precocious puberty has been linked to pineal tumor. The syndrome is actually precocious pseudopuberty because the hypothalamic-gonadal axis is not mature and therefore limited to tumors viz. choriocarcinoma which produces ectopic secretion of β-HCG.

86. α-fetoprotein indicates presence of fetal yolk sac elements and levels are markedly elevated with endodermal sinus tumors, smaller elevations are seen with embryonal cell carcinoma and immature teratomas. β-HCG with choriocarcinoma and low level of same are associated with but not all embryonal cell carcinoma and germinomas.

Biologic markers in germ cell tumor.

Tumour	β-HCG	α-Fetoprotein
Immature teratoma	?	+/-
Germinoma	-	-
Germinoma with syncytiotrophoblastic cells	+	-
Embryonal cell carcinoma	+/-	+/-
Choriocarcinoma	++	-
Endodermal sinus tumor	-	++

87. Modified Chang classification for Medulloblastoma:

T_1 – Tumor <3 cm in maximal diameter, limited to the midline vermis, roof of fourth ventricle or cerebellar hemisphere.

T_2 – Tumor ≥3 cm in maximal diameter including one adjacent structure or partially filling fourth ventricle.

T_{3A} – Tumor ≥3 cm with extension into aqueduct of sylvius, foramen of magende or Luschka with HCP

T_{3B} – Tumor ≥3 cm invading brainstem.

T_4 – Tumor ≥3 cm, involving mid brain or third ventricle.

T_0 – No metastasis.

M_1 – Microscopic tumor cell in CSF.

M_2 – Gross nodular seeding in cerebellar or cerebral sinus arachnoid space in third or lateral ventricle.

M_3 – Gross nodular seeding in spinal sub-arachnoid space.

M_4 – Extraneural metastasis.

Current prognostic factors for medulloblastoma

Factor	Standard or average risk	Poor risk
Extent of disease	Posterior fossa, no brainstem involvement, no metastatic disease	Disseminated with intracranial or spinal disease; extraneural disease
Extent of resection	Near total; <1.5 cm^2 residual	Subtotal; >1.5 cm^2 residual
Age	Older than 3 years	Younger than 3 years
Histopathology	Undifferentiated	Differentiated

90. Frontal lobe tumors can present with a myriad of symptoms. Based on the location of the tumor patient can be elated with features of disinhibition or can be depressed with loss of interest in the surroundings. Generally speaking tumors which elevate the frontal lobe e.g. skull base tumors, elate the patients mood while as tumors which depress the frontal lobes e.g., callosal tumors depress the patients mood.

91. Paraneoplastic cerebellar degeneration is associated with small cell lung carcinoma, ovarian, breast, uterine carcinoma and lymphoma. In breast, ovarian and uterine cancer paraneoplastic syndromes is associated with a circulating autoantibody, designated anti-Yo, **that reacts with Purkinie cell cytoplasm.** PCD has been found in association with other antibodies like anti-Hu, pleocytosis may be present in CSF. MRI may show cerebellar atrophy. Clinically PCD begins with a gait disorder, progressing over weeks to months to involve most cerebellar function and eventually producing severe dysarthria and dysmetria and associated with diplopia and vertigo. Treatment is unsatisfactory.

98. Loss of heterozygosity on chromosome on 22q and deficiency of protein merlin has been with linked with NF-2. NF-2 gene codes for protein called merlin. Merlin is also called schwannomin. Merlin is a protein and not a sphingolipid, it is present in the cell membrane. Merlin is a member of the protein 4.1 family of membrane associated protein.

99. FGF-1 (acidic) and FGF_2 (basic) have been shown to be elevated in astrocytomas. Both these polypeptides play rule in cellular proliferation. PGF-2 has additional angiogenic properties. High expression of FGF-2 is associated with worse outcome in children with high grade gliomas and in adults with astrocytic tumors. FGF-Receptor (FGFR-1) is elevated in malignant gliomas, whereas FGFR-2 expression is lost. FGFR-2 expression predicts malignancy in astrocytomas. FGFR-1 usually occurs in what is called alpha-form. this form is expressed in LGG. In contrast high grade astrocytomas express beta form.

101. Extracellular matrix molecules include:

Collagen – restricted to the mesenchymal component of gliomas.

Fibronectin – expression restricted in glioma blood vessels, can be detected weakly in involved brain.

Laminin – associated with mesenchymal component of glial tumors. Laminin-2 also known as merosin.

Tenascin-C – Expression correlates with degree of anaplasia. It is impregnated extremely in granulation tissue and astroglial scars such as glioma, fibrosarcoma, oteosarcoma, melanoma, mammary carcinoma and squamous cell carcinoma.

Thrombospondin – increased expression in gliomas may have antigenic properties.

Other ECM are: osteopoetin, vitronectin, matrix-metalloproteins, heparin sulphate, proteoglycans, hyaluronic acid.

103. Factors responsible for decreased blood brain permeability include:

Intracellular CAMP, Steroid, Glia derived neurotrophic factor, Basic fibroblastic growth factor, Polyunsaturated fatty acids, Transforming growth factor-F

Factors responsible for increased blood brain permeability include:

ANP, bradykinin, histamine, serotonin, thrombin, glutamate, ATP, ADP, AMP, endothelin-1, adenosine, phospholipase A_2, arachidonic acid, prostaglandins, leukotrienes, interleukin IL-IX, IL-B, IL-6, tumor necrosis factor-α, nitric oxide.

104. Definitive diagnosis of carcinomatous meningitis is made by identification of malignant cells in CSF. The selective sensitivity of this test depends upon the number and volume of CSF specimen examined. CSF-protein determination has historically been the most sensitive indicator of CM and greater than 45mg/dl is seen in 80–90% patients. Lumbar or cisternal CSF is more likely than ventricular fluid to have elevated protein and malignant cells. Approximately 30–57% have lumbar CSF pressure higher than 15 mmH_2. MRI of the brain and spine with gadolinium contrast is the procedure of choice. During the course of disease 70% of patients will have abnormal imaging. Patchy nerve root enhancement, matting of nerve roots of cauda equina, nodular deposits and linear, continuous enhancement of pia-arachnoid of conus medullaris and brainstem (sugar coating) are hallmarks of diagnosis. Sometimes there may be patchy enhancement of leptomeninges over cerebral convexities and in basilar cisterns, insulae, pituitary stalk, cranial nerve roots or superior cerebellar folia.

106. Benign, non-neoplastic, expansile lesion. The solitary lesions are usually found in young persons and are rare after 3rd decade. F:M ratio is 2:1. On imaging studies, the finding of a lytic, loculated lesion with fluid levels caused by layering of blood products within internal cavities is highly suggestive of ABC. MRI is more sensitive than CT. The treatment of choice for aneurysmal bone cyst is gross total excision which is curative when feasible. Preoperative embolization has been reported to be useful adjuvant. Radiotherapy may be helpful.

107. Chordomas are slow growing tumors that arise from notochordal remnants, M:F = 2:1. Clivus and sacrum are common sites. Clival chordomas present with abducent palsy, lower cranial nerve palsy and headache, pituitary dysfunction and torticollis. Untreated patients rarely survive 30-months. Some chordomas may turn frankly malignant with metastatic potential. The classic findings on radiograph of skull is chordomas is an expansile lytic lesion with periosteal elevation. Although slow growing tumor, but local recurrence is challenging to manage. Surgical approaches to clival cordomas are frontorbitozygomatic, extended middle fossa, transmaxillary, transcondylar, anterior basal, transnasal. Heavy particle irradiation has also shown promising results.

109. The clinical manifestations usually centers in one or more three clinical occasions:

First pituitary hyperfunction in the form of several characteristic hypersecretory states. Hypersecretion of PRL, GH, ACTH and TSH. The second type involves pituitary insufficiency and is typically associated with large tumors that compress normal pituitary gland or its stalk. Third one is mass affect with or without presence of endocrinopathy. Headache, visual loss due to compression of anterior visual pathways, and asymmetric bitemporal hemianopia is classic feature. Superior temporal quadrants affected first as tumor grows from below and compresses the inferior nasal fibers which represent the superior temporal fields followed by inferior ones. With continued growth, tumor may infiltrate hypothalamus causing variety of vegetative states like disorders of sleep, alertness, eating, behavior and emotion. Extension to third ventricle causes hydrocephalus. With lateral extension temporal lobe epilepsy or cranial nerve palsy can occur. Pituitary adenomas do not usually present with diabetes insipidus, if a patient presents with DI think of other causes first viz. craniopharyngioma, suprasellar germinoma. In craniopharyngioma patient develops inferior temporal field defects as the tumor grows from superior to inferior direction and compresses the superior nasal fibers first which represent the inferior fields. Suprasellar germinoma may on MRI show drop metastasis, moreover CSF markers should also be looked for.

110. The incidence of brain metastasis and spectrum of metastasizing primary cancers vary with patients age and more common in adults than children. Common metastasis in this group are lung, breast and skin in descending order. In children most common cause is leukemia followed by lymphoma. Osteogenic sarcoma and rhabdomyosarcoma are also common solid brain metastasis in children.

111. About 10% meningiomas are malignant (high grade) which include grade-III meningiomas which are papillary, anaplastic and rhabdoid meningiomas (PAR). Hyperostosis is a characteristic finding particularly in en-plaque meningiomas. The dura matter adjacent to brain may enhance so called dural tail on CT or MRI. Meningiomas arise from arachnoid cap cells while as hemangiopericytomas arise from pericytes. Both the tumors are noted for hypervascularity to the extent that preoperative embolization is not only a good management option but sometimes a necessity. Tumors which have been embolized need to be surgical removed within next 48-hrs as otherwise collaterals develop and defeat the very purpose of the embolization. Common embolizing agents used are gelfoam, NBCA. Lipoidol is the vehicle for the embolizing agents and it also lends radio-opacity to the agent. Other tumor wherein pre-op embolization has made a mark is juvenile nasopharyngeal angiofibroma.

113. ABCs are cystic and osteolytic lesions that affect patients younger than 20-years (benign tumor). Slight female tendency. Usually arise from long bones but 12–30% of cases involve spine. Typically involve posterior elements and thoracic spine is most frequent site of involvement.

ABCs are benign lesions and are classified as type 1(latent), type 2 (active) or type 3 (aggressive) lesions. Strictly speaking, ABCs are not tumors, but in view of their local destructive nature, by convention these lesions have been categorized under tumors. In fact, ABC has been defined by the WHO as 'an expanding lesion with blood-filled cavities separated by septa of trabecular bone or fibrous tissue containing osteoclast giant cells. ABCs can be primary or secondary. Primary ABC is more common. Secondary ABCs are associated with hemangiomas, giant cell tumors and osteoblastoma. ABC is thought to be a reactive lesion produced by a vascular disturbance in bone. Spontaneous regression of the disease is also known. No patient usually dies from the progression of the disease. Preoperative embolization has a role in large vascular ABCs. Treatment is surgical excision. Preoperative embolization is helpful to decrease bleeding, during surgery.

114. Ewing's sarcoma is the second most common primary malignant bone tumor. It is the most common malignant primary spinal tumor in childhood. It is a poorly differentiated tumor and can arise from soft tissue or bone. Peak incidence is seen in 10–20 years of age and 80% of cases occur before the age of 20-years. In spine sacrococcygeal followed by lumbar and thoracic site are common. On radiographs there is mottled appearance with periosteal reaction that results in onion skin appearance. Treatment is chemo-radiotherapy.

117. Pineal region tumors manifest in three clinical ways:

Symptoms of increased ICP. Direct brainstem and cerebellar compression. Endocrine dysfunction.

Diabetes insipidus can occur with a germinoma spreading along the floor of the third ventricle. Such features can occur early even before tumor becomes radiologically visible. Beta-HCG is produced by trophoblastic elements, high levels are found in choriocarcinomas and low levels can be associated with some but not all embryonal cell carcinoma and germinomas.

118. Direct compression of midbrain, particularly at the level of the superior colliculus can cause disorders of extraocular movement classically known as Parinaud's syndrome. The syndrome consists of paralysis of upward gaze, convergence or retraction nystagmus and light-near pupillary dissociation. Dorsal midbrain compression can lead to lid retraction (Collier's sign) or ptosis.

121. The dorsally exophytic brainstem gliomas have good outcome after surgery. The surgical procedure includes identification of floor of fourth ventricle and then the tumor is removed in stepwise fashion.

122. Pain in distribution of trigeminal nerve fibers (90–100%). Facial hypoesthesia – 70%. Diplopia – 20%. Bony erosion on CT-70%. Meningiomas, intracranial aneurysms, trigeminal schwannomas, diastematomyelia are common in females.

124. Intraventricular tumor histology.

Colloid cyst, Craniopharyngioma, Pilocytic astrocytoma, Pineocytoma, Cavernous malformation, Medulloblastoma, Metastasis, Meningioma, Ependymoma, Dermoid/epidermoid, SEGA.

125. Ependymomas WHO grade-II tumor, peak age of incidence is around 3-years with equal incidence in boys and girls. Ependymomas arise from the floor of the 4th ventricle close to vomiting zone hence incidence of vomiting is very high in such tumors even before causing raised ICP. Also keep in mind that MRI in these tumors shows no CSF cleft between the tumor and the ventricular floor. Features of raised ICP supervene later as the tumor grows and blocks the outlet. Sometimes tumor can project through one of the foramen of Magendie and cause lower cranial nerve palsy. In such cases the tumor needs to be differentiated from choroid plexus papilloma which on imaging may show a grape-like configuration. Both tumors show calcification on CT. Hydrocephalus is commoner in CPP as it in addition to the 4th-ventricular outlet, it blocks the distal absorption sites because of the tumor debri.

128. Steroids stabilize the blood brain barrier. They decrease permeability of BBB. They have vasoconstrictive features.

129. The most common sites are liver, lungs, pleura and lymph nodes. Papillary, anaplastic and rhabdoid subtypes belong to WHO-III group and are considered malignant with propensity for metastasis.

132. Meningioma may contain ER, PR, androgen, dopamine D_1 and PG- C, D receptors.

Some meningioma are associated with high systemic levels of CEA or prolactin.

133. Typical angiography features of meningiomas:

Usually supplied by meningeal artery if the tumor arises from convexity dura. In general meningiomas are vascular lesions. Prolonged vascular blush beginning in early arterial phase and persists till late venous phase (called mother-in-law) blush. After tumor penetration, the primary feeding vessel branches in a radial or sunburst pattern. Enplaque meningiomas, especially those associated with planum sphenoidale, clinoids and floor of anterior cranial fossa are generally poorly vascularized.

134. Tuberculum sellae meningiomas account for 5–10% of intracranial meningiomas. Mean age around 40-years. F:M ratio is 3:1. The chiasmal syndrome includes primary optic atrophy with bitemporal field defects with essentially normal sella. The optic atrophy is bilateral but asymmetric.

137. Calvarial metastasis common in decreasing order are- breast, thyroid and kidney.

139. Foster-Kennedy syndrome usually occurs secondary to olfactory grove meningioma characterized by: ipsilateral anosmia, ipsilateral optic atrophy, contralateral papilledema due to raised ICP.

140. Pituitary adenoma tend to enlarge sella while as craniopharyngioma invade sella. J shaped sella suggests optic nerve glioma. Pituitary adenoma produces **waist** sign on imaging. Calcification suggests craniopharyngiomas.

143. Corticosteroids may produce tumor regression in 40% of patients likely through apoptosis and reduced tumor associated edema. So interval CT may detect hypodensity.

145. Hypothalamic hamartomas are rare congential heterotopic lesions that may be asymptomatic or may be associated with precious puberty, behavior disturbances and cognitive impairment. These are epileptogenic and are associated with gelastic seizures.

146. Central neurocytomas represent only 0.1 to 0.5% of all intracranial tumors. Generally occur on lateral ventricles with predilection for left frontal horn. HPE reveals round cells and perivascular rosettes. They are classified WHO grade-II tumors. On CT and MRI – neurocytoma appear hypodense and hyperintense respectively. Most patients present with obstructive HCP.

147. Middle fossa Trigeminal schwannomas grow in interdural space in Meckels cave. They are enveloped by the inner membrane of cavernous sinus. Surgical approaches are:

Pterional trans-sylvian, Subtemporal intradural, Frontotemporal intradural, Extradural approaches. Post-auricular approaches are done for vestibular schwannomas.

148. Sessions grading of juvenile nasal angiofibroma

Stage I: 1A – posterior nares and nasopharyngeal vault.

1B – Posterior nares and /or nasophoyrangeal vault with involvement of at least one paranasal sinus

Stage II: IIA – minimal lateral extension into pterygomaxillary fissure

IIB – tumor fills PMF, displaces posterior wall of the antrum and extends superiorly and erodes bone of orbit.

IIC – Extends into cheek and infra temporal fossa

Stage III: IIIA – erosion of skull base

IIB – Extensive intracranial extension

149. A benign local disease of bone with mononuclear cells and eosinophils. Most commonly found in skull (43.80%), in femur (14.5%). It is regarded as the mildest form of histiocytosis. Parietal bone is the most common involved bone followed by frontal bone. Mostly single lesion are treated with curettage. In younger patients recurrence is common.

150. Fisch classification of glomus jugulare tumors:

a. Tumor limited to middle ear cleft
b. Tumor limited to tympanomastoid area with no involvement of the infralabyrinthic compartment
c. Infralabyrinthic compartment of temporal bone and into petrous apex
d. Tumor with intracranial extension.

151. Kadish staging

Group A - Confined to nasal cavity

B - Extension to PNS

C - Tumor spreading beyond PNS and nasal cavities

UCLA staging

- T_1 - Nasal cavity + PNS (excluding SS and superior ethmoidal cells)
- T_2 - Nasal cavity + PNS including sphenoid sinus with extension into cribriform plate
- T_3 - Invading into orbit or protruding into anterior cranial fossa
- T_4 - Tumor involving the brain

153. Radiotherapy is the single most important adjuvant therapy for medulloblastomas.

154. Rathke's cleft cyst arise from pars intermedia of pituitary, they are lined by single layer of cuboidal cells and arise from remnants of Rathke's pouch, these are low density lesions on CT, 50% may enhance on contrast, MRI appearance is variable.

156. Fiber bundle (arcuate) defects. Lesions of optic nerve between chiasma and the retina. Common causes include vascular lesions, toxins, optic nerve glioma, demyelinating lesions.

157. Glutariaciduria is an inherited disorder in which the body is unable to break down completely the amino acids lysine, hydroxylysine and tryptophan. Excessive levels of their intermediate breakdown products (glutaric acid, glutaryl-CoA, 3-hydroxyglutaric acid, glutaconic acid) can accumulate and cause damage to the brain particularly the basal ganglia. Bilateral sylvian fissure arachnoid cysts is a feature. Patients have macrocephaly also.

Tay–Sachs disease (also known as GM2 gangliosidosis or hexosaminidase A deficiency) is a rare autosomal recessive genetic disorder. Tay–Sachs disease is caused by a genetic mutation in the *HEXA* gene on (human) chromosome 15. Mental deterioration is common and death is early.

Mutations in the *SMPD1* gene cause Niemann–Pick disease types A and B. Hepatosplenomegaly is the presentation.

158. They tend to occur in the midline, either at the pineal region (majority) or along the floor of the third ventricle/ suprasellar region. Germinomas are tumors of young patients with a peak incidence of 10–12 years of age. They are the most common tumor of the pineal region accounting for approximately 50% of all tumors. These are radiocurable.

165. There is compelling preclinical evidence for using the microtubule inhibitory drug mebendazole (MBZ) to treat several molecular subtypes of medulloblastoma, including group 3. As a long-standing antihelminthic drug, MBZ has the advantage of a low-toxicity profile in children compared with other micro- tubule inhibitors such as vincristine and paclitaxel. As a lipophilic agent with a low molecular weight, MBZ has the additional advantage of blood-brain barrier permeability. Previous studies suggest that MBZ acts as an inhibitor of vascular endothelial growth factor (VEGF) receptor 2 (VEGFR2), the primary receptor mediating the effects of VEGF. This study reveals the antiangiogenic effect of MBZ in medulloblastoma preclinical mouse models and its encouraging impact on overall survival. *[Neurosurgery. 2015 Feb;76(2):N15-6]*

167. Bobble-head doll syndrome is a rare neurological movement disorder in which patients, usually children around age 3, begin to bob their head and shoulders forward and back, or sometimes side-to-side, involuntarily, in a manner reminiscent of a bobble head doll. The syndrome is seen in suprasellar arachnoid cyst.

169. Collins' law, known as period of risk for recurrence (PRR), is used as a method for the prediction of recurrence or cure of embryonal tumors including medulloblastomas. The PRR is defined as the age at diagnosis plus 9-months of gestation. According to Collins' law, a patient who has no clinical evidence of recurrence within this time period is considered cured.

175. Lambert–Eaton myasthenic syndrome (LEMS, also Lambert–Eaton syndrome, or Eaton–Lambert syndrome) is a rare autoimmune disorder that is characterized by muscle weakness of the limbs. It is the result of an autoimmune reaction in which antibodies are formed against presynaptic voltage-gated calcium channels, and likely other nerve terminal proteins, in the neuromuscular junction. It is the commonest paraneoplastic syndrome and it occurs commonly in small cell cancer of lung.

3

CHAPTER

Neurovascular

Nayil Khursheed, Uday Singh, Muhammad Sultan

IMPORTANT THEORY

ANEURYSMAL SUBARACHNOID HEMORRHAGE

Epidemiology

Aneurysmal Subarachnoid Hemorrhage (SAH) constitutes the 2nd commonest cause of SAH, after trauma. The incidence of aneurysms in general population is 1% on Digital Subtraction Angiography (DSA) and 5% on autopsy. About 10% of aneurysms bleed, i.e. 10 per 100,000 persons years. Incidence of aneurysms is however affected by geographic and ethnic distribution. It is maximum in Finland and lowest in Middle East. Blacks are twice susceptible than whites. The sex ratio is in favor of females and peak age is 50–60 years.

Risk Factors

Most cases are sporadic, but some risk factors have been identified viz. smoking, alcohol use, hypertension, cocaine abuse. The relative risk of SAH increases if two or more risk factors are present, as the effect is synergistic. Diabetes, hyperlipidemia do not appear to be associated with increased risk of SAH. Role of oral contraception is controversial. Certain inherited conditions like Autosomal Dominant Polycystic Kidney Disease (ADPKD), coarctation of aorta, pseudoxanthoma elasticum, Marfan's syndrome, Ehlers-Danlos syndrome are associated with increased incidence of aneurysms. ADPKD has 4% incidence of aneurysms and multiple aneurysms are common especially middle cerebral artery (MCA) aneurysms. Most aneurysms rupture in morning or evening hours, reflecting a circadian rhythm of rupture. About 1/3rd of aneurysms rupture during sleep. The rate of rupture is lowest in summer and highest in winter.

Clinical Presentation

The commonest symptom is SAH is sudden onset severe headache, often described as the 'worst headache of my life'. Other symptoms include vomiting, altered sensorium, seizures, weakness. SAH is the commonest cause of sudden death due to stroke and about 15% patients die before reaching the hospital. About one third of patients with sudden onset headache have SAH. Signs of meningeal irritation are seen in about half of the patients. Focal deficit is seen in 20%. Retinal hemorrhages are seen in quarter of patients. Many patients (1/3rd) have history suggestive of minor bleed referred to as 'warning leak' or 'sentinel hemorrhage' few weeks back before presenting with a massive aneurysmal bleed. Patients with warning leaks have usually worse outcome. The clinical grading of SAH is done by WFNS (World Federation of Neurological Surgeons) grading (Table 1).

Table 1: WFNS grading for SAH

Grade	GCS score	Deficit
0. (unruptured)	15	Absent
1.	15	Absent
2.	13–14	Absent

Grade	GCS score	Deficit
3.	13–14	Present
4.	7–12	Present or absent
5.	3–6	Present or absent

Etiology and Pathology

Hemodynamic theory: It is supported by the fact that aneurysms commonly develop at arterial bifurcation where vascular stress in maximum, aneurysms are seen in high flow area of AVM, hypertension is a general risk factor for aneurysmal formation.

Genetic theory: This explains the familial evidence of aneurysms and patients with genetically transmitted disease, e.g. ADPKD (autosomal dominant polycystic kidney disease), Marfan's syndrome, Ehler – Danlos syndrome have an increased predisposition of developing aneurysms. However, there is growing evidence that both the above theories play their part and in addition, environmental factors, e.g. smoking, alcohol have a role to play.

Current concept of pathology of aneurysms supports the fact that damage to the internal elastic lamina is the critical pathologic change. However, it is to be borne in mind that in addition to the absence of the elastica, all aneurysms show absence of media.

Imaging

Computed Tomography

Non-contrast CT scan is the initial imaging study in any patient in whom SAH is suspected. CT scan will reveal the extent of blood, hydrocephalus, edema, infarct. Patients in whom CT scan is normal but clinical suspicion of SAH is high need a lumbar puncture to look for xanthochromia. CT classification of SAH is given by Fisher (Table 2). Aneurysms do enhance on contrast however CT slice thickness if (5–10 mm) is likely to miss small aneurysms. Routine contrast CT scan is not advisable to diagnose an aneurysm. CT angiography can detect as small as 2–3 mm aneurysms with a sensitivity of 90%. This investigation can also show the relationship of aneurysm neck in relation to bony landmark, a parameter so useful in surgical planning for supraclinoid aneurysms. Besides this, it can diagnose thrombosed aneurysms also and this is the only investigation which can be done in an unstable patient who requires an urgent craniotomy before a regular DSA can be done.

Table 2: CT scan grading of SAH (Fisher)

Fischer Grade	*Blood on CT Scan*
1	No subarachnoid blood seen
2	Diffuse or vertical layers 1 mm or less thick
3	Localized clot and/or vertical layers >1 mm
4	Intracerebral or intraventricular clot with diffuse or no SAH

Magnetic Resonance Angiography

The reported sensitivity is 86% when compared to DSA. It is basically a tool useful for screening, especially for aneurysms more than 3 mm. Patients who are allergic to iodinated contrast or have renal dysfunction are the most suitable candidates for this type of investigation.

Digital Subtraction Angiography

It is the gold standard for diagnosing aneurysms. Since the incidence of multiple aneurysms is 20% both internal carotid arteries (ICA) and both vertebral arteries (VA) should be visualized. The routine views for anterior circulation are AP, lateral, ipsilateral waters oblique and for posterior circulation are Caldwell and lateral views are worth mentioning.

Treatment

All SAH patients need ICU monitoring, arterial line, central venous access. Double 'H' therapy (i.e. hypervolemia and hemodilution) is instituted before clipping or coiling an aneurysm. Blood pressure of 150 mm Hg systolic is ideal. Isotonic normal saline 3 mL/Kg/hr is the fluid of choice. Since 20% of patients have seizures so prophylactic anticonvulsants are started. Patients are sedated, analgesics are given, calcium channel blocker, i.e. nimodipine is started 60 mg 4 hourly. Role of steroids is controversial. CVP should be around 10 cm H_2O and PCV of 30–33% is ideal. Hyponatremia is commonly seen in SAH which is corrected by 3% hypertonic saline. There is no substitute for good nursing care.

Timing of Aneurysmal Obliteration

The International Cooperative study on the timing of Aneurysm surgery demonstrated that the outcome is best if patients are operated (clipping) between 0 and 3 days after SAH or after 14 days. The outcome in the intervening period is poor as during this period vasospasm is maximum. The major goal in treating a ruptured aneurysm is its obliteration to prevent rebleeding. About 60% of patients who rebleed, die. Untreated, 30% of aneurysm re-rupture within the first month and then at the rate of 3% per year. Rebleeding is maximal on day 1 (4%) and occur at a rate of 1 to 2% per day during the subsequent month.

Acute Intraventricular Hemorrhage and Hydrocephalus

Usually seen in poor grade patients, external ventricular drainage (EVD) has been recommended, however the risk is of increased aneurysm rebleeding because of changes in the transmural pressure of the aneurysm. Studies have revealed that patients who improve within 24 hours of EVD have better outcome. About half of the patients who require an urgent EVD, ultimately need a ventriculoperitoneal shunt.

Role of Endovascular Treatment

Endovascular treatment of aneurysms has gained recent popularity especially since GDC (Guglielmi Detachable Coil) became available. The benefits of endovascular techniques have yet to stand the test of the time. However, several studies have revealed that high-risk surgical candidates or technically challenging complex aneurysms may be better treated by GDC coiling. International Subarachnoid Aneurysmal Trial (ISAT) which was a multicentric randomized trial, has concluded that neurocognitive outcome is better in coiled patients than surgically clipped patients. However, the chance of rebleed is more in the former group.

Vasospasm

60% angiographic and 30% symptomatic. Vasospasm is less in AVM than in aneurysm because of less blood in subarachnoid space in the former.

Causes of delayed neurologic deficit in SAH are-Vasospasm, rebleed, seizure, hydrocephalus, cerebral edema, embolic phenomenon, dyselectrolytemia, hypovolemia.

Risks of triple H therapy- CCF, bleeding abnormalities, rupture of unsecured aneurysm, dyselectrolytemia, cerebral edema.

Nimodipine is a calcium channel antagonist and is basically a dihydropyridine. It also affects platelet aggregation and RBC membrane deformability, hence it improves microcirculation.

Predisposing factors for vasospasm

Fisher grade III has highest incidence. Higher WBC count. Hyponatremia. Hypovolemia.

Female sex. MCA aneurysms. Coexistent hydrocephalus. Poor neurological status.

Modalities to assess vasospasm noninvasively:

Transcranial Doppler, Xenon 133, Xenon CT, PET, SPECT.

Conclusion

Aneurysmal SAH is an important cause of SAH. Most of the cases being sporadic with few patients having genetic and environmental risk factors. It is responsible for 1/3rd of sudden onset headaches. CT scan is the primary investigation which detects blood in subarachnoid space in more than 90% patients. DSA is the gold standard to locate the aneurysm. Ideally aneurysms should be treated within 72 hours of bleed. Clipping of the aneurysms has stood the test of the time, though there is room for coiling of giant and complex aneurysms. Medical management of SAH also contributes a lot in overall outcome of SAH.

Facts about Aneurysmal SAH

About 1% population has aneurysms. Vasospasm kills 7%, causes morbidity in 7%. In SAH, 15–20% die within 2 weeks due to rebleeding. 15% die before reaching the hospital. 30% of SAH's occur in sleep. 30% of SAH have warning bleeds. SAH is complicated by intracerebral bleed in 20–40%, intraventricular hematoma in 15–30% and subdural bleed in 2–4%. Hydrocephalus occurs in 20% of acute SAH. Xanthochromia is seen as early as 6 hours. 50% of patients who rebleed – die. Rebleed – maximum on day 1st (4%) and then @ 1–2%/day for next 4 weeks. Posterior circulation aneurysms have higher chance of rebleed. Highest seizure rate is seen within first week of ictus. Symptomatic aneurysm rupture rate is 6%/year. Large aneurysm is 1–2.5 cm, giant >2.5 cm. Infective aneurysms constitute 2–6% of all aneurysms and in children 10–20%. 5% of patients with infective endocarditis present with bleed. Infective aneurysm – about 50% decrease in size after antibiotics. 10–30% patients develop new aneurysms or increase in size. 90% traumatic aneurysms occurs within 2–3 weeks of injury. 8% pituitary adenomas have associated aneurysms especially growth hormone secreting. Rupture of aneurysms starts at 3 mm size and mass effect starts at 7 mm size. If aneurysm is seen in anterior circulation – 5% chance of another aneurysm in posterior circulation. If 2 aneurysms coexist – proximal usually bleeds. Peak rupture – 6th decade. Before 40 years of age, sex ratio is equal and beyond 40 years females outnumber. Familial aneurysms – rupture at small size. In coarctation of aorta – associated aneurysms rupture occurs in twenties. Pediatric aneurysms – M:F ratio is equal. Damage to internal elastic lamina (IEL) is the key factor in pathogenesis of aneurysms, however it should be noted that besides absent IEL, all aneurysms show absent tunica media. 1% of aneurysms have AVMS, 6–12% of AVM have aneurysms. Hypertension increases the chance of multiple aneurysms two fold. Smoking increases rupture by 4 times. Mortality in patients with missed warning bleeds – 24% in those diagnosed early – 4%.

MCA Aneurysm

Divided into proximal, bifurcation and distal aneurysms. Proximal aneurysm means that 3/4th patients have associated aneurysm. Proximal MCA aneurysms have wide necks, incorporate many vessels. 80% MCA aneurysms are at bifurcation and project inferolaterally. MCA aneurysms pointing medially have the highest risk for intraoperative rupture. MCA is the most frequent site of mirror aneurysm. Patients with proximal MCA aneurysm has 3-fold risk of associated aneurysms than bifurcation or distal MCA aneurysm. 10% MCA aneurysms are giant.

MCA aneurysms mostly have wide necks. Incidence of intracerebral hematoma in MCA aneurysms is 20%. MCA is the most frequent site for giant aneurysms. Larger the size of MCA aneurysm – poor is the outcome. Irregular MCA aneurysm – poor outcome in 33%. Smooth MCA aneurysm – poor outcome in 7%.

ACom Artery Aneurysm

Constitutes 35% of intracranial aneurysms. Males outnumber females. Rarely associated with multiple aneurysms. Least favorable for giant aneurysms. Frequency of dyselectrolytemia is maximum. 99% present with rupture and 1% with mass effect. Anteriorly projecting aneurysms are the easiest technically. Anteriorly projecting aneurysms obscure the opposite A1. Inferiorly projecting aneurysms are most difficult as sac is adherent to perforators; for these aneurysms interhemispheric approach is better.

Giant Aneurysms

60% are partially thrombosed, 60% occur in females, common in anterior circulation. Cause mass effect, SAH in 15–75%, can cause embolic phenomenon. 18% have egg shell calcification and 18% have bone erosion, display target sign and wash-in and washout phenomenon.

Traumatic Aneurysms

Features suggestive are irregular shape, non-bifurcation aneurysms, poorly defined neck, delayed filling and emptying of the aneurysm.

PCom Artery Aneurysm

10% do not cause 3rd nerve palsy. 70% cause 3rd nerve palsy with SAH. 20% cause 3rd nerve palsy without SAH. In 10%, where there is no 3rd nerve palsy, indicates that the fundus is directed laterally towards temporal lobe instead of downwards, so retraction on temporal lobe has to be careful.

Giant Paraclinoid Carotid Aneurysms

These aneurysms encompass: Aneurysms arising from ophthalmic segment, from superior hypophyseal artery and aneurysms arising from superior aspect of carotid artery. The first 2 aneurysms displace the optic nerve medially. All these aneurysms share some common problems as:

Difficult proximal control. Inability to deflate the sac before clipping. Appreciation of exact site of aneurysms. Delicate handling of attenuated optic nerve. For proximal control – best is exposure of carotid in the neck.

Posterior Circulation Aneurysms

Commonest site is basilar bifurcation, commonest direction of fundus is superiorly. Clinical presentation-loss of consciousness, respiratory arrest. 6th nerve palsy– aneurysm at basilar artery – AICA junction. 12th nerve palsy– vertebral artery – PICA junction.

Side of Approach Governed by

Side of dominant vessel. Side of associated hematoma. Projection of aneurysm. During Acom artery aneurysm clipping SSEP from posterior tibial nerves can be used to check ACA perfusion.

Cause of Neurologic Deterioration after Clipping

Seizures. Vasospasm. Infarct. Hyponatremia. Hypotension. Cerebral swelling. Direct injury to vessel and vasospasm. Hydrocephalus. Rebleed.

Mycotic Aneurysm

Etiology – cardiac valves (SABE) – 2–10% of SABE develop infected aneurysms, no neck, distal location. Vasovasorum are present up to M1 and at A1– obstruction of these – ischemia – weakening of the wall - mycotic aneurysm. Immune complexes deposit on vessel wall and cause weakening. MCA is the commonest site.

Management

Antibiotics for 6 weeks– weekly CT angiogram, if no decrease in size or there is increase in size – surgery. For proximal aneurysm – wrapping. For distal aneurysms – excision. Neuronavigation has a role in localization.

Cirsoid Aneurysm

Present in subcutaneous tissue, usually in front or just behind the ear. Genesis: congenital or trauma. Nidus – artery, veins, no capillaries. Artery – usual, scalp arteries may communicate via emissary vein with intracranial vessels. Pericranial component is very important, as unless it is removed – recurrence is the rule. Clinical presentation – palpable mass, headache, tinnitus, pressure on carotid will decrease the size of the swelling. Diagnosis- CT and DSA.

D/D – Hemangioma, sinus pericranii, lymphangioma, dermal lipoma, encephalocele, neurofibroma.

Treatment – surgical excision. Embolization – transarterial/transvenous. Direct injection of sclerosant.

SAH of Unknown Source

Incidence of vasospasm is low. 80% fare better while only 50% in aneurysmal SAH fare better. Rebleed rate: 40% over next 3 months and then 0.8%/year for next 3 years. Shunt required in 3% patients.

Aneurysms in AVM

Perata classification

Type I : Dysplastic aneurysm, aneurysm located at some distance from AVM and appears unrelated to major inflow vessels

Type II : Aneurysm in proximal portion of feeders

Type III : Aneurysm in middle portion of feeders

Type IV : Intranidal aneurysms

Incidence of intracerebral hematoma is 2 fold than SAH. Incidence of vascular anomalies in cerebellar bleeds is 5–10%. Prevalence of bleed in AVM is 2–4% bleed year. AVM with only one draining vein will be associated with a larger hematoma than AVM's with 2 draining veins. 7% of AVM have associated aneurysm. AVM with aneurysm – 7% bleed rate/year. Commonest site of blood in aneurysmal SAH is subarachnoid space, 30% bleed in ventricles, 40% in parenchyma. MCA rupture – temporal lobe hematomas in 55%.

Arteriovenous Malformations

Mc Cormick classification

AVM – 50%

Cavernoma – 20%. Telangiectasias – 10%. Venous angioma – 10%. Venous varix – 10%

AVM

Large arteries and large veins and vascular nidus, consisting of dilated tortuous vessels. No capillary bed. High flow A-V shunt. Poor tissue perfusion. No intervening brain parenchyma. Patients with AVM who present with seizures, bleed rates – 33%. Patients with AVM who present with bleed, re-bleed rates – 51%. Temporal and occipital lobe AVM – bleed rates are more as compared to other locations Occipital AVM – known to cause migrainous attacks, visual symptoms. Posterior fossa AVM's are located deep and present with bleed. Cortical AVM's present with seizures. In children, bleed in AVM is 7 fold commoner than seizure. AVM's are common in MCA region. AVM's can cause intellectual decline due to steal phenomenon. In neonates, other presentation is high-output cardiac failure. AVM in pregnancy tends to rebleed more. Bleed from angiographically occult AVM is not so devastating. Morbidity and mortality is same in pregnancy as in non-pregnancy. Embolization is one of the modalities of treatment. Embolization has no effect on seizures. High surgical mortality is seen if, size >6 cm, age >50 years, evidence of steal on DSA, involvement of MCA or PCA perforators. 1/10th of AVMs are located in the posterior fossa.

Radiosurgery for AVMs

If volume of the lesion is 1 cc – cure rate is 88% if 8 cc cure rate is – 60%. Overall cure rate – 80%. 2 years gap between treatment and resolution of the lesion. 4% patients have permanent neurodeficits after radiosurgery.

Cavernomas

Slow flow, hence calcifications are seen. No intervening brain parenchyma. Sinusoid like capillaries, average size is 5 mm. Normal arteries and veins. 10% calcified. MRI – popcorn appearance. PET can differentiate cavernoma from tumor. Risk of bleeding in cavernoma – 0.25% @ year. High-risk of expansion and bleed in cavernoma occurs during pregnancy. Radiosurgery for cavernomas: Results are unfavorable.

Capillary Telangiectasia

Dilatation of capillaries. Normal intervening brain. Normal arteries and veins.

Venous Angiomas

Abnormally dilated veins, but which are physiologically competent. Caput medusae on angiography. Usually seen in deep white matter. Posterior fossa venous angiomas, tend to bleed.

Usually associated with cavernoma and in case of bleed it is the cavernoma which bleeds and not the venous angioma. Treatment is removal of clot and cavernoma but venous angioma is left alone. Removal of normally draining venous angiomas may cause venous infarction.

Carotid Cavernous Fistula

Causes – congenital (rare)

Acquired – trauma, atherosclerosis, hypertension, pseudoxanthoma elasticum, Ehler-Danlos syndrome, Marfans syndrome, fibromuscular dysplasia, sinus thrombosis.

Fistulas that drain anteriorly have predominantly eye signs, while as those which drain into sphenoparietal or petrosal sinuses they have minimal eye signs but cortical and brainstem dysfunction are seen. Further fistulas that drain into the cortical veins have higher chance of bleed.

When anterior intercavernous sinus is patent, ocular symptoms may be contralateral or bilateral

Occasionally the fistula may thrombose spontaneously (10–70%)

Characteristic angiographic features

Direct opacification of cavernous sinus. Early filling of ophthalmic veins. Diminished opacification of the distal arterial system. MRA shows flow voids in superior ophthalmic vein and dilatation of intracavernous sinuses.

Goals of Treatment

Preserve vision. Eliminate bruit. Restore the orbit and its contents. Avoid cerebral ischemic complications.

Surgical Goal

Occlude the fistula. Preserve the ICA.

Urgent treatment is needed in case of:

Progressive visual loss. Corneal exposure. Cortical venous drainage. Epistaxis. Medically intractable headache. Intolerable bruit.

Treatment of CCF

Type A: Intra-arterial occlusion of fistula is the treatment of choice. If it fails, direct surgery and packing of cavernous sinus to induce thrombosis.

Type B: Intra-arterial balloon carries risk of embolization and ischemia, so transvenous balloon occlusion via superior ophthalmic vein or inferior petrosal sinus.

Type C: Intra-arterial balloon occlusion

Type D: Trans-arterial occlusion of ECA branches – wait – will decrease the flow – and hence induce thrombosis, if still flow is maintained, then transvenous approach for ICA branches.

Direct surgery, if embolization fails. Direct surgical packing through inferior petrosal sinus if fistula is posterior and through superior ophthalmic vein if fistula is anterior. If inferior petrosal sinus is patent, then Parkinson triangle is opened to reach cavernous sinus. If superior ophthalmic vein is not patent, then cavernous sinus is opened via anteroinferior triangle.

Spinal AVMs are Classified Under 3 Groups

a. Dural AVM
b. Intradural AVM
c. Cavernoma

Intradural AVMs can be subclassified into spinal cord AVMs and perimedullary AVMs. The former is of juvenile and glomus type. All spinal AVM can be diagnosed by myelo/DSA except cavernoma. Cavernomas can be diagnosed by MRI, however MRI is not as suitable as myelo/DSA for other lesions.

	Dural AVF	Intradural AVF
Age	>40 years	<40 years
Male : Female	M > F	M = F
Symptom profile	Chronic worsening of symptoms	Acute presentation secondary to bleed
SAH	0%	50%

Overall 90% of patients are females. Signs and symptoms are LBA, radiculopathy, myelopathy

Site of AVM – lower dorsal or lumbar. Lesions are thought to be acquired. Dural branch of spinal ramus supplies the nidus – blood drains into coronal plexus via radial veins and then via medullary veins. Higher venous pressure causes myelopathy. 15% patients have sudden symptoms and 85% have chronic symptoms.

Cavernomas

Computed tomography (CT) scan-isodense with minimal enhancement. MRI – Popcorn appearance. Histopathology – gliotic tissue with macrophage laden with hemosiderin, familial cavernomas are associated with mutation on chromososome – 7q, risk of rupture – 0.6% @ year.

Indications for surgery – recurrent bleed, progressive neurological deficit, intractable seizures

Radiosurgery – usual dose is 32 cGy.

Indications for observation are:

a. Asymptomatic lesions
b. Symptomatic in deep location where you feel that surgery will give more deficits, MRI is done 6 monthly for 2 years and if the lesions are stable after every 1 year.

AVM requires treatment when it causes

Progressive neurological deficit. Bleed. Intractable seizures. Severe headache. Disabling bruit. Hydrocephalus.

Indications of Embolization

To reduce the size of AVM to make it amenable for radiosurgery. To coil intranidal aneurysm. Residual AVM after surgery or radiosurgery. For palliation in large AVMs to decrease steal phenomenon. Before radiosurgery to decrease the risk of bleed till the lesion gets obliterated fully. To reduce headaches in AVM's with ECA supply. High-flow AVM's are less suitable to radiosurgery, hence it is an indication for embolization followed by radiosurgery.

Indications of Preoperative Embolization

To obliterate intranidal aneurysms, fistula, venous varix. To obliterate deep feeders, not accessible at surgery. Reduce the size of nidus. In the past n-butyl-2-cyanoacrylate (NBCA) was used as an embolizing agent. It is soft compressible, has superior nidal penetration and lower recanalization rate. Newer agents are onyx.

Timing of surgery after embolization is 1–3 weeks, early surgery causes NPBP, late surgery will cause recruitment of collaterals.

Preradiosurgery Embolization

Goals are

Decrease the nidus size. Occlude intranidal aneurysms, fistulas, varices. Large AVM can be compartmentalized and made amenable to radiosurgery. To occlude dural support of AVM as radiosurgery cannot target these vessels as they are close to bone and scalp.

Palliative Embolization

AVM which are giant and hence cannot be operated, in such cases aim is to eliminate intranidal aneurysms, venous varices, AV fistulas, etc. Improvement occurs in bleed rates, seizures and headaches.

Angiographic features demonstrating successful angiographic obliteration of AVM:

Disappearance of nidus, feeding artery and draining vein. Normal circulation time

Radiosurgery for AVMs

At 1-year radiosurgery – 40% obliteration rate and there is 80%, obliteration rate at 2 years, with average dose of 25 Gy for <3 cm size. For >3 cm, obliteration rate is 60% at 2 years. Deep seated AVMs respond better than peripheral AVM's.

Moyamoya Disease

Bimodal age, 1st and 4th decade. Common in Japan. Moyamoya – puff of smoke in Japanese

Symptoms are

In children–Ischemia / bleed. In adults – bleed / ischemia. Seizures, focal deficits. Bleed is usually parenchymal, ventricular or subarachnoid hemorrhage. Bleed is secondary to associated aneurysms on collaterals.

Investigations

CT/MRI – multiple ischemic areas, bleed, cortical atrophy

DSA – stenosis of ICA – MCA – ACA – PCA, increased collateralization of thalamogeniculate, lenticulostriate, choroidal artery (puff of smoke).

Treatment

Vasodilator therapy. Encephalomyosynangiosis (EMS). STA-MCA bypass. Encephaloduroarteriosynangiosis (EDAS)

Angiographic Points

Colliculocentral point – where the precentral cerebellar vein (PCV) exits from the precentral cerebellar fissure, it lies halfway on Twining line. Choroidal point – 2.5 cm down a line from the midpoint of Twining line to opisthion. Copular point – where tonsillar vein joins near pyramid and forms the inferior vermian vein.

Angiographic Signs of Hydrocephalus

Stretching of thalamoperforating vessels. Reduced distance between medial and lateral posterior choroidal arteries. Increased distance between posterior choroidal arteries and parieto-occipital and calcarine branches. Increased sweep of pericallosal artery. Change in venous angle.

Veins which Opacify on Angiogram Early

Thalamostriate vein, caudate vein, internal cerebral vein, cortical veins except vein of Trolard, dural sinuses, vein of Trolard.

CRANIAL AVM

Vascular abnormality constituted by a complex, tangled web of afferent arteries and draining veins linked by an abnormal dysplastic intervening capillary bed. In contrast with an AVF which has direct fistulous connection without intervening nidus.

Angioarchitecture

Composed of: (a) Arterial feeder, (b) Nidus (c) Draining vein and (d) Intervening gliotic neural parenchyma. Arterial feeder (s) May be single/multiple, pial/perforating/dural, Direct feeders supply as terminal branch and indirect feeders supply en passage.

Nidus

The AVM nidus is a compact tangle of dysplastic, thin-walled vessels of varied length connecting feeding arteries to draining veins. An AVM nidus can either be globular or conical in shape and may be compact or diffuse. Within the nidus, arterial blood is shunted directly into draining veins without passage through a normal, high-resistance arteriolar– capillary network.

AVM-associated Aneurysms

Type I: unrelated dysplastic /incidental, *Type II:* flow related on proximal vessel, *Type III:* on distal small feeding vessel, and *Type IV:* intranidal aneurysm.

Hemodynamics

The velocity of blood flow is considerably higher through AVMs than through normal brain parenchyma. As a result of the abnormal hemodynamic condition, feeding arteries and draining veins become progressively dilated and tortuous. AVMs could be compared to vascular "sponges", which consume large volumes of blood, depriving the brain of normal circulation (steal phenomenon).

Etiology

Initially thought to be congenital. May be due to aberrant vasculogenesis and angiogenesis in 40–89 mm length embryo. Failure of the embryonic vascular plexus to fully differentiate and develop a mature capillary bed in the affected area. Developmental theory has been challenged. New AVM in angiography negative patients have been found. It is likely that a combination of congenital predisposition and extrinsic factors lead to their generation.

AVM Syndromes

Sturge–Weber syndrome or encephalotrigeminal angiomatosis a cutaneous, facial angioma in the distribution of the trigeminal nerve, and an ipsilateral, parietal–occipital vascular malformation.

Rendu–Osler–Weber syndrome (hereditary hemorrhagic telangiectasia) is an autosomal-dominant syndrome of multiple visceral, mucosal and cerebral vascular malformations.

Wyburn Mason (Bonnet Blanc-Dechaume syndrome) or mesencephalo-oculo-facial angiomatosis corresponds to the association of unilateral retinal angiomatosis and a cutaneous hemangioma in an ipsilateral trigeminal distribution with an AVM located in the midbrain.

Natural History

AVMs are dynamic, i.e., they undergo continuous subtle anatomic and hemodynamic changes. A cerebral AVM becomes clinically evident when the host's capacity to effectively compensate has reached its threshold. Enlargement of brain AVMs is observed in young patients (under 30 years of age), and especially in childhood. Spontaneous obliteration of cerebral AVMs is rare; only 50 cases have been reported in the literature. Several factors appear to be associated with spontaneous occlusion of cerebral AVM: single draining vein (84% of cases of occlusion),solitary arterial feeder (30%), and small size of the nidus (<3 cm in 50%). Based on autopsy findings AVM is found in cerebral hemisphere in 60 to 70%, cerebellum and brainstem 11 to 18% and deepseated 13 to 16%.

Presentation

Hemorrhage, Seizures, Headache, Neurological deficits, Asymptomatic picked in routine imaging and in pediatrics-hydrocephalus and heart failure.

Hemorrhage

Most common and found in 32–82%. It may be parenchymal, intraventricular or SAH. Patient presents with sudden onset severe headache. Vasospasm is rare (around 1–2%). Most AVMs are located subpially.

Factors Increasing the Risk of Bleeding

Nidus

82% small AVMs (less than 3 cm), 29% medium-sized AVMs (3–6 cm) and 12% large AVM (greater than 6 cm). Large AVMs can more often present in other ways than hemorrhage (seizures, deficits, headache).

Location

Some authors suggest that AVMs in deep locations such as in the basal ganglia or in the periventricular or intraventricular space, have an increased risk of bleeding. Can be partly explained as they are unlikely to have other presentation. Other factors deep venous drainage, venous stenosis, single draining vein and feeding artery pressures are associated with increased bleeding and arterial stenosis decrease bleeding risk. Annual rate of bleeding for one hemorrhage is 2–4% per year and declines to pre-hemorrhage rates over 5-years. Recurrent hemorrhage occurs in 6 to 18%.

Seizures

It is the 2nd most common clinical presentation of a cerebral AVM. Nearly three-quarters of patients experience a seizure at some point during their life. AVM-related seizures may be caused by: a) overt intracranial hemorrhage, b) from hemosiderin deposition following recurrent micro-hemorrhages, c) secondary to venous hypertension, d) ischemia following steal. In majority of cases, seizures are partial or complex partial and controlled on medications.

Headaches

Chronic headache is the initial symptom in 7%–48%. Migraine-like headaches commonly are associated with occipital lobe AVMs fed by the posterior cerebral artery.

Neurological Deficits

Focal neurologic deficits such as hemiparesis, aphasia without hemorrhage are the initial symptom in 1%–40% of patients. May be due to: vascular steal, mass effect, venous hypertension or perifocal edema.

Imaging

Imaging has several roles and goals: Main are to establish the diagnosis of brain AVM in various clinical situations, make a pre therapeutic evaluation of the AVM to help in decision-making, to treat the AVM in a sole therapy or in association with surgery or radio surgery and to perform post-therapeutic evaluation. CT is usually the first imaging modality used to rule out hemorrhage. AVM is suspected in young patients, if hematoma has lobar topography and if hyperdense serpiginous structures (calcifications) are seen. Parenchymatous calcifications are observed in 20% of cases, related to intravascular thrombosis or evolution of an old hematoma. MRI is currently used in case of un-ruptured AVM or to find the underlying lesion in case of lobar hematoma days or weeks after the bleeding. On T_1-weighted images with gadolinium, vessels are enhanced. The size and the anatomic location of the nidus are precisely delineated by MRI. Magnetic resonance angiograms (MRAs) can reveal the anatomy of the AVM non-invasively. Functional MRI can assist in treatment planning by defining the functionality of adjacent brain. Selective angiography still always is necessary to make a decision regarding the treatment. The exact and therapeutically relevant anatomic and functional information still has to be obtained by angiography.

Classifications

(A) Luessenhop-Gennarelli (1977), (B) Spetzler-Martin (1986), (C) Garretson, (D) Nataf and (E) Vienna classification

Spetzler-Martin Grading

Size; Small (<3 cm) –1, Medium (3–6 cm) –2 and Large (>6 cm) –3.

Cortical eloquence (sensorimotor, language, visual, thalamus, hypothalamus, internal capsule, brain stem, cerebellar peduncles, and deep cerebellar nuclei).

Deep venous drainage: Yes –1 and No –0

AVM grade = sum (size + eloquence + deep component)

The Spetzler and Martin (1986) classification was established to grade AVMs according to their degree of surgical difficulty and the risk of surgical morbidity and mortality. There are 5 grades; Grade I, II, III, IV and V. Further classified into; Low grade AVM, High grade AVM and Inoperable lesions. Drawbacks of S-M grading definition of eloquence, lack of consideration for nidus compactness, not useful for posterior fossa AVM, only applicable for surgical outcome and grade III in homogeneity.

Nataf Grading

Five angiographic parameters were considered to be determinants of the bleeding risk, leading to a four-grade classification.

Grade I: no risk factor

Ia: with venous recruitment

Ib: without venous recruitment

Grade II: venous stenosis or venous reflux

Grade III: deep venous drainage only

Grade IV: intra- or juxtanidal aneurysm

In the series mentioned, there were 13% of hemorrhages in grade Ia, 38% in grade Ib, 48% in grade II and 90% in grade III and IV.

Vienna Classification

Gr 0, Gr I, Gr II, Gr III Feeders Pial + perforators

No. of feeders 1–2, >2

Nidus (cm) <2 cn, 2–4 cm and > 4 cm

The algorithm is similar to that of Spetzler and Martin for use in arteriovenous malformation surgery, allowing the comparison of surgical and endovascular feasibility.

Management options are AVM microsurgery, embolization, radiosurgery and combination of these.

Microsurgery

Not every AVM is amenable to or best treated with surgery. Factors associated with increased surgical risk are large size, deep venous drainage, deep location, diffuse nidus, feeders from deep perforating system.

Microsurgical Principles

Surgical AVM excision should be an elective procedure, even in patients with ruptured AVMs. Preopsteroids, anti-convulsants and antibiotics need to be given. Wide craniotomy and dural opening should be done. When the nidus is below the surface, an arterialized draining vein (red vein) can be followed to the AVM. Localization may be assisted with ultrasound or frameless stereotaxy. Spiral nidus dissection layer by layer. At least one major draining vein should be preserved till the end of dissection. At the end of dissection this vein becomes bluish proving that feeders have been eliminated. Complete AVM excision should be documented by post op angiogram.

Surgical complications may be in the form of intra op-rupture, post retraction edema, new onset seizures, retrograde thrombosis of feeding vessels, resection of eloquent brain and normal perfusion pressure breakthrough. Risk of surgery is quite well estimated by the Spetzler-Martin grading system, with a favorable outcome in 97%–100% grade I, 95% grade II, 88% grade III, 73% grade IV, 57% grade V.

Embolization

Firstdescribed in 1960 by Luessenhope and Spence. It is one of the rapidly evolving technique. Embolic agents (silk, NBCA, histoacryl, onyx) and delivery systems (balloons with calibrated leaks, flow-guided micro catheters, over the wire micro catheters) have undergone drastic modifications. Initially used as an adjunct to microsurgery or radio surgery and in some cases as a stand alone treatment modality. Embolization may be curative embolization, palliative embolization, partial (targeted embolization), pre-operative embolization and pre-radio surgery embolization. Onyx is innovative and promising material and is non-adhesive and available in ready to use vials, it is composition of EVOH (ethylene vinyl alcohol copolymer), DMSO (dimethyl sulfoxide) and tantalum. It is easily injected, nonadhesive, prolonged injection times are common.

Complications

Gluing of micro catheter, perfusion pressure break through phenomenon.

Radiosurgery

Currently GK (cobalt-60), Linac or proton beams are used. Following bleed, part of nidus may be hidden or compressed by clots hence it is rational to wait till resolution or first evacuate it. Radiation dose causes endothelial damage, smooth muscle cell proliferation, progressive sclerosis and subsequent thrombosis of nidal channels over time. he success of stereotactic radiosurgery depends on AVM size and the radiation dose delivered. Factors influencing obliteration rate are AVM volume, target determination (complete nidus), angioarchitecture and hemodynamics, AVM location (hemispheric better) and radiation dosage. Drawbacks of radiosurgery are risk of bleed during latent period, unknown individual radio sensitivity and neurologic deficits related to radiosurgery.

POSTERIOR CIRCULATION ANEURYSMS: SURGICAL MANAGEMENT

Occur in fifth to sixth decade. Account for 15% of all intracranial aneurysms. Common in females. Most commonly occur at basilar apex followed by origins of SCA and PICA. PCA and AICA aneurysms are very rare.

Clinical Presentation: Subarachnoid hemorrhage, intraventricular hemorrhage, single or multiple cranial nerves palsies, local mass effect, hydrocephalus and long tract signs. Diagnosis is by NCCT for location of SAH and diagnosis, bony details of posterior fossa. Four vessel DSA, vessel of origin and relation to other vessels and presence and location of vasospasm. Re-bleeding rate 10% (thrice that of anterior circulation aneurysms). Mortality of untreated patients 63% against 11% of surgically treated patients. Management options include-Clipping, Endovascular and bypass procedures.

Subtemporal Approach: Supine position with head tilted to facilitate temporal lobe retraction, temporal craniotomy is done, temporal lobe retracted upwards till cerebral peduncles and field centered on third nerve and temporal lobe resection indicated if required. Merits include easy proximal control, excellent visualization and easy dissection of perforators, anterior and posterior directed aneurysms can be tackled easily and fenestrated clips can be placed well. Demerits include narrow field, access to contra-lateral P1 is difficult, temporal lobe damage, intra-operative bleeding is difficult to control and III nerve palsy is very common.

Trans-sylvian Approach

Pterional craniotomy, OZ osteotomy to improve superior view, bone removal (if required): sphenoid ridge, anterior clinoids, dorsum sellae, clivus and medial petrous apex followed by wide opening of sylvian fissure. Merits include familiarity with approach, proximal control is straight forward, wide exposure is possible, both P1 can be exposed for temporary trapping. Demerits are exposure of posteriorly located perforators is difficult. Distal clip blade is difficult to visualize and anteriorly or posteriorly directed aneurysms difficult to tackle. This approach is the most favored approach for laterally tilted aneurysm and high located basilar top.

PAVEL-Pterional Approach via Extended Lateral Corridor

Performed from surgeons dominant side and sylvian fissure dissected thoroughly. Field centered on Cr III and mesial temporal lobe elevated up. Posterior dissection is performed behind and below ipsilateral P1.

Basilar Trunk Aneurysms

Operative approaches are Transpetrosal approach, Retrolabyrinthine, Translabyrinthine, Transcochlear, Combined supra and infratentorial, Extended middle fossa approach, Transoral approach.

Transpetrosal Approaches

Approach the basilar trunk from lateral side and ENT surgeon's assistance is required for temporal bone drilling.

Retrolabyrinthine exposure: bone posterior to semicircular canals is removed and hearing is preserved.

Translabyrinthine exposure: semicircular canals are removed and hearing is sacrificed and 7th nerve is preserved.

Transcochlear: Hearing and seventh nerve both are sacrificed and maximum bone is removed.

Extended middle fossa approach: was popularized by Kawase and temporal craniotomy is done followed by extradural mobilization of temporal lobe. Anterior petrous apex drilling of Kawase's triangle. Approach the aneurysm from superior and anterior trajectory. The advantage is hearing is preserved.

Combined supra-infratentorial approach: Two maneuvers-posterior mobilization of sigmoid sinus, division of tentorium and superior petrosal sinus divided. The Vein of Labbe is preserved. Provides access from foramen magnum to dorsum sellae and there is minimum need for brain retraction.

Trans oral approaches: Obsolete these days and was associated with high incidence of complications like CSF leak and meningitis.

Aneurysms of Vertebral Artery, PICA and Vertebrobasilar Junction

Exposures: Midline suboccipital, far lateral, extended far lateral and combined.

Far Lateral Approach

Most commonly utilized for PICA aneurysms, distal vertebral aneurysms and PICA- Vertebral junction aneurysms.

Position-lateral decubitus, neck flexion and neck rotation with ipsilateral lateral flexion. Hockey stick or S shaped incision, paramedian suboccipital craniotomy half to two third of condoyle and posterior arch of C1 with rim of foramen magnum. Advantages offered are extra lateral angle of visualization and minimal brainstem retraction and vertebral artery is visible early in the exposure.

Extended far lateral approach: Superior occipital bone is removed and transverse- sigmoid junction is exposed and CPA is entered.

Combined approach: Supra and infratemporal combined approach for basilar trunk is combined with far lateral approach. Obsolete these days with availability of endovascular methods.

Midline Suboccipital Craniotomy

Indications-bilateral vertebral aneurysm or distal PICA aneurysms, bypass procedures, however it does not provide good access to anteriorly located aneurysms.

Ligation: When both Pcom are large in size, when balloon occlusion suggests good collateral circulation, gradual compression can be used and vertebral artery tolerates ligation very well if opposite vertebral is not aberrant.

Revascularization procedures. When ligation is not feasible so also the endovascular management. High morbidity and mortality associate with the procedure and needs team approach including endovascular surgeon and neurosurgeon.

Hypothermic cardiac arrest: last resort. Aneurysm shrinks and become amenable to manipulations and is associated with high morbidity and mortality.

Timing of surgery: Early surgery

Advantages are; reduces the risk of rebleed, better management of vasospasm and mortality is decreased (8%)

Main disadvantages are; more friable aneurysm, more intraoperative rupture and more damage to vital structures.

CAVERNOMAS

Cerebral cavernous malformation (CCM), cavernous hemangioma, cavernous angioma, cryptic vascular malformation, occult vascular malformation are the synonyms.

Developmental abnormalities that affects the blood vessels supplying the brain. Dilated sinusoidal channels lined by single layer endothelium without intervening brain parenchyma. These can occur anywhere in the CNS, these are angiographically occult vascular malformations.

Epidemiology

Prevalence around 0.5% and 5–10% of all cerebrovascular malformation. 80% are supratentorial. Familial CCM accounts around 20–30%. Increased prevalence in Mexican American families. 30–50% are asymptomatic. Age at first diagnosis: <20 years: 25–30%, 20–40 years: 60% and >40 years age group 10–15%. Bimodal presentation in pediatric 3–11 years and in adults 2nd to 4th decade. 20–30% of cavernomas may be associated with venous anomaly.

Genetics

Usually sporadic (80%). Three autosomal dominant genes (7p/7q/3q) associated with familial form. The precise function not known, CCM1 on 7q chromosome and expresses KRIT1, CCM2 on 7p chromosome and expresses MGC4607 and CCM3 on 3q chromosome and expresses PCD10.

Pathology

Mulberry appearance, soft/hard consistency, usually 1–5 cm. Enlarged capillaries with abnormal gap between endothelial cells with thin collagenous wall and lack of smooth muscle/elastic fibers. Capillaries are immediately adjacent to each other, with no intervening neural tissue. No feeding arteries or draining veins. May be associated venous anomaly. Blood flow is less. Blood degradation products (hemosiderin staining) and gliotic reaction in the adjacent brain.

Clinical Presentation

Approx 50% asymptomatic. Seizure in (40–80%). Males more commonly presents with epilepsy and chronic intractable epilepsy is found in almost half. Sudden onset neurological deficits caused by hemorrhage, commonly observed in thalamic and brain stem CCM. Prior hemorrhage, female sex and pregnancy are the risk factors for rebleed. Most common presentation is seizure.

Natural History

Subclinical hemorrhage seen in all and clinical hemorrhage in 12.1%. Annual hemorrhage rate 0.5 to 1% and rebleed rate of 4.5%. The epileptic risk is correlated to the localization, more frequent for temporal and frontal lesions (1.5 to 2.4% each year). Lesion may arise de novo, may grow / shrink / remain unchanged.

Radiology

CT scans may show focal hyperdensity, reflecting calcification or recent hemorrhage and intravenous contrast may show faint enhancement. On MRI T2WI show reticulated core of lesion "popcorn" appearance with a lucent halo surrounding a lesion. This pathognomonic appearance is produced due to repeated hemorrhages and hemosiderin deposition around the lesion. No peri-lesional edema. Gradient sequences are more sensitive for detection of small lesions. T1WI demonstrates blood products. Axial T2WI shows the circumferential within the lesion (hemosiderin ring). Cerebral DSA demonstrate no vascular abnormalities.

Differential Diagnosis

Hemorrhagic metastasis viz melanoma, glioma e.g. oligodendroglioma and pleomorphic, Hemorrhagic telangiectasia (Osler Weber Rendu disease)/multiple metastasis.

Management options are: Medical treatment, stereotactic radiotherapy or gamma knife and surgical resection (gold standard).

Medical Management

Offered to asymptomatic, incidentally detected lesions, surgically inaccessible lesions and unfit for surgery. Regular follow up MRI to assess increase in size or new hemorrhages. Medical treatment is limited to control of seizure activity. Patients are refrained from strenuous exercises, anticoagulant use, avoid pregnancy.

Surgical Treatment

No re-bleeding from completely excised CCM. 75–88% of patients become seizure free after complete resection. Intractable epilepsy may become well controlled. Complete cure can be assured. Demerits are; in brainstem and thalamic CM, surgical treatment may lead to high surgical mortality and morbidity. If lesion is in the eloquent area, then functional imaging along with cortical mapping should be done. Frameless stereotaxy is considered in small and deep seated lesions.

Surgical Technique

Surgical technique depends on the location of lesion, presence of associated venous malformations and presence of overt hematoma. Position and approach based on location, trans-sulcal approach is preferred. Lesion should be localized after opening the dura. Intraoperative sonography, or stereotaxy can be used. Surface lesion appear as purple-blue mulberry like structure surrounded by area of hemosiderosis. The cortical venous drainage pattern should be inspected. Lesion is initially shrunk with bipolar coagulation. The surrounding gliotic brain (pseudo capsule) offers a plane of dissection. Cotton patties are used for preservation of plane of dissection. Complete resection is to be attempted. Resection bed to be inspected for satellite lesion. Associated venous anomaliesare seen in approximately 24% patients of CCM. These venous anomalies are the normal veins draining brain. Every effort is made to preserve them. These may be the only veins supplying the brain. Coagulation of these may result in venous infarcts and increases the morbidity of surgery. Surgical excision options include lesionectomy alone, lesionectomy and excision of abnormal tissues and lesionectomy and removal of abnormal area remote from the cavernoma. Special Considerations should be given to intractable epilepsy and includes pre op. work up to localize source of seizure. If the location is non-eloquent, surrounding hemosiderin stained brain may be resected because of possible epileptogenicity.

Optic Pathway CM

May present with acute / subacute visual disturbances and may mimic SAH on CT. Urgent decompression for chiasmal apoplexy. Pterional or subfrontal route. CM may affect any part of optic pathway, lesionectomy is usually attempted and mostly successful.

Pineal CM

EVD / Shunt to lower ICP. Special Considerations <1% of CM. Present with features of raised ICP, ocular symptoms, neuroendocrine. Interhemispheric transsplenial, sub occipital transtentorial and supra cerebellar infratentorial approach depending on location of CM.

Multiple CM

Multiple in 50% cases and treatment at addressing symptomatic lesion. Large sized, hemorrhage, seizure focus. Familial CM are at risk for the formation of de novo CM.

Dural-based CM

Commonly found in middle fossa, CP angle, tentorium and convexity. Present with headache and they rarely bleed. It may mimic meningioma. Enhance strongly and homogenously on Gd MRI. Preoperative embolization/SRS or EBRT is advisable for highly vascular CM. Postoperative morbidity as high as 38%.

Brainstem CM

Of all CNS cavernoma, 9–35% are found in brain stem. Acute onset focal neurological deficits are the most common presentation. The waxing and waning of symptoms mimic multiple sclerosis. Hemorrhage rate is 30 times more than that for supratentorial CMs. Rebleeding rate is as high as 35%.

Gamma Knife Therapy in CCM

Radiation injury to endothelial cell causes release of growth factors and fibroblast proliferation. This causes hyperplasia of smooth muscles cells and occlusion of lumen. Coagulation necrosis of cavernoma and obliteration of vessels is also a proposed mechanism.

Indications: Surgically inaccessible lesions like thalamic, brainstem or deep seated lesion, lesions presented with minor hemorrhage, multiple lesions and patients preference.

Merits: Reduction of rebleed rates, halting of growth of lesion, volume control and seizure control. Demerits; radiation edema and transient or permanent deficits and lower efficacy of treatment.

Morbidity: Perilesional edema was found in 27% with transient morbidity of 20.5% with permanent morbidity of 4.5%. Rebleed common in patients who presented with bleed, larger lesion volume and prescription dose less than 13 Gy. Edema was common with prescription dose > 13 Gy.

SPINAL AVMs

Introduction

Vascular malformations of spinal cord are a rare clinical entity, representing 5% of all primary spinal cord lesions, with arteriovenous malformations (AVM) and cavernous malformations being the most common. They are relatively heterogeneous with distinct angiographic pattern and associated with specific etiology, pathophysiology, natural history and even a different therapy.

Historical Perspective

In 1888 Gaupp: 1st to describe a spinal dural AVM from a postmortem study.

In 1910 Krausse: 1st attempted to resect the lesion.

1914 Sir Charles Elsberg: 1st successful therapeutic operation for a spinal AVM.

1926 Foix and Alajouanine reported the syndrome of subacute necrotic myelopathy associated with rapidly progressive onset of paraplegia and subsequent death.

In 1960 with introduction of selective spinal angiography vascular anatomy of spinal AVMs became more clear.

Vascular Anatomy

Arterial Anatomy

1. **Medullary arteries:** Two arterial networks (a) Anterior, (b) Posterior and both system supplied by medullary artery.
2. **Radicular arteries:** Supplies dorsal / ventral nerve roots.
3. **Dural arteries:** Dural root sleeves and spinal dura.

Venous Drainage

Spinal cord drained by radial veins which carry blood from parenchyma to surface where they empty into the sulcal vein and coronal venous plexus in pia materon the cord and via medullary vein to epidural venous plexus.

Classification

Niimi and Berenstein (1999)

a. Spinal vascular lesion-spinal dural AVF, spinal extradural and paraspinal AVF.
b. Spinal cord vascular lesion-AVF / AVM metameric / non-metameric
c. Spinal cord telangiectasia
d. Cavernous vascular malformation

Anson and Spetzler (1992)

Type I: Dural (intradural or extradural) AVF (also referred to as Type I spinal AVM or as "angioma racemosum venosum," nidus, or true AVM).

Type II: Glomus AVMs

Type III: Juvenile AVMs (nidus usually intramedullary)

Type IV: Direct spinal AVF

Extradural AVF: Rare vascular lesion and abnormal communication between an extradural radicular artery and epidural venous plexus. Progressive myelopathy / radiculopathy occasionally epidural hematoma. Diagnosis with MRI angiography

Treatment: Extradural AVF treated by endovascular treatment with embolization of arterial feeder.

Intradural Dorsal AVF: Type-1

Type-I spinal AVM also known as spinal dural AVF. Most common type AVF 80–85%. Pathophysiology - low flow fistula between dural branch of radicular artery and intramedullary vein. age at presentation – middle age (40–60 year). Male 90% and > female 10%. Most common site – thoracic spine.

Progressive myelo-radiculopathy or cauda equina syndrome is usual presentation. Aggravated by raised intra-abdominal pressure and sub arachnoid hemorrhage is rare manifestation. Acute deterioration unlikely, two sub type

Type-1a: Single arterial feeder

Type-1b: Two or more arterial feeder

Diagnosis

Angiography

Reveals expanded radiculomeningeal arteries, a vascular conglomerate in the region of the intervertebral neural foramen shunted into the expanded perimedullary veins. Nidus characterized by slow blood flow. The blood flow in spinal cord arteries is also slower.

Treatments

Goal: isolation and obliteration of the fistula and draining veins. Best treated surgically: Direct surgical ligation of arterial feeder and caries low morbidity and high success rate. Embolization of the feeding vessel, via endovascular techniques is less invasive carried in same sitting.

Dural AVMs

Two variants of surgical technique:

1. Occluding the malformation in the dural leaf of the spinal nerve root or cutting off the feeding vessels immediately outside the root.
2. Occluding the radicular vein, which provides retrograde blood shunting from the AVM into the perimedullary veins.

Intradural Ventral AVF: Type IV

Rare lesion, not true AVM but instead pial AVF. First describe by Djindjian and coworker as perimedullary AVF. Heros and associates introduced the term Type IV.

Direct fistula between anteriorn spinal artery and draining vein.

Merland's sub classification

IV-A: Smallest shunt, slow blood flow, less venous hypertension

IV-B: Larger shunt, higher blood flow and greater degree hypertension

IV-C: Giant, very high degree blood flow, with significant hypertension.

Usually present at younger age and manifests as progressive myelopathy due to compression, venous hypertension or hematoma. SAH and acute neurological deterioration may occur.

Treatments

IV-A: Surgery

IV-B: Embolization

IV-C: Combination of endovascular ablation, followed by surgical excision of retained elements.

Intramedullary AVM

Also known as type-2 AVMs, glomus AVM, classic AVM, angioma racemosum arteriovenous. True AVM of spinal cord closely resemble intracranial AVMs.

15–20 % of all spinal AVM. Incidence is equal in males and females. Usually present earlier in 2nd or 3rd decade of life. Associated with other vascular anomalies (13%–37%). Site: uniform distribution cervical (30%), thoracolumbar (70%). Clinical presentation is acute (35%) due to hemorrhage and progressive myelopathy (50%) and two type: 1) compact, 2) diffuse have been described.

Diagnosis is by MRI and shows: Hematomyelia /cord expansion /SAH. Spinal angiography shows multiple feeding vessels from anterior and posterior spinal artery and high pressure, relatively low resistance and high blood flow.

Management

a. Embolization followed by surgery
b. Radiosurgery for residual / non embolized lesion

Two ways of nidus resection: In first isolate the vessels near the nidus and coagulate, then dissect the nidus and resect and in second one the vessels are cut off in the nidus itself during its separation, and resection of the nidus.

Extradural-Intradural: AVM Type-III

In this are included juvenile AVMs and metameric AVMs and these lesions are extremely rare. It is complex lesion involving skin, vertebra, and spinal cord.

Congenital lesions are inborn errors of vascular embryogenesis. Anatomically lesion is fed by multiple enlarged medullary artery via anterior and posterolateral spinal artery and have a voluminous arteriovenous nidus that completely fills the thecal sac. Nidus has neural tissue within its interstices. The incidence is equal in males and females and onset is at young age. These lesions are uniformly distributed along spinal axis and are associated with other vascular anomalies. Pain and progressive myelopathy related to compression and arterial steal is the usual presentation.

Treatment

Primary extradural localization: Endovascular approach. Mainly intradural location and spinal cord compression: combination of endovascular and microsurgical methods.

Conus AVMs: Conus AVM are location specific and have feature of both AVMs and AVFs. They can be both perimedullary and intramedullary with diffuse border. They present with progressive myeloradiculopathy and occasional SAH. Spinal angiography s/o multiple arterial feeder, more than one nidus, and complex venous drainage.

Treatment – combination of endovascular and surgical approach because of the possible pelvic disturbances.

Embolic Agents used are:

Particulate materials

- Polyvinyl alcohol (150–250 micro lts)
- Gelfoam
- Sponge microparticulate
- Balloon occlusion
- Liquid agents
- N-butyl cyanoacrylate

Ethylene vinyl alcohol copolymer

COBB SYNDROME

Consists of metameric AVMs of spinal canal. These lesions, first described by Cobb, demonstrate varying involvement of dura, vertebrae, muscle and skin. Superficial angiomatosis is a part of this syndrome. Neurological symptoms depend on type, extent and location of the lesion. Complete cure is very difficult.

MOYAMOYA DISEASE

A chronic occlusive cerebrovascular disease affecting arteries around the 'circle of Willis' & formation of extensive collaterals at the base of the brain. Presents with ischemic and hemorrhagic symptoms. First described in Japan-Takeuchi & Shimizu (1957). Spontaneous occlusion of the ' circle of Willis'- Kudo (1968). Moyamoya means 'puff of smoke'. Coined by Suzuki and Takaku in 1969.

Epidemiology: Highest incidence in Japan (0.35/ lakh). Incidence in Western countries-1/10th of Japan. Females are more commonly affected than males 2:1 ratio. Bimodal age distribution: larger peak in 1st decade and smaller peak around 30–49 years. 10–15% have familial form.

Etiology

Multifactorial: Genetic predisposition and environmental stimuli

Genetic loci: Chromosome 3, 6, 8 & 17.

Associated conditions include Grave's disease/thyrotoxicosis: Leptospirosis and tuberculosis: Aplastic anemia, Fanconi anemia, sickle cell anemia, and lupus anticoagulant: Apert syndrome, Down syndrome, Marfan syndrome, tuberous sclerosis, Turner syndrome, NF-1, Hirschsprung's disease: Atherosclerosis, coarctation of aorta, fibromuscular dysplasia & hypertension: head and neck irradiation.

Pathophysiology: There is smooth muscle hyperplasia of vessel wall and luminal thrombosis and fibro-cellular thickening of intima and attenuation of media. Disruption of internal elastic lamina. No evidence of inflammation or arteriosclerosis.

Site: Supraclinoidal ICA, ACA & MCA. Rare involvement of PCA & BA and extra-cranial involvement.

Most commonly involved are pediatric population and manifest with ischemic symptoms in 70–80% cases and occurs in watershed areas. Precipitating factors are hyperventilation and dehydration.

Features: Hemiparesis, speech disturbance, hemorrhage which can be IVH, intraparenchymal or subarachnoid, cognitive impairment, seizure, subtle deficits like developmental delay, syncope, personality changes, visual disturbance, headache and choreiform movements. Sources of bleed are fragile collateral vessels, micro aneurysms in the circle of Willis, periventricular pseudo aneurysms and saccular aneurysms in vertebrobasilar system.

Imaging

Angiography: Gold standard.

MRI & MRA: steno-occlusive carotid lesion and basal Moyamoya.

Plain CT: helps in acute stage.

Cerebral blood flow studies: Xenon enhanced CT, PET, SPECT.

Angiography (Suzuki and Takaku staging)

Stage 1: Narrowing of carotid fork

Stage 2: Initiation of Moyamoya

Stage 3: Intensification of Moyamoya

Stage 4: Minimization of Moyamoya

Stage 5: Reduction of Moyamoya

Stage 6: Disappearance of Moyamoya

Types: Basal Moyamoya, Ethmoidal Moyamoya and Vault Moyamoya

Management: No definite treatment available.

Medical treatment: not effective. Aspirin, anticoagulants, calcium channel blockers and steroids have been tried.

Surgical management: The main aim is augmentation of cerebral blood flow and improve cerebral hemodynamics. Methods are direct revascularization and Indirect revascularization. Indication for revascularization are symptomatic patients with good neurological status, infarction <2 cm on CT & all previous hemorrhages resolved completely, angiographic stage II to IV.

Direct revascularization: Indicated when donor & recipient vessel diameter >1 mm. Immediate selective perfusion of ischemic area and there is chance of hyper perfusion syndrome and usually done in adults. The Direct revascularization procedures are STA-MCA bypass, STA-ACA bypass and STA-PCA bypass.

Indirect revascularization: Aimed at stimulating neovascularization but extent of revascularization unpredictable and is useful in pediatric population. Encephalomyosynangiosis (EMS): implantation of temporalis muscle on lateral brain surface and secured to dura. Encephaloduroarteriosynangiosis (EDAS): dissected STA is laid onto the cortical surface. Ribbon EDAS: pedicle of galea inserted into inter-hemispheric fissure. Autogenic omentum transplantation as free graft.

Follow-up

Clinical evaluation & angiography after 6 months and angiography after 1 year. MRA annually from second year.

Assessment of revascularization

Qualitative:

Matsushima grading on DSA:

Grade A: Good revascularization- >2/3rd of MCA territory

Grade B: Fair- 1/3 to 2/3rd of MCA territory

Grade C: Poor- slight or no collateral formation

Qualitative:

Doppler grading after EMS:

Grade 1: No vessel formation

Grade 2: 1–4 vessel formation

Grade 3: >4 vessel formation

Prognosis

Benign course in 75–80% and rebleeding occurs in 30–65%. Revascularization reduces rebleeding and TIAs. Unilateral disease progresses to bilateral involvement in 7–27%.

STENTS

Intracranial stents, initially launched in 2002, were developed to provide additional support and re-modelling of the aneurysm neck, and the concept of parent artery reconstruction was further advanced with flow-diverting stents introduced in 2008. The development of intracranial stents has revolutionized the endovascular management of complex intracranial aneurysms and the proportion of aneurysms allocated to endovascular therapy ranges from 10% to 90%. Many previously untreatable cerebral aneurysms (i.e. fusiform or dissecting aneurysms or aneurysms with a wide-necked profile) are now within the scope of endovascular treatment, but many limitations remain. Stent-assisted coil embolization is a feasible endovascular treatment method for ruptured wide-necked intracranial aneurysms which are difficult to treat surgically or with balloon assisted embolization. Stent-assisted embolization is beneficial also for the treatment of wide-necked recurrent or residual intracranial aneurysms, although stability and permanent occlusion of the aneurysm is unlikely if the aneurysm exceeds 20 mm in diameter, the recurrent diameter of the aneurysm exceeds 10 mm, or if mass effect is present with the recurrent aneurysm. Flow-diverting stents, on the other hand, offer another valuable tool in the endovascular treatment of complex cerebral aneurysms. Many previously untreatable aneurysms may be successfully treated with a flow-diverting stent.

Advantages

Intracranial stents have several advantages in the treatment of cerebral aneurysms. In addition to disturbing the inflow jet to the aneurysm sac and thus promoting aneurysm thrombosis, the presence of the stent reduces the risk of coil protrusion and provides a physical matrix for possible endothelial growth across the aneurysm neck.

Limitations

There are, however, also many limitations in stent-assisted coiling. The reconstruction of very wide-necked or fusiform aneurysms with coils may be difficult and even accessing the aneurysm sac after stenting may prove challenging. The dual antiplatelet therapy necessitated by the stent may be problematic especially in the setting of acute subarachnoid hemorrhage, and even when adequate occlusion has been initially achieved with stent-assisted embolization, aneurysms remain prone to coil compaction and recanalization. Flow-diverting stents, on the other hand offer fascinating opportunities for the treatment of segmentally diseased vessels and complex cerebral aneurysms.

The concept of flow redirection and curative vessel reconstruction represents a paradigm shift in the treatment philosophy for endovascular aneurysm therapy. However, many uncertainties remain with this relatively new form of aneurysm treatment, including, the lack of long-term knowledge of the risk of arterial stenosis after stent deployment. These are:

The fate of perforating vessels crossed by the device, the duration of post-procedural antiplatelet medical therapy and optimal patient selection. There are several advantages in using stents in the management of intracranial aneurysms: in addition to reducing the risk of coil protrusion into the parent artery, an intracranial stent provides a physical matrix for possible endothelial growth across the aneurysm neck and disturbs the inflow jet to the aneurysm sac, thus promoting aneurysm thrombosis. Possibly due to this flow reduction and decrease in the shear stress in the aneurysm sac, deployment of an intracranial stent seems also beneficial with respect to reducing the recanalization rate of cerebral aneurysms. In wide necked aneurysms located at arterial bifurcations, narrowing of the bifurcation angle and additional support to the aneurysm neck may also be provided by the 'Y-stent' technique, whereby dual stents are deployed sequentially into each arterial branch.

TYPES OF STENTS-NEUROFORM, ENTERPRISE, FLOW DIVERTERS, COVERED STENTS, WEB, ONYX

Enterprise/Neuroform

The Neuroform stent (Boston Scientific/Target Therapeutics, Fremont, CA, USA), a flexible, self-expanding, nitinol stent specifically designed for use in the cerebral vasculature, became available for aneurysm treatment in November

2002. Dedicated to intracranial usage, this flexible, self-expanding, open cell stent is available in diameters of 2.5–4.5 mm and lengths of 10–30 mm. It is made up of 6–8 linked radiolucent cells comprised of a nickel–titanium alloy (nitinol) with a high degree of elasticity, deformity and shape memory. It has four radiopaque markers at each end and 6.5–9.5% metal surface coverage. However, this flexible open cell design does make it more prone to migration or herniation into the aneurysm. In addition, its open cell design provides a weaker scaffold for coil support with some cases of coil herniation. It cannot be easily retrieved.

Enterprise Stent

Succeeding the Neuroform stent with FDA approval in 2007, the Enterprise stent (Cordis) is a closed cell nitinol design, affording a stronger scaffold, minimizing coil prolapse and also allowing for stent recapture and repositioning after up to 70% deployment. This allows for the 'semi-deployment' technique where the stent is partially deployed during coiling of the aneurysm to allow for subsequent retraction and repositioning for optimal final stent positioning after coiling. Although it has a similar percentage of metal surface coverage as the Neuroform, its closed cell design provides a stronger radial force for aneurysm neck scaffolding. It is available in only one diameter, 4.5 mm, and four lengths—14 mm, 22 mm, 28 mm and 37 mm. Although all of the conventional intracranial stents are laser-cut nitinol stents, the features of the stent vary depending on the profile and structure of the stent. It is generally accepted that stents with open cell design (i.e. adjacent cells formed by the strands of the stent are not interconnected) conform adequately also in tortuous vessels while stents with closed cell design (i.e. with adjacent cells interconnected) are usually re-sheathable and may have superior scaffolding across the aneurysm neck.

Flow Diverter

The efficacy of flow-diverting stents was first demonstrated in several animal studies. Flow-diverting stents have a dense mesh geometry and a very high metal-to-surface coverage which induces stronger turbulence and flow reduction than that induced by conventional intracranial stents, potentially inducing thrombosis in the aneurysm sac. While the metal surface coverage of conventional intracranial stent is usually around 10 %, the dense mesh of flow diverting stents provide a metal surface area coverage of 35 to 55%, depending on the stent size and parent vessel diameter. There are reports of hemorrhagic and thromboembolic events associated with flow-diverting stents, limiting the use of flow-diverting stents mostly to the endovascular treatment of complex intracranial aneurysms. The latest reports on flow-diverting devices have had variable and even somewhat conflicting results. Efficacy and favorable safety profile of flow-diverters has been shown in several well-designed studies.

Embolization with Liquid Embolic Agent

(Onyx; ev3 Neurovascular, Irvine, CA, USA) has also been used to treat cerebral aneurysms, with reportedly similar morbidity and mortality rates to those of other current endovascular techniques. When the material comes into contact with blood it precipitates and forms a soft polymer cast, which solidifies over a period of 10 minutes. In addition allowing theoretically nearly 100% volumetric occlusion of the aneurysm sac (as opposed to the optimal occlusion rate of 30 % with coil embolization). Onyx induces reportedly intense neo-endothelialization reaction which may lead to complete aneurysm exclusion from the circulation. During Onyx injection, a remodeling balloon is typically inflated in the parent artery to protect it against leakage of the liquid embolic agent. The balloon must be intermittently deflated to allow cerebral reperfusion, Onyx embolization conventionally involves repetitive cycles of balloon inflation and deflation.

INTRASACCULAR FLOW-DISRUPTION TREATMENT

The WEB (Woven EndoBridge Cerebral Aneurysm Embolization Device; Sequent Medical, Aliso Viejo, CA, USA) is an intrasaccular ellipsoid braided-wire embolization device designed to provide blood flow disruption at the level of the aneurysm ostium.

Covered stents (stent-grafts) in the treatment of intracranial aneurysms.

MULTIPLE CHOICE QUESTIONS

1. **The commonest cause of subarachnoid hemorrhage is:**
   a. Aneurysm b. AVM
   c. Trauma d. Vasculitis
   Ref. Greenberg, 4th/e, p814

2. **The commonest cause of aneurysmal bleed is:**
   a. A com artery aneurysm
   b. ICA bifurcation aneurysm
   c. MCA aneurysm
   d. Basilar top aneurysm
   Ref. Schmidek and Sweet, 4th/e, p1181

3. **Most severe vasospasm is seen in:**
   a. Fisher I SAH b. Fisher II SAH
   c. Fisher III SAH d. Fisher IV SAH
   Ref. Greenberg, 4th/e, p824

4. **Unilateral headache is usually found in which aneurysmal rupture?**
   a. MCA aneurysm
   b. A com aneurysm
   c. Superior cerebellar aneurysm
   d. P com aneurysm
   Ref. Youmans, 5th/e, p1960

5. **Following are the surgical procedures for MoyaMoya disease, except:**
   a. STA-MCA bypass
   b. Carotid endarterectomy
   c. Encephalo-synangiosis
   d. Encephalomyosynangiosis
   Ref. Youmans, 5th/e, p1718-20

6. **Following are the diseases associated with high risk for cerebral venous thrombosis, except:**
   a. Wegner's granulomatosis
   b. Cogan's syndrome
   c. Ankylosing spondylitis
   d. Behcet's disease
   Ref. Youmans, 5th/e, p1723-4

7. **All the following are true about 'cord sign', except:**
   a. It is a hyperdense cortical vein on imaging
   b. May be seen normally in pregnancy
   c. May be seen in dehydrated individuals
   d. May be seen when hemoglobin is elevated
   Ref. Youmans, 5th/e, p1724

8. **The commonest cause of intracerebral hematoma above 70 years is:**
   a. Hypertension
   b. Congophilic angiopathy
   c. Aneurysmal bleed
   d. AVM
   Ref. Greenberg, 4th/e, p882-3

9. **Following are associated with high incidence of aneurysms, except:**
   a. Chiari malformation
   b. Pseudoxanthoma elasticum
   c. Autosomal dominant polycystic kidney disease
   d. Marfan's syndrome
   Ref. Neurosurgery Clinics, Vol 9th/ p425

10. **The frequency of cardiac wall motion abnormalities in aneurysmal SAH is:**
    a. 70% b. 50%
    c. 80% d. 1%
    Ref. Neurosurgery Clinics, Vol 9th/ p599

11. **What should be the minimum Lindegaard's ratio for middle cerebral artery to qualify for vasospasm?**
    a. > 2 b. > 3
    c. > 5 d. >10
    Ref. Youmans, 5th/e, p1850

ANSWERS

1. c. **2.** a. **3.** c. **4.** a. **5.** b. **6.** c. **7.** b. **8.** b. **9.** a. **10.** b. **11.** a.

12. **Normal velocity of blood in middle cerebral artery is:**

a. up to 20 cm/sec
b. up to 50 cm/sec
c. up to 70 cm/sec
d. up to 120 cm/sec

Ref. Youmans, 5th/e, p1850

13. **The recommended dose of oral nimodipine for aneurysmal SAH in adults is:**

a. 30 mg 6 hrly.
b. 40 mg 4 hrly
c. 50 mg 6 hrly
d. 60 mg 4 hrly

Ref. Youmans, 5th/e, p1852

14. **Which of the following aneurysms causes maximum incidence of electrolyte disturbances?**

a. P com artery aneurysm
b. Basilar top aneurysm
c. A com artery aneurysm
d. DACA aneurysm

Ref. Schmidek and Sweet, 4th/e, p1181-3

15. **Which of the following aneurysm has maximum incidence of seizures?**

a. DACA aneurysm
b. MCA aneurysm
c. SCA aneurysm
d. A com artery aneurysm

Ref. Youmans, p1960

16. **Blister aneurysms arise from:**

a. ICA
b. ECA
c. A com artery
d. Basilar top

Ref. Indian Journal of Cerebrovascular Surgery 2005;1(1):26-35

17. **Following are the various embolizing/coiling agents for vascular malformations, except:**

a. Onyx
b. Polyvinyl alcohol
c. Gelatin sponge
d. Methyl methacrylate

Ref. Youmans, 5th/e, p2057-77

18. **Giant aneurysms are aneurysms which are:**

a. $\geq$ 1 cm
b. $\geq$ 2 cm
c. $\geq$ 2.5 cm
d. $\geq$ 5 cm

Ref. Youmans, 5th/e, p2079

19. **GDC for coiling of aneurysms is made of:**

a. Titanium
b. Platinum
c. Steel alloy
d. Silver

Ref. Greenberg, 4th/e, p835

20. **Mycotic aneurysms are:**

a. Fungal aneurysms
b. Bacterial aneurysms
c. Infectious aneurysms
d. None of the above

Ref. Youmans, 5th/e, p2101-3

21. **The commonest site of traumatic pseudoaneurysms of middle meningeal artery is:**

a. Frontal
b. Temporal
c. Parietal
d. None of the above

Ref. Turkish Journal of Neurosurgery 2012; 22(2):239-41

22. **Which chromosome is associated with mutation in cavernoma?**

a. Chromosome 1
b. Chromosome 3
c. Chromosome 5
d. Chromosome 7

Ref. Youmans, 5th/e, p2299-301

23. **Medusa head appearance on imaging is seen in:**

a. Venous angioma
b. Meningioma
c. Cavernomas
d. Telangiectasia

Ref. Greenberg, 4th/e, p873

ANSWERS

12. d. **13.** d. **14.** c. **15.** b. **16.** a. **17.** d. **18.** c. **19.** b. **20.** c. **21.** b. **22.** d. **23.** a.

24. Spetzler-Martin grade for cerebral AVM's takes into account all the following, except:

a. Size of the lesion
b. Venous drainage
c. Number of feeders
d. Eloquence of the cortex

Ref. Greenberg, 4th/e, p871

25. All the following phakomatosis have cutaneous manifestations, except:

a. Tuberous sclerosis
b. von Hippel Landau syndrome
c. Neurofibromatosis-1
d. None of the above

Ref. Greenberg, 4th/e, p292

26. Normal pressure breakthrough phenomenon is seen after surgeries for:

a. Aneurysm b. AVM's
c. Meningiomas d. Carotid artery

Ref. Schmidek and Sweet, 4th/e, p1370

27. Embolic agent of choice for AVM's is:

a. Gelfoam b. Onyx
c. GDC coil d. None of the above

Ref. Neurosurgery 1998;43(5):1164-72

28. What percentage of AVM's have co-existent intracranial aneurysms?

a. 3% b. 7%
c. 11% d. 24%

Ref. Greenberg, 4th/e, p870

29. Obliteration of AVM's after radiosurgery usually takes:

a. 2 months b. 2 years
c. 5 years d. 10 years

Ref. Youmans, 5th/e, p4078

30. Which of the following types of spinal AVM's is the most common?

a. Type I b. Type II
c. Type III d. Type IV

Ref. Youmans, 5th/e, p2363-5

31. Acute hydrocephalus in aneurysmal SAH is defined as ventriculomegaly in:

a. First 3 days after SAH
b. First 7 days after SAH
c. First 14 days after SAH
d. First 21 days after SAH

Ref. Neurosurgery Clinics, Vol 9th/ p531

32. The incidence of hydrocephalus is least in which of the following aneurysms?

a. A com b. P com
c. MCA d. Basilar

Ref. Youmans, 5th/e, p1959-69

33. The commonest site of ICA aneurysm is:

a. P com segment
b. Anterior choroidal segment
c. Ophthalmic segment
d. Cavernous segment

Ref. Greenberg, 4th/e, p842

34. The commonest direction of P com artery aneurysm is:

a. Medial
b. Superolateral
c. Superomedial
d. Posterolateral

Ref. Greenberg, 4th/e, p842

35. Which of the following subtypes of MCA aneurysms is the most common?

a. Proximal
b. Bifurcation
c. Distal
d. Equally all segments are affected

Ref. Youmans, 5th/e, p1959-68

36. Which of the following aneurysm sites is favored for mirror aneurysms?

a. DACA aneurysms
b. P com artery aneurysms
c. MCA aneurysms
d. Superior cerebellar artery (SCA) aneurysms

Ref. Youmans, 5th/e, p1959-68

Neurovascular (MCQs)

ANSWERS

24. c. **25.** b. **26.** b. **27.** b. **28.** a. **29.** b. **30.** a. **31.** c. **32.** c. **33.** a.
34. d. **35.** b. **36.** c.

37. Giant aneurysms are located most commonly on:

a. A com artery
b. MCA
c. Basilar artery
d. ICA

Ref. Youmans, 5th/e, p1959-68

38. The incidence of visual field defects is highest in:

a. A com artery aneurysms
b. Basilar top aneurysms
c. MCA aneurysms
d. DACA aneurysms

Ref. Youmans, 5th/e, p1959-68

39. Which of the following aneurysms is commoner in men than in women?

a. P-com artery aneurysm
b. MCA aneurysm
c. A-com artery aneurysm
d. Basilar top aneurysm

Ref. Schmidek and Sweet, 4th/e, p1214-18

40. Which aneurysm site is the least common for giant aneurysms?

a. DACA
b. A com artery
c. PCA
d. Vertebrobasilar artery

Ref. Schmidek and Sweet, 4th/e, p1214-8

41. Which of the following types of circulation at circle of Willis is the commonest?

a. Type I
b. Type II
c. Type III
d. Type IV

Ref. Osborn, 1st/e, p145

42. The maximum incidence of intracranial aneurysms is seen in:

a. India
b. Sweden
c. South Africa
d. Finland

Ref. Neurosurgery Clinics, Vol 9th/ p436

43. The risk of re-rupture of untreated aneurysm is:

a. 3–4% per year
b. 7% per year
c. 10% per year
d. None of the above

Ref. Greenberg, 4th/e, p822

44. All the following are true about AVM's, except:

a. It consists of large arteries and veins
b. Nidus consist of dilated tortuous vessels
c. It is usually a high flow shunt
d. There is high tissue perfusion

Ref. Youmans, 5th/e, p2147-55

45. A young alcoholic, hypertensive sustained a heady injury. On X-ray, there was a depressed fracture of temporal bone for which he was operated upon and discharged. About 1 month later, patient reports to the emergency room with history of sudden onset of loss of consciousness. His CT scan shows a large extradural hematoma on the side of previous surgery. The most likely cause of this hematoma is:

a. Alcohol induced coagulopathy and spontaneous bleed
b. Bleed from traumatic pseudoaneurysm of middle meningeal artery
c. Unrecognized trauma to head and hematoma formation
d. Uncontrolled hypertension

Ref. Turkish Journal of Neurosurgery 2012; 22(2):239-41

46. All the following are bad prognostic factors for venous thrombosis, except:

a. Neonates
b. Involvement of superficial venous system
c. Old age
d. Presence of coma

Ref. Youmans, 5th/e, p1723-30

47. Which of the following is/are predisposing factors for cortical venous thrombosis?

a. Behcet's disease
b. Ulcerative colitis
c. Protein C and S deficiency
d. All the above

Ref. Youmans, 5th/e, p1723-30

Answers

37. b. **38.** c. **39.** c. **40.** b. **41.** a. **42.** d. **43.** a. **44.** d. **45.** b. **46.** b. **47.** d.

48. The most sensitive test to detect subarachnoid hemorrhage is:

a. Spectrophotometry
b. CT angiogram
c. MR angiogram
d. Digital subtraction angiogram

Ref. Postgraduate Medical Journal 2005;81: 470-3

49. All the following features are true about traumatic lumbar puncture, except:

a. The sample does not clot
b. The RBC: WBC ratio is normal
c. The CSF pressure is normal
d. Xanthochromia is absent

Ref. Greenberg, 4th/e, p99

50. All the following about spinal hemorrhage are true, except:

a. Intradural spinal AVM type II is a cause of spinal hemorrhage
b. Spinal subdural bleed is commoner than spinal epidural bleed
c. Vertebral body tumors can also cause spinal hemorrhage
d. Patient presents with acute myelopathy

Ref. Greenberg, 4th/e, p224-5

51. All the following about anterior spinal artery syndrome are correct, except:

a. The common level involved is the mid cervical cord
b. Fox-Alajouanine syndrome is one of the causes
c. Clinically patient may have dissociated anesthesia
d. Overall prognosis is poor

Ref. Greenberg, 4th/e, p766

52. The commonest sinus which gets involved in venous thrombosis is:

a. Superior sagittal sinus
b. Inferior sagittal sinus
c. Transverse sinus
d. None of the above

Ref. Youmans, p1723-30

53. All the following are predisposing factors for cortical vein thrombosis, except:

a. Sickle cell anemia
b. Polycythemia
c. Dehydration
d. Volume overload

Ref. Youmans, 5th/e, p1723-30

54. Aneurysmal bleed causes:

a. Communicating hydrocephalus
b. Non-communicating hydrocephalus
c. Both 'a' and 'b'
d. None of the above

Ref. Greenberg, 4th/e, p823

55. The best MRI sequence to diagnose cavernoma is:

a. Gradient MRI
b. Diffusion weighted images
c. Fluid attenuation inversion recovery
d. Magnetic resonance spectroscopy

Ref. AJNR 1996;17:987-94

56. In benign perimesencephalic SAH, blood on CT scan is usually seen in:

a. Prepontine cistern
b. Chiasmatic cistern
c. Interhemispheric cistern
d. None of the above

Ref. Greenberg, 4th/e, p857

57. A 45-year-female presents with proptosis of right eye. On examination, there is restriction of eye movements also. Her thyroid hormone profile is normal. Upon auscultation a bruit is heard over the globe. The most likely diagnosis is:

a. Hemangioma of orbit
b. Orbital cellulitis
c. Optic nerve hemangioblastoma
d. Carotid-cavernous fistula

Ref. Greenberg, 4th/e, p877

ANSWERS

48. a. **49.** a. **50.** b. **51.** a. **52.** a. **53.** d. **54.** c. **55.** a. **56.** a. **57.** d.

58. All the following conditions are indications for surgical treatment of mycotic aneurysms, except:

a. Fungal aneurysms
b. Aneurysms not responding to antibiotic therapy
c. Aneurysm which is located distally
d. Associated hematoma causing mass effect

Ref. Neurosurgery Clinics, Vol 9th/ p577-85

59. All the following statements about n-butyl-2-cyanoacrylate are true, except:

a. n-butyl-2-cyanoacrylate is a liquid embolic agent
b. It has high viscosity
c. It hardens immediately
d. It can be injected through microcatheter

Ref. Seminars in Interventional Radiology 2004;21(1):59-66

60. The following factor is/are good prognostic factors for successful radiosurgery in arteriovenous malformations:

a. Less draining veins
b. Young age
c. Hemispheric location
d. All the above

Ref. Youmans, 5th/e, p2126-8

61. The mechanism of obliteration of AVMs after radiosurgery is:

a. Direct necrosis of the nidus
b. Intimal hyperplasia with vessel narrowing and occlusion
c. Induction of thrombosis within the nidus and subsequent fibrosis
d. Induction of calcification within the nidus

Ref. Youmans, 5th/e, p2270

62. Following statements are true about direct AVF's:

a. All subtypes, i.e. Cognard type I, II and III cause subarachnoid bleed
b. Only type I causes subarachnoid bleed
c. Only type III causes subarachnoid bleed
d. Only type II and III cause subarachnoid bleed

Ref. Youmans, 5th/e, p2171-3

63. All the following are indications for surgery in brainstem cavernoma:

a. Presence of mass effect
b. Multiple bleeds
c. Progressive neurological
d. All the above

Ref. Youmans, 5th/e, p2323-7

64. In which of caroticocavernous fistula, there exists direct communication between ICA and the cavernous sinus:

a. Type A
b. Type B
c. Type C
d. Type D

Ref. Youmans, 5th/e, p2343-8

65. All the following features viz. vascular disease involving the cerebral vessels, Xenon-CT shows low CBF, EEG reveals rebuild phenomenon, association with posterior circulation aneurysms, association with primary pulmonary hypertension:

a. Fibromuscular dysplasia
b. Autoimmune vasculitis
c. Down's syndrome
d. MoyaMoya disease

Ref. Youman's 1715-17

66. The posterior circulation aneurysms have more chances of rupture than anterior circulation aneurysms. It is exactly:

a. 2 times more
b. 3 times more
c. 4 times more
d. 5 times more

Ref. Youman's p1788

67. A massive subarachnoid bleed is defined as:

a. >1000 ml
b. >150 ml
c. >200 ml
d. >250 ml

Ref. Youman's 1813

Answers

58. a. **59.** b. **60.** d. **61.** b. **62.** d. **63.** d. **64.** d. **65.** d. **66.** c. **67.** b.

68. All the factors are predisposing factors for vasospasm, except:

a. Thick subarachnoid status
b. Poor neurologic grade
c. Pre-existing hypertension
d. Hypokalemia

Ref. Youman's p1842

69. The following are the measures to reduce infarct size during temporary clipping in aneurysm surgery, except:

a. Increase systolic blood pressure by 10% of baseline
b. Reduce core body temperature to 33°C
c. Give barbiturates to cause burst suppression of EEG
d. Administer oral 5-amino-levulinic acid

Ref. Youmans p1522

70. During endovascular coiling of ruptured intracranial aneurysm:

a. Heparin is contraindicated
b. Heparin is given intravenously in a dose of about 50 IU/Kg
c. Heparin is given intra-arterially in a dose of about 50 IU/Kg
d. Heparin is given subcutaneously in a dose of 80 IU/Kg

Ref. Interv Neuroradiol. 2012;18(1):89-96

71. During femoral artery puncture for diagnostic angiography, the needle should puncture the artery:

a. About 2-3 cm below the inguinal ligament
b. About 6 cm below the inguinal ligament
c. About 2 cm above the inguinal ligament
d. None of the above

Ref. Br J Radiol. 1990;63(752):602-4

72. All the following statements about brain cavernomas are true, except:

a. These are congenital in nature
b. Bleed rates are 5% per year and rebleed rates are about 35% per year
c. Deeper seated cavernomas have higher changes of bleed than superficial
d. These do not grow in size

Ref. Neurosurgery 2013;72(4):573-89

73. During Diamox challenge test, the:

a. CBF may increase in normal area and reduce in areas liable for infarct
b. CBF may decrease in normal area and increase in areas liable for infarct
c. CBF decreases in both normal area of brain and in areas liable for infarct
d. CBF increases in both the areas

Ref. Neurosurgery focus 2011;11(5):1-5

74. Following are the sites for aneurysms which occur at non-branching sites of vessels:

a. A_1-segment
b. Dorsal wall aneurysms
c. Spinal artery
d. All the above

Ref. World Neurosurg. 2015 Oct;84(4):1178, e11-3

ANSWERS

68. d. **69.** d. **70.** b. **71.** a. **72.** d. **73.** a. **74.** d.

EXPLANATION

1. The commonest cause of SAH is trauma. Other etiologies of SAH are: Ruptured intracranial aneurysm (75–90%), Cerebral AVM (4–57%), Vasculitis and vasculopathies, rare causes include pituitary apoplexy, cocaine use, coagulation disorders.
2. The single most common site of aneurysms presenting with SAH. Hypothalamic dysfunction is common in Acom aneurysms which includes electrolyte disturbances. CT scan: blood in anterior interhemispheric fissure and chiasmatic cistern (star sign) in most of the cases. Associated with intracerebral hematoma in 63% cases. IVH is seen in 79% cases. Frontal lobe infarcts occur in 20% cases.
3. Fisher grade
   1. No subarachnoid blood detected
   2. Diffuse on vertical layers <1 mm thick
   3. Localized clot and/or vertical layer ≥1 mm
   4. Intracerebral or intraventricular clot with diffuse or no SAH

   "Vertical Layer" refers to blood within "vertical subarachnoid spaces including interhemispheric fissure, insular cistern, ambient cistern.
4. Unilateral headache is usually found in MCA aneurismal ruptures. Other features in these aneurysms include loss of consciousness at the outset, high incidence of seizures, hemiparesis, visual field defects.
5. MoyaMoya disease is a rare chronic, cerebrovascular disease → stenosis → occlusion of the bilateral ICA at their terminal portion and subsequent development of collaterals at the base of the brain. MoyaMoya – Japanese for "Puff of smoke" (appearance of collateral vasculature at base of brain on angiogram). Female: male = 1:8. Bimodal presentation, pediatric and adults. Superficial temporal arteries and renal arteries are sometimes shown to be affected by similar pathology, so MMD can be considered systemic. In children ischemic attacks are common and in adults intracranial bleeding is the usual presentation. Infarctions are observed in cortical and subcortical regions mainly in the watershed territories but basal ganglia and thalamus are usually spared. Bleeding in adults is mainly intraventricular or periventricular and not subarachnoid. Annual re-bleeding rate is 7%, often occurs at varying sites. Main causes of intracranial bleeding are: rupture of dilated and stressed perforating arteries containing microaneurysms, rupture of microaneurysms in the periventricular region, especially around superolateral wall of lateral ventricle. On MRI sulcal hyperintensity and ivy sign are suggestive of this entity, besides this T2-sequence detects microbleeding. Xenon-enhanced CT, SPECT, PET → can measure regional CBF and metabolic distribution. Reduced CBF and cerebrovascular reactivity to CO_2 on acetazolamide are seen.
6. CVT is a pathological condition accompanying thrombosis of cortical and deep cerebral veins and dural sinuses. Causes include hypercoagulable states → dysfunction of protein C, protein S, antithrombin III, plasminogen 3, Factor V mutation and prothrombin (factor II) gene mutation, Lupus anticoagulants + anticardiolipin antibodies, Behcet's disease, inflammatory bowel disease, Wegner's granulomatosis, Cogan's syndrome, Infections – cavernous and transverse sinus thrombosis associated with otitis, staphylococcus is the most frequent pathogen, neoplasms, puerperium, OC pills. 40% cases of CVT are idiopathic.

   Clinical findings: headache → most common and often earliest symptoms. Focal neurological defects are present in 50–75% cases, In some patients complaints are present for days to weeks and symptoms can be fluctuating or progressive. Clinical features also vary according to site and extent of thrombosis. Thrombosis in SSS transverse sinus → isolated intracranial hypertension, If thrombosis extends to cortical veins → focal deficits and seizures may occur, bilateral deficits are late signs of SSS thrombosis. Transverse sinus thrombosis → associated with otalgia, otorrhea, cervical tenderness and adenopathy from infection. Cavernous sinus thrombosis -eyelid edema, chemosis, retro-orbital pain and exophthalmos, paralysis of III, IV, V1, V1 and V2 nerves. Thrombosis of deep venous system- patient may have akinetic mutism, coma. Cortical vein thrombosis without sinus involvement - can manifest as stroke syndrome. Cerebellar vein thrombosis → rare and often lethal.

Diagnosis

CT scan → dense vein or cord signs (20% of patients on non-enhanced scan), Cord signs and the dense triangle sign correspond to spontaneously hyperdense cortical vein or sinuses respectively, can be seen during first 1 to 2 weeks, falsely positive in neonates, dehydrated individuals.

Dense triangle: also known as delta signs - thrombus occupies SSS. On contrast enhanced CT, the empty delta sign consists of peripheral dural leaf enhancement along with a central non-opacified thrombus, occurs in 10 to 30% of patients with SSS thrombosis. CT can also show hemorrhagic infarctions as a result of poor drainage secondary to CVT. MRI/MRA/MRV → modality of choice for detecting CVT. Cerebral angiography → only in cases where MRI is uncertain or when intervention is desired, non-visualization of all or part of sinus during venous phase of angiogram, in cortical vein thrombosis, there is sudden non-visualization of occluded vein which may be surrounded by dilated collateral "corkscrew vessel".

8. Intracerebral hemorrhage is the 2nd most common form of stroke. Cerebral amyloid angiopathy (CAA) involves cerebrovascular amyloid deposition and is classified according to the amyloid protein involved. Sporadic amyloid β-protein (Aβ)-type CAA is the most common subtype found in older individuals. CAA-associated vasculopathies lead to development of hemorrhagic lesions viz. lobar intracerebral bleed, cortical microhemorrhage, and cortical superficial siderosis, ischemic lesions (cortical infarction and ischemic changes of the white matter), and encephalopathies that include subacute leukoencephalopathy caused by CAA-associated angiitis. Pathologically, CAA is seen mainly in the leptomeningeal and cortical vessels of the cerebral lobes and cerebellum. The frontal lobe is the most affected, whereas CAA is uncommon in the basal ganglia, thalamus, brainstem, and white matter. Pathologically the vessels display hyaline degeneration, microaneurysmal dilatation, and fibrinoid necrosis. Unenhanced CT is the diagnostic study of choice.

Risk factors: Age – increases after age 55 years, Gender – more common in men, previous CVA, alcohol consumption, street drugs – cocaine, amphetamines, phencyclidine, liver dysfunction.

9. The role of inheritance in the development of intracranial aneurysm is well established for disorders such as autosomal dominant polycystic kidney disease and connective tissue disorders such as Ehler-Danlos type IV, Marfan syndrome and pseudoxanthoma elasticum. Other conditions include fibromuscular dysplasia, arterovenous malformations including moyamoya disease, coarctation of aorta, Osler-Weber-Rendu syndrome, atherosclerosis, bacterial endocarditis.

10. Cardiac changes include EKG changes in over 50% of cases of SAH and include: broad or inverted T-waves, Q-T prolongation, S-T-segment elevation or depression. U-waves, premature atrial or ventricular communication, SVT, bradycardia. Takotsubo cardiomyopathy also can occur in which transient hypokinesia of the left ventricle is known to happen. Possible mechanism is supposed to be hypothalamic ischemia which leads to increased sympathetic tone and resultant catecholamine surge which may produce subendocardial ischemia or coronary artery vasospasm.

12. TCD (transcranial Doppler) works on the principle that as an artery narrows, blood flow velocity within it increases. Velocity in MCA greater than 120 cm/sec is indicative of some degree of vasospasm and those greater than 200 cm/sec is consistent with severe vasospasm. Because other factors can influence velocity including blood pressure and overall mean cerebral blood flow, therefore Lindegaard ratio i.e., velocity of blood in MCA/ICA came into place: ratio> 3 → consistent with vasospasm.

Mean MCA velocity	Lindegaard ratio	Interpretation
<120	<3	Normal
120–200	3–6	Mild vasospasm
>200	>6	Severe vasospasm

13. Nimodipine administered orally or via nasogastric tube 60 mg every 4 hourly and continued for 3 weeks is standard treatment of patient with aneurismal SAH. It prevents increases in intracellular calcium by blocking dihydropyridine-sensitive (L-type) calcium channels, hence limits the cytotoxic effect of increased calcium.

Nimodipine does not reduce vasospasm as was concluded by BRANT (British Aneurysmal Nimodipine Trial). It can cause temporary depression of blood pressure in which case dose can be reduced. If possible, given more frequently – (30 mg every 2 hours). Other side effects are headache and intestinal pseudo-obstruction (Ogilvies syndrome).

17. Embolic agents

- Cyanoacrylates
- Onyx
- Polyvinyl alcohol

1. **Cyanoacrylates:** Low viscosity, delivered quickly and infusion <1 min, High resistance to immune-biodegradation, intensive inflammatory response - vessel occlusion. N-Butyl-2-cyanoacrylate (NBCA) is the embolisation material of choice. Mixed with low viscosity oil contrast media with or without tantalum or tungsten powder for radiological visualization. NBCA polymerizes immediately on contact with free hydrogen ion, but catheter is rinsed with dextrose to prevent initiation of such polymerization.
2. Onyx → Onyx is a biocompatible non-adhesive liquid embolic agent and is comprised of EVOH (ethylene-vinyl alcohol) copolymer dissolved in DMSO (dimethyl sulfoxide), and suspended micronized tantalum powder to provide contrast for visualization under fluoroscopy. It permits more time for operator control over the volume and rate of delivery.
3. **PVA (polyvinyl alcohol):** It is a particulate agent (50 to 1000 μm), recanalization rates are higher than cyanoacrylates.

18. Minimum diameter of at least 25 mm. Giant intracranial aneurysms have a relatively morbid natural history. More than 50% of patients suffer from rupture of these aneurysms and mortality is >60%. The majority of giant aneurysms are located in the MCA and ICA regions. The MCA region is the commonest site for giant aneurysms. Most of the giant aneurysms have a distinct angioarchitecture i.e., fusiform shape, intraluminal thrombus. Many perforators and sometimes big branches also get incorporated into the aneurysms making therapy difficult. These aneurysms constitute 2 to 5% of all intracranial aneurysms, Patient becomes symptomatic in 4th to 6th decade. Clinical signs and symptoms include: SAH – 1/3rd of patients, Mass effects – 2/3rd of patients. If the aneurysm is in Acom region it presents as visual field defects, dementia, mental disturbances, epilepsy, Posterior circulation – multiple cranial nerve dysfunction, hemiparesis, partially thrombosed aneurysm → thromboembolism to distal vasculature.

19. GDC (Guglielmi detachable coil) for coiling of aneurysms is made of platinum soldered to a wire. When current is passed through it there is ionization at the junction and release of coil from the wire which is withdrawn.

20. Infectious aneurysms → Mycotic aneurysms, underlying infections are bacterial and not fungal as mycotic would suggest. Incidence is 2 to 6% in adults, 10% in children, 80% patients have endocarditis (left sided valve disease) cerebral infarction is most common – 31% patients, in 1 to 4% patients with infective endocarditis → infectious intracranial aneurysm is clinically diagnosed.

Extravascular infections: meningitis, cavernous sinus thrombophlebitis, cerebral abscess, subdural empyema, osteomyelitis of skull and sinus infections → can extend into arterial wall → arteritis → aneurysms formation. From meningitis → infectious aneurysm occur → proximally, from embolic infections → distal. Fungal or true mycotic aneurysm → immunocompromised states. Prolonged steroid use, exposure to broad spectrum antibiotics.

Most bacterial aneurysms arise as a result of intravascular embolism, nearly all fungal aneurysm find their origin in extravascular space."True" mycotic aneurysms → large and more fusiform with higher association of occlusion of the vessel than bacterial aneurysm. Adventitia and muscularis are infiltrated initially by polymorphonuclear leukocytes, then intimal proliferation occurs. Fungal infections → aspergillosis, directly invade blood vessel wall, release elastase → digest elastic tissue → leads to intramural growth → fusiform aneurysm.

Antibiotic treatment → can alter the natural course (dynamic cycle of formation, enlargement, regression and resolution – make aneurysm tough, fibrotic and less likely to rupture. Antibiotic therapy should be started immediately in patients suspected of any infection intracranial aneurysms and continued for 4 to 6 weeks.

Relative indications for intervention/antibiotic therapy:

1. Proximal cerebral aneurysm – whenever sacrifice of parent vessel not possible.
2. Aneurysm where obliteration will result in seizure, neurological deficit
3. Regression/aneurysm or antibiotic therapy
4. Fungal aneurysm

Surgery and endovascular:

Indications:

1. Presence of symptomatic mass effect
2. Ruptured aneurysm
3. Enlargement of aneurysm on antibiotic therapy
4. Neurological deterioration on antibiotic therapy

Clipping is frequently not possible because of friable nature, so excision of aneurysm along with short segment of parent vessel → usually for distal aneurysm, for proximal aneurysms-excision with revascularization

22. It is now established that genetic mode of inheritance of familial CCM (cerebral cavernous malformation) is autosomal dominant with a high degree of penetrance. Genetic linkage analyses have mapped three CCM loci of chromosome 7.

23. Venous angiomas are low pressure vascular, malformation, Demonstrated on angiography as a starburst pattern – or sunburst or spokes of wheel: caput medusa. Other angiograph features: a long draining vein, draining an excessive amount of brain tissue.

Treatment: In general, should not be treated as they are venous drainage of normal brain.

26. Two main theories have been postulated to explain this phenomenon. On one hand, normal perfusion pressure breakthrough phenomenon" is based on the loss of cerebral vessel autoregulation due to the chronic vasodilation of perinidal microcirculation. However there are recent objections to this assumption. On the other hand, the "occlusive hyperemia" deals with thrombotic and venous obstruction phenomena that may also generate such manifestations.

30. Spinal AVMS may present with sudden subarachnoid hemorrhage, i.e. coup de poignard or gradually progressing myelopathy, i.e. Foix-Alajouanine syndrome. Symptoms such as paraparesis, gait difficulty, sphincter dysfunction and even sensory loss may be present. Symptoms may vary from months to years. The diagnosis of this syndrome is difficult as it not common. It can be confused with intramedullary tumor or polyneuropathy. The diagnosis of spinal AVMs is primarily based on imaging which includes digital subtraction angiography (DSA), CTA, and MRA. DSA is the modality of choice as it visualizes smaller vessels in detail.

54. Factors contributing to acute hydrocephalus are blood interfering with CSF flow through sylvian aqueduct, fourth ventricle outlet or subarachnoid space (non-communicating). Factors contributing to chronic hydrocephalus are due to the permanent impairment of arachnoid granulations (communicating).

55. Gradient MRI detects blood better (blooming effect).

57. Carotid-cavernous fistula

Classic triad: Chemosis, pulsatile proptosis, ocular bruit

- Type A (direct) high flow shunts between ICA and cavernous sinus.

  Traumatic/spontaneous.
- Indirect (dural) → most are shunts, from dural arteries

  Type B – between meningeal branch of ICA and cavernous sinus.

Type C – between meningeal branch of ECA cavernous sinus.

Type D – between meningeal branch of ICA and ECA.

61. The primary mechanism of AVM obliteration after radiosurgery involves hyperplasia of vascular intima with progressive narrowing and ultimately occlusion. Such obliteration takes place over 2–3 years' period.

63. Cavernomas

Conservative management: observation with repeated neuroimaging for patients whose symptom completely resolve after an acute hemorrhagic event or for patients with incidentally discovered lesion. Patient to be told that risk of hemorrhage from:

Incidentally discovered - <1%, Seizure – risk – 2% to 3%, Pregnancy → increased risk of hemorrhage, Patients should not restrict their activities or exercises based on theoretically increased risk.

Anticoagulants are not contraindicated. Patients with CM in non-eloquent location, hemorrhage rates are extensively low.

Surgical indication:

CM in ventricular system (therefore no tamponade effect on bleeding)

CM in Brainstem or thalamus

Contraindications

Medical problems, Multiple lesions.

4 CHAPTER

Spine

Humam Nisar, Nayil Khursheed

IMPORTANT THEORY

Ossified Posterior Longitudinal Ligament (OPLL)

The posterior longitudinal ligament is composed of bundles of collagen fibers intermingled with occasional fibroblasts and rare blood vessels. Some ligaments contain matrix vesicles in the vicinity of degenerated cells. Hydroxyapatite crystals are frequently precipitated within the matrix vesicles. These findings are similar to the fine structure of the early stage of calcification in normal and pathological calcifying tissues described previously. The calcification process of the posterior longitudinal ligament suggests that matrix vesicles originate from degenerated cells, and acquire hydroxyapatite crystal deposits. Some eventually coalesce to form a large calcifying mass. Ligament cells from patients with OPLL have osteoblast-like characteristics. Several genes and proteins have emerged over the years as promising targets for future investigation and intervention: NPPS, COL11A2 and COL6A1, and BMP–2 and TGFβ. In short OPLL is believed to arise because of endochondral bone formation.

Chordoma

Chordoma is a rare malignant bone tumor that arises from ectopic rests of notochordal tissue. Restricted to the axial skeleton, it has a predilection for the sacrum (50%), skull base (35%), and the mobile segments of the spine (15%). Sacral chordoma occurs almost twice as frequently in men compared with women and is uncommon in individuals younger than 40 years of age.

Chordomas are typically slow growing but locally aggressive. Significant extra-compartmental growth is often seen by the time of diagnosis. Most sacral chordomas present as surgical Stage IB with anterior extension into the pelvis. The tumor often displaces but does not invade the rectum, because the tough periosteum and presacral fascia resist the transgression of disease. Metastasis is usually a late event. Local recurrence of sacral chordoma is associated with a 21-fold increased risk of tumor-related death. *Neurosurgery focus 2003;15(2):Article 9*

Differential Diagnosis of Causes of Neck Stiffness

A. Neurogenic causes: 1. Neural cause: involvement of 11th cranial nerve with or without other cranial nerve involvement. 2. Basal irritation of dura, basal meningitis, subarachnoid hemorrhage, tumors originating or irritating the posterior fossa basal dura.

B. Non-neurogenic causes: 1. Primary muscular causes: may or may not be associated with torticollis. 2. Periosteum and bony end plate involvement of cervical vertebrae in CV junction and subaxial cervical spine: infective pathology (Grisel syndrome: infectious or inflammatory processes of the head and neck region, such as sinusitis, otomastoiditis, and retropharyngeal abscess, osteomyelitis), tumors, degenerative (osteoarthritis), ankylosing spondylitis, rheumatoid arthritis. 3. Facet joint involvement (at CV junction and subaxial spine): trauma (fall, road side, chiropractic exercises), infective (tuberculosis), tumors pathology (lymphoma, metastasis, chordomas, osteoblastoma, plasmacytoma, chondrosarcoma, neurofibroma, etc), congenital (Klippel Feil anomaly, AAD, Basilar invagination). 4. Degentrative changes, OPLL, spondylosis, disc bulge, and trauma. Infective pathology: tuberculosis, extradural abscess. 5. Others: cervical lymphadenitis, cervical abscess, tumors of SCM.

Syringomyelia

Syringomyelia is a generic term referring to a disorder in which a cyst or cavity forms within the spinal cord. This cyst, called a syrinx, can expand and elongate over time, destroying the spinal cord. The damage may result in pain, paralysis, weakness and stiffness in the back, shoulders, and extremities. Syringomyelia may also cause a loss of the ability to feel extremes of hot or cold, especially in the hands. The disorder generally leads to a cape-like loss of pain and temperature sensation along the back and arms. Each patient experiences a different combination of symptoms. These symptoms typically vary depending on the extent and, often more critically, to the location of the syrinx within the spinal cord. Signs of the disorder tend to develop slowly although sudden onset may occur with coughing, straining, or myelopathy.

Pathogenesis

Cerebrospinal fluid normally flows in a pulsatile manner throughout the subarachnoid space which envelops the spinal cord and brain, transporting nutrients and waste products. The cerebrospinal fluid also serves to cushion the brain. Excess cerebrospinal fluid in the central canal of the spinal cord is called hydromyelia. This term refers to increased cerebrospinal fluid that is contained within the ependyma of the central canal. When fluid dissects into the surrounding white matter forming a cystic cavity or syrinx, the term syringomyelia is applied. As these conditions coexist in the majority of cases, the term syringohydromyelia is applied. However physicians use the terms interchangeably. The movement of the cerebrospinal fluid within the subarachnoid space is a result of the phase difference in influx and outflow of blood within the cranial vault. The total fluid flow between the brain and spine per cardiac cycle is approximately 1-cc in a healthy adult. Since the brain is contained within the nearly rigid cranial cavity, the cerebrospinal fluid pulsation moves into the more compliant spinal canal having nearly zero net flow during each cardiac cycle.

It has been observed that obstruction of the cerebrospinal fluid spaces in the subarachnoid space can result in syrinx formation. A number of pathological conditions can cause an obstruction of the normal cerebrospinal fluid spaces. These include Chiari malformation, spinal arachnoiditis, scoliosis, spinal vertebrae misalignment, spinal tumors, spina bifida, and others. The reasons that blockage of the cerebrospinal fluid space within the subarachnoid space can result in syrinx formation are not known. Moreover, it is unclear if syrinx fluid originates from bulk movement of cerebrospinal fluid into the spinal cord, from bulk transmural movement of blood fluids through the spinal vasculature into the syrinx, or from a combination of both. Once a syrinx has formed, pressure differences along the spine have been proposed to be one mechanism causing fluid movement within the cyst, possibly resulting in damage to the spinal cord. Generally, there are two forms of syringomyelia: congenital and acquired. In addition, one form of the disorder involves a part of the brain called the brainstem. When syrinx affect the brainstem, the condition is called syringobulbia).

Congenital

The first major form relates to an abnormality of the brain called an Chiari malformation. This is the most common cause of syringomyelia, where the anatomic abnormality causes the lower part of the cerebellum to protrude from its normal location in the back of the head into the cervical or neck portion of the spinal canal. A syrinx may then develop in the cervical region of the spinal cord. Because of the relationship that was once thought to exist between the brain and spinal cord in this type of syringomyelia, physicians sometimes refer to it as communicating syringomyelia. Here, symptoms usually begin between the ages of 25—40 and may worsen with straining or any activity that causes cerebrospinal fluid pressure to fluctuate suddenly. Some patients, however, may have long periods of stability. Some patients with this form of the disorder also have hydrocephalus, in which cerebrospinal fluid accumulates in the skull, or a condition called arachnoiditis, in which a covering of the spinal cord—the arachnoid membrane—is inflamed. Some cases of syringomyelia are familial, although this is rare.

Acquired

The second major form of syringomyelia occurs as a complication of trauma, meningitis, hemorrhage, a tumor, or arachnoiditis. Here, the syrinx or cyst develops in a segment of the spinal cord damaged by one of these conditions. The syrinx then starts to expand. This is sometimes referred to as non-communicating syringomyelia. Symptoms may appear months or even years after the initial injury, starting with pain, weakness, and sensory impairment originating at the site of trauma. The primary symptom of post-traumatic syringomyelia (PTS) is pain, which may spread upward from the site of injury. Symptoms, such as pain, numbness, weakness, and disruption in temperature sensation, may be limited to one side of the body. Syringomyelia can also adversely affect sweating, sexual function, and, later, bladder and bowel control. A typical cause of PTS would be a car accident or similar trauma involving a whip-lash injury. What can make PTS difficult to diagnose is the fact that symptoms can often first appear long after the actual cause of the syrinx occurred, e.g. a car accident occurring and then the patient first experiencing PTS symptoms such as pain, loss of sensation, reduced ability on the skin to feel varying degrees of hot and cold, a number of months after car accident.

Symptoms

Syringomyelia causes a wide variety of neuropathic symptoms due to damage of the spinal cord. Patients may experience severe chronic pain, abnormal sensations and loss of sensation particularly in the hands. Some patients experience paralysis or paresis temporarily or permanently. A syrinx may also cause disruptions in the parasympathetic and sympathetic nervous systems, leading to abnormal body temperature or sweating, bowel control issues, or other problems. If the syrinx is higher up in the spinal cord or affecting the brainstem as in syringobulbia, vocal cord paralysis, ipsilateral tongue wasting, trigeminal nerve sensory loss, and other signs may occur. Rarely, bladder stones can occur in the onset of weakness in the lower extremities. Classically, syringomyelia spares the dorsal column/medial lemniscus of the spinal cord, leaving pressure, vibration, touch and proprioception intact in the upper extremities. Neuropathic arthropathy, also known as a Charcot joint, can occur, particularly in the shoulders, in patients with syringomyelia. The loss of sensory fibers to the joint is theorized to lead to damage of the joint over time.

Diagnosis: MRI is safe painless, and informative and has greatly improved the diagnosis of syringomyelia.

Treatment

Surgery

Surgery is the only viable treatment for syringomyelia. Not all patients will advance to the stage where surgery is needed. Evaluation of the condition is necessary because syringomyelia can remain stationary for long periods of time, and in some cases progress rapidly. Surgery of the spinal cord has certain, characteristic risks associated with it and the benefits of a surgical procedure on the spine have to be weighed against the possible complications associated with any procedure. Surgical treatment is aimed at correcting the condition that allowed the syrinx to form. It is vital to bear in mind that the drainage of a syrinx does not necessarily mean the elimination of the syrinx-related symptoms, but rather is aimed at stopping progression. In cases involving an Arnold-Chiari malformation, the main goal of surgery is to provide more space for the cerebellum at the base of the skull and upper cervical spine without entering the brain or spinal cord. This often results in flattening or disappearance of the primary syrinx or cavity, over time, as the normal flow of cerebrospinal fluid is restored. If a tumor is causing syringomyelia, removal of the tumor is the treatment of choice and almost always eliminates the syrinx. Surgery results in stabilization or modest improvement in symptoms for most patients. Delay in treatment may result in irreversible spinal cord injury. In some patients it may also be necessary to drain the syrinx, which can be accomplished using a catheter, drainage tubes, and valves. Shunts are used in both the communicating and non-communicating forms of the disorder. First, the surgeon must locate the syrinx. Then, the shunt is placed into it with the other end draining cerebrospinal fluid (CSF) into a cavity, usually the abdomen. By draining syrinx fluid, a shunt can arrest the progression of symptoms and relieve pain, headache, and tightness. Without correction, symptoms generally continue. The decision to use a shunt requires extensive discussion between doctor and patient, as this procedure carries with it greater risk of injury to the spinal cord, infection, blockage, or hemorrhage and may not necessarily work for all patients. Draining the syrinx more quickly does not produce better outcomes, but a shunt may be required if the fluid in the syrinx is otherwise unable to drain. In the case of trauma-related syringomyelia, the surgeon operates at the level of the initial injury. The syrinx collapses at surgery but a tube or shunt is usually necessary to prevent re-expansion.

Other Treatments

Surgery is not always recommended for syringomyelia patients. For many patients, the main treatment is analgesia. Physicians specializing in pain management can develop a medication and treatment plan to ameliorate pain. Medications to combat any neuropathic pain symptoms such as shooting and stabbing pains (e.g. gabapentin or pregabalin) would be first-line choices. Opiates are usually contraindicated for pain of neuropathic origin and would not be a drug of choice for management of this condition. Facet injections are not indicated for treatment of syringomyelia.

Drugs have no curative value as a treatment for syringomyelia. In the absence of symptoms, syringomyelia is usually not treated. In addition, a physician may recommend not treating the condition in patients of advanced age or in cases where there is no progression of symptoms. Whether treated or not, many patients will be told to avoid activities that involve straining. Since the natural history of syringomyelia is poorly understood, a conservative approach may be recommended. When surgery is not yet advised, patients should be carefully monitored by a neurologist or neurosurgeon. Periodic MRI's and physical evaluations should be scheduled at the recommendation of a qualified physician.

LUMBAR DISC DISEASE AND LUMBAR SPONDYLOSIS

Lumbar Disc Herniation

Anatomy: It is the largest mobile segment of spine. The normal disk is composed of nucleus pulposus surrounded by the annulus fibrosus. The annulus has more collagen and is therefore tougher than the more gelatinous center. Surrounded by 12 lamellae, fibers in lamellae are at 60 degree to vertical and run in opposite directions. This arrangement increases strength and elasticity. The annulus is fused to the epiphyseal ring above and below by Sharpey's fibers along with the ALL & PLL.

Pathogenesis: Normally degeneration involves equal loss of nucleus pulposus and annulus fibrosus leading to narrowed disc space. Degenerated AF only causes bulging disc. Loss of AF>NP leads to increased centrifugal forces and may tear AF causing extrusion. After the excess nucleus has herniated, disc becomes stable as forces on NP and AF are in balance. If loss is more in nucleus only then intradiscal gas formation occurs. Most common is posterolateral herniation because PLL is strongest in the midline.

Nerve root affected in posterolateral L4–L5 disc protrusion is L5 and far lateral protrusion causes - L4 root compression. Depending on location, disc prolapse may be central and paracentral (15%), posterolateral (70–80%) & extreme lateral (15%).

Clinical presentation and history: Back pain increasing gradually (over days to weeks) or suddenly followed by radicular pain. Disc herniation in absence of sciatica is uncommon-1 in 1000. Pain relief seen on flexing knees and thigh and exacerbation with coughing, sneezing and straining. Bladder symptoms seen in 1–18% cases which presents as reduced bladder sensation, difficulty in straining.

Straight leg-raising test: To differentiate Sciatica from Hip pathology (sensitivity 80%, specificity 40%). It tests L5 and S1 most, L4 less and proximal roots little. Positive test: leg pain or paraesthesia in the distribution of pain at less than 60 degree. May be positive in lumbosacral plexopathy. Crossed SLRT is SLR on painless leg causes contralateral limb pain (sensitivity is 25%, specificity 90%). Reverse SLRT: Prone patient, palm at popliteal fossa and knee is flexed till pain starts. It is positive in L2, L3, L4 root compression.

Cram test: Raise symptomatic leg with knee flexed, then extend knee which triggers pain. Other signs in evaluation for lumbar radiculopathy are: FABER test: flexion, abduction and external rotation of hip triggers pain. Positive in hip diseases e.g Sacroiliitis.

Radiographic evaluation: Plain radiographs, flexion and extension Views: Some spine tumors, instabilities, malalignments, and congenital anomalies can be identified best with plain radiographs. Should have plain films on all patients prior to surgery. MRI is the most common investigation, very sensitive in delineating the pathology. Far lateral discs are best evaluated with this test. In reoperations, MRI can delineate the full extent of scar tissue and, with moderate reliability, differentiate it from recurrent disc herniation. CT scan myelography : Indicated for evaluating patients who have severe spondylotic changes, claustrophobia & severe pain so that patient can not lie for long time. CT delineates bony structures better than MRI.

MANAGEMENT

Nonsurgical treatment: All patients with sciatica and disc herniations deserve a trial of medical therapy except patients presenting with cauda equina syndrome or profound motor deficits. Counseling and education about the disease is important. Bed rest, anti-inflammatory agents with analgesic, Muscle relaxants which aid in relieving associated muscle spasm are helpful. After 7–14 days, slow mobilization is started. Once the patient has recovered from radicular pain, physical therapy can be instituted. Return to work (either limited or full) is important at this point.

SURGICAL TREATMENT

Indications: 1. cauda equina syndrome 2. Progressive motor deficit e.g. foot drop 3. A patient with persistent bothersome sciatic pain, despite conservative management, for a period of 6–12 weeks (a time period that varies from surgeon to surgeon) patient presenting with a profound motor deficit of varying duration

Contraindications: A patient with unrelenting back pain: Patients who have back pain after a bout of sciatica has resolved are not good candidates for operative treatment. A patient who is not provided adequate conservative treatment, when diagnosis is uncertain associated diabetic plexopathy.

Surgical options: 1. **Microdiscectomy:** Small incision, Advantage: cosmesis, shorter hospital stay, Lower blood loss, Minimally invasive

2. **Intradiscal procedures:** Considered most controversial procedure. Concept is to remove disc material from center and ↓↓ intradiscal pressure. Only 10–15% surgical candidates are fit.
3. Percutaneous endoscopic discectomy 4. Automated percutaneous lumbar discectomy, Nucleotome is required. It is less effective than chymopapain. 1-year success-37% approx. 5. Intradiscal endothermal therapy. 6. Laser disc decompression, it places a laser fiber into the disc, is a blind procedure and can effect the nerve root. It is not very effective and not done often anymore. 7. Chemonucleolysis, intradiscal chymopapain is injected. It is done for soft discs. Complications can be anaphylaxis, neurologic injury, vascular injury.

Chemonucleolysis is indicated in (a) Contained herniation (outer margin of annulus intact), appropriate level and best for L4-5 while as difficult at L5-S1. It is not recommended in presence of severe neurological deficits. Advantage: Epidural scarring is avoided. Small incision or only puncture is done. Less post operative pain and hospital stay.

Surgical outcome in disc disease: depends on patient profile also, adversely affecting outcome are ; atypical symptoms, equivocal imaging, very long duration of symptoms, workers compensation claims, litigation, drug and alcohol dependence, smoking, obesity, concurrent medical problems.

Complications: Intraoperatively; Operate on wrong level, bleeding due to malpositioning, major vessel injury –visible bleeding in less than 10%, CSF leak should be repaired immediately, Infections-Usually skin infections, discitis can cripple a patient who is recovering, fever, severe localized pain and recurrent symptoms and ↑ESR. Increased neurologic deficit is usually mild and is due to excessive retraction of the root. If a nerve root is mistaken for a disc herniation & is removed, the resultant injury can be severe. Failed Back Syndrome is seen after discectomy in 8–25% cases.

Lumbar spondylosis: Encompasses degenerative disc disease with associated vertebral osteophytosis, ligamentous disease, facet joint disease & neurologic complications. Usually begins by 45-years. Frequent cause of low back & leg pain & is primary cause of LCS.

Lumbar canal stenosis: Verbiest first described in 1950, 2 types seen: Congenital – usually short pedicles and sagittal diameter <10 mm. Second is acquired type: Previously normal individuals with APD < 12 mm. Acquired changes due to thickened laminae, arthritic facets, infolding of yellow ligament, protruding disc.

Pathophysiology: Radiculopathy and neurogenic claudication due to direct mechanical compression or due to ischemia of nerve roots. Standing/walking increase lordosis exaggerating by infolding of yellow ligament. Sitting and bending forwards reverses lordosis, increases blood flow, relieves complaints.

Lateral recess syndrome: Lateral recess is bordered anteriorly by vertebral body, laterally by pedicle, posteriorly by superior articular facet of lower vertebra. Usually do not develop symptoms of nerve compression. Typically have radicular symptoms in a specific dermatomal pattern. Often have pain at rest, at night & with Valsalva maneuver.

Patients are younger (mean age 41 years) than patients with central canal stenosis. Evaluation is by high resolution CT (lateral recess height <3 mm) and MRI. Treatment: Trial of conservative management is initially preferred if no response then laminectomy and one third medial facetectomy is usually done.

BIOMECHANICS OF THE SPINE

What is *Biomechanics*?

In the context of the spine: "Biomechanics is the study of the consequences of application of external "forces on the spine." This concept allows the laboratory study of biomechanics of the spine particularly in vitro.

The vertebral column, Basic anatomy: Vertebral column consists of 33 vertebrae (7 cervical, 12 thoracic, 5 lumbar, 5 sacral and 4 coccygeal). A typical vertebra consists of a cylindrical body and a dorsal arch. The dorsal arch consists of pedicle, lamina, pars interarticularis and spinous process. The vertebral column has four natural curvatures in sagittal plane; 2 primary curvatures (thoracic and lumbosacral kyphosis) and 2 secondary curvatures (cervical and lumbar lordosis). Curvatures are maintained by variation in the inter-vertebral disc heights and vertebral body dimensions. Center of gravity of the spinal column passes from the dens of axis to the promontory of sacrum.

Regional Characteristics of the Vertebral Column

The cervical column: Cervical vertebrae are smaller, laminae are narrow and overlap, the pars interarticularis in the cervical spine have been termed the lateral masses. The superior and inferior facets pull out from the pars superiorly and inferiorly. The cervical facets from C2-3 to C6-7 are oriented approximately at 45 degrees with respect to the horizontal and coronal orientation of the facets is also seen.

Thoracic spine: Thoracic vertebrae are somewhat heart shaped. Uniquely, they possess costal facets at the junction of the body and transverse process for articulation with ribs. Transitional features: Upper thoracic (T_{1-4}) resemble cervical, lower (T_{9-12}) resemble lumbar. Spinous processes of T_1, T_2, T_{11} and T_{12} are horizontal; T_3, T_4 and T_9, T_{10} are oblique; T_5-T_8 spinous processes overlap considerably and are long and vertical. The thoracic facets are oriented along a coronal plane. At the thoracolumbar junction the facets assume a more sagittal orientation.

Lumbar spine: Lumbar vertebral bodies are the largest and typically increase in diameter as one descends. The bodies of L1-2 vertebrae are deeper dorsally, that of L4-5 deeper ventrally while L3 is transitional while L3 is transitional. Fifth lumbar vertebra represents the transition from lumbar to sacral spine. L5 body is taller ventrally contributing to the lumbo-sacral angle. The lumbar articular facets are oriented obliquely in the sagittal plane limiting axial rotation of the spine.

Sacrum and Coccyx: Sacrum is triangular, concave and having a relatively smooth pelvic surface. Dorsal surface is formed by the fusion of costal ligaments and transverse processes of sacral vertebral elements. The fused bodies are demarcated by transverse lines that end laterally in four pairs of ventral sacral foramina.

Intervertebral discs: 23 Inter-vertebral discs are interposed between the vertebral bodies. Most rostral is C2-3 disc and distally is L5-S1 disc. They account for one third to one fifth of the height of vertebral column. A disc comprises off our concentrically arranged components: (a) Outer alternating layer of collagen fibers forming the peripheral rim of annulus fibrosus (b) Fibrocartilage component that forms a major portion of the annulus (c) Transitional region where annulus and nucleus merge (d) Central nucleus pulposus (NP) which is a mucoprotein gel.

Age-related disc changes: with aging loss of water content of NP and disc height is seen, number and size of collagen fibers decreases. Structural organization of the discs permits them to tolerate compression, shear, torsion and bending forces and bending forces. During the axial loading stress causing failure, the first component to fail is the vertebral end plate, due to herniation of the nucleus pulposus into the end plate.

Ligaments: These are; The longitudinal ligaments – Anterior & Posterior, Ligamentum flavum, supraspinous ligament, interspinous ligament, intertransverse ligament and capsular ligaments.

Anterior longitudinal ligament: From occiput to sacrum covering a fourth to third of the ventral circumference of vertebral bodies. Consisting of three layers, deepest layer binds the edges of discs extending between adjacent vertebrae, middle layer binds vertebral bodies and discs over three levels and superficial layer extends over four or five levels. High collagen content prevents hyperextension and over distraction. Posterior longitudinal ligament begins at

C2 as the tectorial membrane and extends upto sacrum. Fibers spread out at the disc level and narrow in the middle of vertebral body. The ligament is much thinner over the vertebral body than over the disc. It is multilayered with maximum thickness in thoracic region.

Ligamentum flavum or yellow ligament (flava = yellow). It has high elastin content, and is one of the most elastic tissues in body. They are broad paired ligaments which connect the lamina of adjacent vertebrae, extend from C1-2 level to L5-S1, arise from ventral surface of caudal lamina and attach to dorsal border of adjacent rostral lamina. They have high elasticity and assume their original size once a flexed spine straightens or extends. They loose their elasticity with age and impinge upon the dura when slack.

Capsular ligaments: Attach to vertebra adjacent to articular joints. They are perpendicular to the plane of facets and primarily prevent distraction of the joint.

Intertransverse ligaments: They are seen only in thoracic and upper lumbar spine. They pass between the transverse processes and attach to the deep muscles of the back.

Interspinous and supraspinous ligaments: Interspinous ligaments attach from base to tip of each spinous process. Supra-spinous ligaments attach at the tips of spinous processes. Ligament is weakest in cervical region and becomes progressively stronger caudally.

Spinal motion: Degrees of freedom is a useful concept in the description of motion of vertebral column. There are a number of unique independent motion vectors that one vertebra can have with respect to another. Six degrees of freedom are, three translational & three rotational, along three axes.

Significance of facet joint orientation: In cervical spine, facets are oriented 45 degree to horizontal, almost in the coronal plane. In thoracic spine, the orientation is intermediate allowing axial rotation. In the lumbar spine, rotation is prevented by relatively sagittal orientation of the facets while flexion and extension is free.

Coupling: Defined as obligatory movements of the spine (translations and rotations) that accompany a primary motion. Principal motion is defined as the motion produced in the plane of the force and any associated out of phase motion is coupled.

Instantaneous axis of rotation: Defined as the axis perpendicular to the plane of motion and passing through the points within or outside the body which is static during the motion. Example, when opening a door, the axis of rotation passes through the hinges

Functional Biomechanics of the Spine

Paramount concept of spinal stability is ability of spine to maintain its pattern of displacement under physiologic loads without producing incapacitating pain, deformity and neurological deficit.

Theories of Spine Stability

Two-column concept: Anterior column includes vertebral body, ALL, PLL. Posterior column includes posterior ligamentous complex (PLC): Interspinous, supraspinous, ligamentum flavum and apophyseal joints. It was advanced by Holdworth who stressed upon the integrity of posterior ligamentous complex in maintaining stability. Unstable fractures involve disruption of PLC and one component of anterior column.

Three-column concept: it has better agreement with clinical observations regarding spinal stability. Anterior column: anterior wall of vertebral body, ALL and anterior annulus, Middle column: PLL, posterior annulus fibrosus, posterior wall of vertebral body & posterior column: posterior ligamentous complex. For instability 2 out of the 3 columns must be damaged.

MANAGEMENT OF METASTATIC TUMORS OF THE SPINE

About 5-10% of all cancer patients have spinal metastasis. Spine is the most common site of bony metastases. Median survival with spinal metastasis (SM) is 3 to 18 months. The highest incidence of SM is found in the 40–65 age-group as this is the period of highest cancer incidence. Vertebral and/or epidural (extradural) involvement is seen in 90–95% of spinal mets. Intradural extra-medullary and intramedullary seeding of systemic cancer is unusual. Leptomeningeal disease occurs in about 10% of patients. Primary tumors most likely to metastasize to the vertebral column are breast

(16–37%), prostate (9–15%), lung (12–15%), kidney (3–6%) & thyroid (4%). Metastases from prostate, breast, melanoma, and lung commonly cause spinal metastases in 90.5, 74.3, 54.5, and 44.9% of patients. Risk for neurological deficits due to epidural spinal cord compression varies with the site of primary disease: 22% with breast cancer, 15% with lung cancer, 10% with prostate cancer, Metastatic spinal disease arises in any of three locations: vertebral column (85%), paravertebral region (10 to 15%) & rarely the epidural or subarachnoid and intramedullary space. The posterior half of the vertebral body is involved first, with the anterior body, lamina, and pedicles are usually affected later. Multiple lesions at non-contiguous levels occur in 10–40%. 10% patients have an unknown primary (in 50% lung will be the primary source). Most metastatic lesions are osteolytic. Only 5% of metastases have an osteoblastic response. Pathways of spread are arterial route, venous routes through the Batson plexus, direct invasion through the inter-vertebral & lymphatics. Presentation is night pain or pain when recumbent is a classic feature of spine malignancy (85–96%). Pain almost always precedes the loss of neurological function. Pain: Tumor related is nocturnal and mechanical due to vertebral destruction. Motor dysfunction is the second most common (35–75%).

Diagnosis: Baseline neurologic examination to grade the patient. X-ray has limited role as 30–50% of vertebral body needs to be destroyed before involvement can be seen. Bone scans are highly sensitive, identifies areas of increased bone deposition. So, easily detects osteoblastic metastases but can only detect osteolytic lesions if there is a significant bone repair occurring. CT scan sensitivity and specificity of CT to detect bony involvement ranges between 90 and 100%. MRI whole spine (about 15% patients will have other lesions) has the greatest sensitivity (98.5%) and specificity (98.9%) with overall accuracy of 98.7%. CT myelography –when MRI can not be done or when an MRI is not available. It can cause neurological worsening if done in presence of high-grade block rostral to the puncture.

Classification and grading: American Spinal Injury Association Impairment (ASIA) Scale:

A (complete): No motor or sensory function is preserved through below the lesion.

B (incomplete): Sensory but no motor function is preserved below the neurological level.

C (incomplete): Motor function is preserved below the neurological level, and most key muscles below the neurological level have a muscle grade <3.

D (incomplete): Motor function is preserved below the neurological level, and most key muscles below neurological level have a muscle grade ≥3.

E (normal): Motor and sensory function are normal.

Gait Scale: Grade Description: 1. Normal, 2. Gait with assistance, 3. Paresis without gait function but still able to move legs, 4. Paraplegia.

MANAGEMENT PRINCIPLES

Surgery, Radiation, Chemotherapy

Early intervention: as neurological outcome after treatment is primarily dependent on the neurological status before treatment.

Recommended: Surgical decompression and fixation in presence of neural compression in patients with life expectancy > 5–6 months, competent immune and nutritional status, incomplete neurological deficit, and a radioresistant tumor or a tumor that failed to respond to previous treatment.

Treatments: Medications Steroids-Used in metastatic disease causing spinal cord dysfunction. Rationale-reduces vasogenic edema, protects against lipid peroxidation and hydrolysis, enhances blood flow, prevents ischemia and intracellular calcium accumulation, stabilizes lysosomal membranes, attenuates inflammatory response, and supports cellular energy metabolism. Dosage-Loading doses 10–100 mg, followed by 4 to 24 mg QDS. Treatments: Medications, Sorensen et al compared high-dose dexamethasone followed by RT with RT alone- 81% patients in the steroid group were ambulatory after treatment compared with 63% in the control group. *[Eur J Cancer 1994; 1:22].*

Bisphosphonates: Work by inhibiting osteoclast activity and thus decreasing bone resorption also have direct tumoricidal effect. Many RCTs evaluated the use of bisphosphonates in the prevention of skeletal-related events (SREs), defined as pathologic fracture, spinal cord compression, RT or Surgery for bone metastases, or hypercalcemia. Bisphosphonates showed to decrease the number of and time to an SRE in prostate cancer, breast cancer, multiple myeloma, lung cancer, and renal cell carcinoma.

Hormone Therapy: Most commonly for breast and prostate cancer. Breast cancer-selective estrogen receptor modulators (SERM) such as tamoxifen, and aromatase inhibitors such as letrozole, anastrozole, and exemestane have been shown to be effective. Prostate cancer-androgen suppression with GnRH agonists and/or flutimide are effective. Even if the primary tumor is responsive to hormone therapy, metastases may not possess the same hormone receptors, therefore, may be unresponsive to hormone therapy.

Surgery for radioresistant tumors (sarcoma, lung, colon, renal cell, breast), obvious spinal instability, clinically significant neural compression secondary to retropulsed bone or from spinal deformity, intractable pain unresponsive to non-operative measures, radiation failure (progression of deficit during treatment or spinal cord tolerance reached). Complications (11%)-wound infection/dehiscence and spinal instability. Decompressive laminectomy is prone to failure because in most cases the tumor is ventral to the thecal sac. Laminectomy can cause/ worsen preexisting spinal instability leading to progressive deformity & pain & neurological compromise. Laminectomy is done when pathology is strictly confined to the lamina and spinous process.

Ambulatory outcome after various treatments: Posterior Decompressive Laminectomy Alone (Mean success-30%), Radiation Alone (Mean success-47%), PDL and Radiation (Mean-47%). Success is defined as the ability to walk after the operation (i.e., gait was maintained, improved, or regained as a result of the laminectomy).

Radiation: Indications: Radiosensitive tumors (lymphoma, multiple myeloma, small cell lung carcinoma, seminoma of testes, neuroblastoma, Ewing's sarcoma), Survival <3–4 months, Inability to tolerate an operation, multilevel or diffuse spinal involvement.

Stereotactic radiosurgery: Indications: No consensus, Limited (i.e. 1–3 metastases), <2 contiguous vertebral bodies involved, Limited and/or controlled systemic disease, Good performance status, Anticipated survival > 3 months. Stereotactic RT for long-term pain control- 86%, Tumor control- 90%, 84% of patients with neurological deficits experienced some clinical improvement.

Intramedullary spinal cord metastases, Rare < 5% patients, Most common source- lung carcinoma (esp. SCLC). When to suspect? — patient with h/o malignancy and new onset of unilateral motor or sensory impairments. Brown-Sequard syndrome: 30–45%. Hallmark - rapid progression of neurological symptoms (primary intramedullary tumors-slow growing and present with a gradual progression of symptoms) 75% patients progressed to full neurological deficit within 1-month of the initial development of neurological symptoms. Intramedullary metastases are generally a late finding. Average survival is less than 1 month. General recommendation-Sensitive tumors-XRT. Resistant tumors-microsurgical resection (often discrete, well circumscribed tumors) combined with treatment of the primary tumor and other secondary metastases.

SPINAL DYSRAPHISM EVALUATION AND MANAGEMENT

Spinal dysraphism: Group of congenital abnormalities resulting from defective closure of the neural tube in the spinal region of neuraxis. It encompasses all forms of spina bifida. Classified into spina bifida aperta: Open communication of neural tube with environment. Spina bifida cystica: myelomeningoceles. Spina bifida occulta: Covered with normally developed skin.

Myelomeningoceles: Disorder resulting from defective primary neurulation. Incidence is 0.4 per 1000 live births. It is racially variable, 85% caudal thoraco-lumbar spine, 10% in the thorax and the rest cervical.

About 80–90% are associated with hydrocephalus and Chiari-malformation. Late neurological deterioration can also occur.

Recommendations for dietary folate supplementation.

Prenatal Diagnosis: Maternal serum alpha-feto protein: initial screening test. High resolution fetal ultrasonography can also demonstrate hydrocephalus and Chiari-II abnormality (Lemon and Banana sign). Maternal serum acetylcholinesterase levels are very specific as AFP can increase in other developmental anomalies of the gut and kidneys.

Preoperative Evaluation

Motor evaluation – Distal most voluntary motion evaluated. Limb abnormalities documented. Anal tone and anal reflex evaluated. Ventricular size documented with preop USG and NCCT head. Observe for symptoms of Chiari II. Renal evaluation as 90% have neurogenic bladder. All should have pre-op renal ultrasound for detecting renal anomalies.

MMC repair: Timing within 72 hours. Delayed repair – high risk of meningitis/ventriculitis/shunt infection. Mortality 13%. Obtain placode culture. VP shunt placement along with MMC repair recommended if signs of hydrocephalus at birth.

Surgical procedure: Patient positioned is prone. Contact of Povidone iodine solution with neural placode to be avoided. Goal of surgery-Protect the functional tissue in the neural placode, Prevent CSF loss, minimize risk of meningitis by reconstructing neural tube and coverings, prevention of fecal contamination of wound, nurse in Trendlenberg's, Observe for HCP – shunt if HCP present.

Complications: Superficial wound dehiscence, meningitis, symptomatic Chiari malformation- ensure functioning shunt or hindbrain decompression.

Occult spinal dysraphism is congenital spinal defects covered by intact skin. Lesions include fatty filum terminale, lipomyelomeningocele, split cord malformations type-I and II, inclusion lesions (dermoid, dermal sinus tract), neurenteric cyst, myelocystocele.

Lipomas of Cord

Classification: Type-I (Dorsal lipoma), Type-II (Transitional lipoma), Type-III (Terminal lipoma).

Dorsal lipoma (Type-I) have fibrolipomatous stalk tethering cord proximal to conus. Usually at middle lumbar to lumbo sacral level. Dorsal spinal cord dysraphic at site of attachment of lipoma. Site of attachment medial to the dorsal root entry. Normal spinal cord distal to myeloschisis. Roots lie within the subarachnoid space.

Caudal or terminal lipomas (Type-III); Directly from conus medullaris or filum terminale. It is largely or wholly intradural, nerve roots are entangled in the lipoma, lipoma cord interface is caudal to the dorsal root entry zone.

Filum may be fatty, thickened and sometimes attached to subcutaneous tissue (sacral dimple).

Transitional lipomas share the characteristics of both Type 1 and type 2.

They have no normal spinal cord distal to lipoma attachment. Initially dorsal roots may be separate but caudally become enmeshed into the lipoma. Frequently asymmetric attachment to cord.

Indication for surgical repair; neurological or urologic symptoms.

Goals of surgery are; Detethering of spinal cord, decompression of the cord by removing as much lipoma as possible, preservation of the functional tissue. Surgical principles are- Relationship between the lipoma-cord interface and dorsal roots to be established, conservative excision of the lipoma to avoid injury to the cord/ exiting roots.

Complications of surgical repair are: Early – CSF leak/ pseudomeningoceles, Late – retethering of the cord. Upto 20% cases may demonstrate retethering. Diagnosis is primarily clinical.

Lipoma of the terminal filum should be suspected if the lipoma is > 2 mm thick on MR imaging, frequent association with sacral/gluteal cleft dimples, may be associated with VATER association, imperforate anus, cloacal exstrophy and other urogenital abnormalities. Sometimes association with sacral agenesis, reflects defective secondary neurulation.

Split cord malformation are longitudinal developmental splitting of the cord over one or multiple levels. Type-I split – separate dural sheaths for the two hemicords separated by intervening osseous/ fibrocartilaginous septum. Type II split – single dural sheath, hemicords separated by fibrotic bands. Both types may be present simultaneously at different levels. SCM more common in females (M : F = 1:3). Average age of presentation is 4–6.5 years. Cutaneous stigmata most specifically hairy patch. Orthopedic deformities including scoliosis are also commonly seen. Clinical course similar to other patients with tethering of spinal cord. In Type I – Bony septum prevents ascent of spinal cord. In Type II – Fibrous bands tether the cord to the dural sheath. Coexistent neuroepithelial cysts, lipomas, dermoids and syrinxes are also found.

Operative management include surgical detethering of cord by excision of the bony spur/ division of the fibrous bands. Caution exercised to avoid damage to the hemicords during excision of the spur.

Neurenteric cysts: are persistent neurenteric canal communicating between yolk sac and amniotic cavity. May be intradural, extramedullary mucosa lined cysts. Formed from persistent tracts communicating with respiratory and gut epithelia. Associated with vertebral anomalies. MRI- demonstrates non-enhancing intradural extramedullary cyst. Presentation usually in late years (50–60 years). May also present in pediatric age group. Most common location is cervico–thoracic. Usually postero-lateral surgical approach. Complete excision of cyst has long term symptom free survival.

Dermal sinus tracts: Abnormal tracts communicating between the skin and intraspinal compartment. Most common is lumbosacral location. May occur anywhere from nasion to coccyx in midline. May be accompanied by other cutaneous stigmata. Tract terminates within thecal sac mostly. Half may have associated dermoids, epidermoids, teratoma at termination. Potential pathway for spread of infection. Repeated episodes of meningitis with atypical organisms. Operative repair consists of complete excision of the track under prophylactic antibiotic cover. Gram positive and gram negative coverage.

Anterior meningoceles: are herniation of meninges and CSF in ventral location. Commonly in presacral and lumbosacral region. Female predominance. Currarino's triad-anorectal abnormalities, presacral mass, sacral bony abnormalities. Presacral tumor may be epidermoid, dermoid or teratoma. Meningitis by atypical organisms may also occur. Posterior surgical approach to repair the dural defect and detether the cord.

Myelocystoceles are terminal dilatation of the central canal that herniates through defective posterior elements. Surgical repair attempted because of the resultant tethering of spinal cord, Repair done within 6 months. Per-operative trumpet shaped distended conus often adheres to the superficial fat. Detethering may be difficult.

MULTIPLE CHOICE QUESTIONS

1. The Dens-Basion interval to diagnose atlanto-occipital subluxation is:

a. >2 mm
b. >3 mm
c. >5 mm
d. >10 mm

Ref. Youmans, 5th/e, p4929-31

2. Dublin method is used to diagnose:

a. Atlantoaxial subluxation
b. Atlanto-occipital subluxation
c. Basilar invagination
d. Platybasia

Ref. Youmans, 5th/e, p4929-31

3. All the following about ossified posterior longitudinal ligament (OPLL) are true, except:

a. Usually seen in Japanese
b. Presents as myelopathy
c. Usually affects C6 level
d. Based on segments involved it is divided into 4 sub-types

Ref. Youmans, 5th/e, p4475-81

4. All the following statements about disks are true, except:

a. Lumbar disks have greater height anteriorly than posteriorly
b. The nucleus pulposus is supplied by blood vessels via small perforations in the central cartilaginous end plates
c. Loss of nutrient supply contributes to the progressive desiccation and degeneration of the disks
d. Torsion and bending loads are less dangerous to the disc than compression

Ref. Youmans, 5th/e, p4507-8

5. All the following about methylprednisolone succinate (MPS) therapy are true, except:

a. It is contraindicated if the spinal injury is >8 hours
b. The loading dose is 30 mg/Kg for injuries within 6 hours and 60 mg/Kg for injuries within >6–8 hrs
c. The maintenance dose is 5.4 mg/Kg/hr
d. The duration of maintenance is more for injuries sustained within 6–8 hrs. than within 6 hrs

Ref. Journal of Neurosurgery 1998;89:699-706

6. The normal Atlanto-dental (AD) interval in children, adult females and adult males respectively are:

a. 5,4 , 3 (mm's)
b. 6, 5, 3 (mm's)
c. 3, 4, 5 (mm's)
d. 4, 3, 2 (mm's)

Ref. Greenberg, 4th/e, p545

7. Chamberlains line joins:

a. Anterior and posterior lips of foramen magnum
b. Hard palate to the anterior edge foramen magnum
c. Hard palate to the posterior edge of foramen magnum
d. Dorsum sella to the inion

Ref. Greenberg, 4th/e, p549

8. Grisel's syndrome may be the sequelae of the following, except:

a. Tonsillitis
b. Mastoiditis
c. Otitis media
d. Trauma to cervical spine

Ref. Youmans, 5th/e, p3337

9. Chiari malformation is associated with basilar invagination in:

a. 25%–30% cases
b. 40%–50% cases
c. 60%–70% cases
d. 100% cases

Ref. Greenberg, 4th/e, p74

ANSWERS

1. c. **2.** b. **3.** c. **4.** d **5.** b. **6.** a. **7.** c. **8.** d. **9.** a.

10. All the following are true about os odontoideum, except:
a. It is an independent bone cranial to the axis
b. It is of two varieties
c. It causes atlantoaxial dislocation
d. The gap between the free ossicle and the axis usually extends below the level of superior facets of axis
Ref. Greenberg, 4th/e, p773-4

11. All the following about odontoid fracture are true, except:
a. There are 3 types of fractures
b. In type I, fracture line passes through tip of the dens
c. In type II, fracture line passes through neck of the dens
d. All the fracture types are unstable
Ref. Youmans, 5th/e, p3341

12. All the following about trans-odontoid screw are true, except:
a. Trans-odontoid screw is recently the treatment of choice for C2 fractures (type II)
b. Disruption of transverse alar ligament is an absolute contraindication to trans-odontoid screw
c. Severe osteopenia is a relative contraindication to the procedure
d. Fractures that slope obliquely and anteriorly are ideal for this type of procedure
Ref. AO Spine manual p-265-6

13. Hangman's fracture is:
a. Comminuted fracture of C_1
b. Bilateral fractures through pars interarticularis of C_3
c. Traumatic spondylolisthesis of C_2 over C_3
d. Fracture of odontoid and C_2 body
Ref. Greenberg, 4th/e, p770

14. Hangman's fracture is best classified by which grading system:
a. Levine Edward
b. Denis
c. White and Punjabi
d. None of the above
Ref. Greenberg, 4th/e, p771

15. All the following about spinal injuries are true, except:
a. In burst fractures, usually the anterior and middle column are disrupted
b. All burst fractures are unstable
c. Chance fractures are a type of flexion-compression loading
d. Flexion-compression fractures are Type-C burst fractures
Ref. Youmans, 5th/e, p4992-4

16. Ossified posterior longitudinal ligament (OPLL) is commonest at:
a. C3 level
b. C4 level
c. C5 level
d. C6 level
Ref. Youmans, 5th/e, p4475-9

17. The rule of thumb is that for cervical spinal subluxation, the amount of weight for traction per vertebra is:
a. 2 lbs b. 3 lbs
c. 5 lbs d. 7 lbs
Ref. Youmans, 5th/e, p4892

18. Spence's rule states that the overhang from the lateral masses of C1 on each side should not exceed:
a. 3.9 mm b. 4.5 mm
c. 6 mm d. 6.9 mm
Ref. Greenberg, 4th/e, p773

19. The ideal surgical procedure for D12/L1 PIVD is:
a. Laminectomy and discectomy
b. Costotransversectomy and discectomy
c. D12 and L1 corpectomy with discectomy
d. Percutaneous chemonucleolysis
Ref. Greenberg, 4th/e, p204

ANSWERS

10. d. **11.** d. **12.** d. **13.** b. **14.** a. **15.** b. **16.** c. **17.** c. **18.** d. **19.** b.

20. The goals of spinal instrumentation are:
a. Early ambulation
b. Prevent late deformities
c. Prevent chronic pain
d. All the above
Ref. Youmans, 5th/e, p4899-4905

21. At what value of cross-sectional canal area a patient starts having intermittent claudication?
a. 50 mm^2 b. 75 mm^2
c. 100 mm^2 d. 150 mm^2
Ref. Schmidek and Sweet, 4th/e, p2210

22. All the following procedures are meant for lumbar canal stenosis, except:
a. Interlaminar decompression
b. Trumpet laminectomy
c. Titanium mesh cage implantation
d. Transforaminal arthoscopic decompression
Ref. Schmidek and Sweet, 4th/e, p2207-17

23. All the following statements regarding spinal cord injury are true, except:
a. Younger patients have better outcome
b. Dorsal spinal injuries fare better than cervical injuries
c. Spinal shock may persist from days to weeks
d. Bulbocavernous reflex is the first reflex to recover after spinal shock
Ref. Greenberg, 4th/e, p754-6

24. In cervical spinal injuries with subluxation, all the following statements are true, except:
a. Traction of 5 pounds per vertebra should be added
b. A compressive force of 50 pounds should be applied to the Gardner-Well tongs applied to the skull
c. For producing extension of the cervical spine, the tongs should be applied anterior to the line perpendicular from the tragus
d. Over-distraction is one of the complications of cervical traction
Ref. Youmans, 5th/e, p4892-4

25. In which of the following conditions, cervical traction is contraindicated?
a. Atlantoaxial dislocation
b. Occipitocervical dislocation
c. C_4–C_5 grade III subluxation
d. None of the above
Ref. Youmans, 5th/e, p4932

26. Clay Shovler's fracture classically is defined as:
a. Avulsion fracture of C-7 spinous process
b. Fracture of the anterior inferior C_5 body
c. Fracture of the anterior column of C_4 body
d. None of the above
Ref. Greenberg, 4th/e, p777

27. The formula to calculate the appropriate drop height in feet for execution in judicial hanging is:
a. 1240 ÷ weight of the body in pounds
b. 2240 ÷ weight of the body in pounds
c. 3260 ÷ weight of the body in kilograms
d. 4760 ÷ weight of the body in pounds
Ref. Neurosurgery Focus 2011;14(2):198-208

28. The difference in the mechanism of Hangman's fracture between judicial hanging and motor vehicle accidents is that:
a. In former, it is hyperextension and distraction and in latter, it is hyperextension and compression
b. In former, it is hyperextension and compression and in latter, it is hyperextension and distraction
c. In former, it is hyperflexion and distraction and in latter, it is hyperextension
d. None of the above
Ref. Neurosurgery Focus 2011;14(2):198-208

29. All the following statements about whiplash injury to the cervical spine are true, except:
a. It is also called cantilever injury
b. It is an acceleration-deceleration injury
c. It is a hyperextension-hyperflexion injury
d. The injury most often affects C_1–C_3 spinal area
Ref. Greenberg, 4th/e, p755

ANSWERS

20. d. **21.** c. **22.** c. **23.** b. **24.** b. **25.** b. **26.** a. **27.** b. **28.** a. **29.** d.

30. In which of the following conditions, the disc space is least involved:

a. Potts spine b. Brucellosis
c. Metastasis d. Pyogenic infection of spine

Ref. Greenberg, 4th/e, p340-4

31. The following statement best depicts judicial hanging:

a. The knot is subaural and the drop height is long
b. The knot is submental and the drop height is long
c. The knot is submental a nd the drop height is short
d. The knot is subaural and the drop height is short

Ref. Neurosurgery Focus 2011;14(2):198-208

32. The usual mode of death in judicial hanging in the past used to be:

a. Medullary injury
b. Cervical cord injury
c. Asphyxia
d. Diminished venous return from neck veins and consequent raised 1CP

Ref. Neurosurgery Focus 2011;14(2):198-208

33. A 25-year-old motorcyclist met with an accident. On arrival in Emergency room his BP was not recordable. He was complaining of pain in the lower dorsal spinal area. He was paraplegic. The most likely cause of hypotension would be:

a. Neurogenic shock b. Spinal shock
c. Cardiac failure d. None of the above

Ref. Greenberg, 4th/e, p754-7

34. A 55-year-diabetic-female reports with fever of 4 days duration and progressive quadriparesis of 2-days' duration. Her MRI reveals an enhancing mass along the dura extending from C_4 to D_3. The vertebral bodies and disks are normal. The most likely diagnosis is:

a. Subdural pyogenic empyema
b. Pyogenic epidural abscess
c. Tubercular epidural abscess
d. Brucellar epidural abscess

Ref. Greenberg, 4th/e, p644

35. A 13-year old boy stock-breeder by occupation reports with history of progressive paraparesis of one week's duration. Imaging reveals a dorsal spinal abscess. The most likely causative organism responsible is:

a. Mycobacterium tuberculosis
b. Brucella melitensis
c. Staphylococcus aureus
d. Cryotococcus neoformans

Ref. Surgical Neurology 2006;66(2):141-6

36. Which of the following surgical procedures is/are meant for atlantoaxial dislocation?

a. Brook's fusion
b. Gallie's fusion
c. Sontag and Dickman fusion
d. All the above

Ref. Greenberg, 4th/e, p415-7

37. A 45-year-old male reports with progressive quadriparesis. MRI cervical spine reveals tonsillar descent of 3 mm and cervical cord syrinx extending from C_3 to C_6. The next best step is to do:

a. Foramen magnum decompression
b. Foramen magnum decompression with syringo-subarachnoid shunt
c. Contrast MRI dorsolumbar spine
d. Syringopleural shunt

Ref. Youmans, 5th/e, p1053-60

38. A severe posterior ligamentous injury is suspected if an X-ray shows that:

a. The interspinous distance is > 5 mm
b. The interspinous distance is >7 mm
c. The interpedicular distance is widened
d. The interpedicular distance is narrowed

Ref. Youmans, 5th/e, p4991

39. Which of the following statements is true?

a. Fracture of spinous process is a minor fracture
b. Fracture of spinous process is a stable fracture
c. Fracture of transverse process is a minor and stable fracture
d. All the above

Ref. Greenberg, 4th/e, p777

Answers

30. c.	31. b.	32. c.	33. b.	34. b.	35. b.	36. d.	37. c.	38. b.	39. d.

40. Which of the following statements is/are correct?

a. Fracture of anterior column of vertebra only qualifies for wedge compression
b. Fracture of anterior and middle column of vertebra qualifies for a burst fracture
c. Fracture of anterior, middle and posterior column qualifies for an unstable burst fracture
d. All the above

Ref. Youmans, 5th/e, p4979-82

41. All the following statements about odontoid fractures are true, except:

a. Type II odontoid fractures are the commonest C_2 fractures
b. Type I odontoid fractures are usually unstable
c. Anterior odontoid screw fixation is the ideal surgical procedure for Type II odontoid fractures
d. Severe osteopenia is a relative contraindication to odontoid screw fixation

Ref. Greenberg, 4th/e, p773

42. All the following statements about redundant nerve root syndrome of cauda equina are true, except:

a. It is common in females
b. Myelogram will reveal serpentine filling defects
c. Intermittent claudication is one of the symptoms
d. At surgery alternate coiling and uncoiling of the nerve root is seen

Ref. Turkish Neurosurgery 2009;18(2):204-6

43. Lhermittes sign is seen in:

a. Multiple sclerosis
b. Cord compression
c. Syringomyelia
d. All the above

Ref. Bickerstaff, 6th/e, p226

44. Anesthesia over Achilles Tendon is seen in:

a. Diabetic neuropathy
b. Ossified posterior longitudinal ligament (OPLL)
c. Tabes dorsalis
d. Amyotrophic lateral sclerosis

Ref. www.wikepedia.org accessed on 27-09-2012

45. All the following statements about Basilar impression are true, except:

a. The tip of the odontoid lies above Mc Raes line
b. It is seen in rickets, Hurler's syndrome and osteogenesis imperfecta
c. The outcome after surgery is better than outcome for congenital basilar invagination
d. It causes myelopathy

Ref. Youmans, 5th/e, p3341-2

46. Radiological differential diagnosis of os odontoideum is:

a. Ossiculum terminale
b. Clival segmentation
c. Fracture tip of odontoid
d. All the above

Ref. Youmans, 5th/e, p3341

47. All the following statements are true about primary syrinx of cord, except:

a. The cavity contains fluid with low protein content
b. There is no contrast enhancement of the wall
c. The wall is thick
d. There are no associated anomalies

Ref. Greenberg, 4th/e, p227-8

48. The symptom which is relieved best after surgery for Chiari malformation with syringomyelia is:

a. Spasticity
b. Headache
c. Dysesthesias
d. Sphincter disturbances

Ref. Schmidek and Sweet, 4th/e, p1959-61

49. Transverse alar ligament gives stability to:

a. Lumbosacral junction
b. Sacrococcygeal junction
c. Cervicothoracic junction
d. Atlantoaxial junction

Ref. Craniovertebral junction anomalies, p6-8

ANSWERS

40. d. **41.** b. **42.** a. **43.** d. **44.** c. **45.** c. **46.** d. **47.** d. **48.** b. **49.** d.

50. An elderly male reports with headache of 2 months' duration. His MRI shows bilateral chronic subdural hematoma. It also reveals a small retroclival lesion which is hypo-intense on T_1W images. There is no contrast enhancement of the lesion. Lesion is most likely:

a. Clival osteoma
b. Brainstem glioma
c. Basilar artery aneurysm
d. Ecchordosis physaliphora

Ref. AJNR 2004;25:1851-5

51. All the following statements are true, except:

a. Nucleus pulposus consists of type I collagen
b. Annulus fibrosus consists of type II collagen
c. The major component of nucleus pulposus is water
d. 'a' and 'b'

Ref. Youmans, 5th/e, p4185-6

52. Which of the following statements regarding neurenteric cyst is false:

a. These derive from remnants of neurenteric canal
b. These are intradural intramedullary lesions
c. The usual age of presentation is 5th to 6th decade
d. Vertebral body anomalies may be associated.

Ref. Youmans p3272

53. Following are the components of currarino triad, except:

a. Anorectal malformation
b. Scimitar sacrum
c. Dermal sinus tract
d. Presacral mass

Ref. Youmans p3278

54. All the following statements about Dandy-Walker syndrome are true, except:

a. The triad includes cystic dilatation of the 4th ventricle, hyperplasia or aplasia of cerebellar vermis, supratentorial hydrocephalus
b. The commonest associated CNS anomaly is corpus callosal agenesis
c. Cardiac defects are the most common non-CNS anomaly
d. Dual shunt elevates symptoms in 40% of the patients

Ref. Youmans p3286-87

55. All the following statements about screws is correct, except:

a. The entry point of C_2 pedicle screw is more lateral than for a transarticular screw
b. In C_2 pars-interarticularis screw, the risk of vertebral artery injury is more than in C_2 pedicle screw
c. In case of high riding anomalous vertebral artery C_2 crossed translaminar screw is a good option
d. Potential complication of crossed translaminar screw is cortical breach and CSF leak

Ref. p476-77 (Mchales C. Bambakidis, Curtis A, Dickman et al Thieme

56. Which of the following statements about lipomyelomeningoocele are correct?

a. In type-I lipoma or dorsal lipomas, the cord-lipoma interface is discrete and the cord below the dural defect is normal
b. In type-II lipoma or transitional lipomas, the cord-lipoma interface is variable and the cord below the dural defect is not normal
c. Type-III lipomas arise directly from the conus or filum. These lipomas are intradural
d. All are correct

Ref. Youman p3232

57. Dissociated sensory loss is a feature of:

a. Central cord syndrome
b. Anterior cord syndrome
c. Posterior cord syndrome
d. None of the above

Ref. Bickerstaff p190

Spine (MCQs)

ANSWERS

50. d. **51.** d. **52.** b. **53.** c. **54.** d. **55.** b. **56.** d. **57.** b.

Self Assessment & Review of Neurosciences

58. Following statements are true about lumbar interbody fusion, except:
a. Anterior lumbar interbody function (ALIF) has more risks of vascular injury than PLIF
b. Posterior lumbar interbody function (PLIF) has more chances of adjacent segment disease (ASD) as compared to ALIF
c. Root injury is more in TLIF than ALIF
d. Lumbar interbody fusions are not indicated for traumatic listhesis

Ref. JNS 2011;14:488-96

59. One of the clinical markers of CVJ anomaly is:
a. Trombone tongue
b. Palatal myoclonus
c. Lingual dyskinesia
d. None of the above

Ref. JNS 2006;5(6):550-3

60. In a patient of Chairi type-II malformation decompensation of neurological status may be secondary to:
a. Development of hydrocephalus
b. Development of syrinx
c. Development of tethering
d. All the above

Ref. Youman's p2255

61. All the following statements regarding operated Chiari type-I patients are true, except:
a. Motor and sensory deficits are not likely to improve
b. Apnea improves markedly
c. Headache and neck pain improve
d. Patients with smaller posterior fossa volumes improve more than with normal posterior fossa volumes

Ref. Youman's p3359

62. The likelihood of improvement of symptoms in Chiari Typ-II malformation after surgery follows this pattern:
a. Sleep apnea >cyanotic spells >Stridor
b. Cyanotic spells >sleep apnea >Stridor
c. Stridor >cyanotic spells >sleep apnea
d. Stridor >sleep apnea >cyanotic spells

Ref. Youman's p3305

63. The most common non-fatal injury to spine is:
a. Whiplash injury
b. C_4/C_5 subluxation
c. Hangman fracture
d. C_2 fracture

Ref. Greenberg p755

64. In which of the following conditions applying cervical traction is a contraindication?
a. Type-I occipitoatlantal subluxation
b. Type-II occipitoatlantal subluxation
c. Type-III occipitoatlantal subluxation
d. None of the above

Ref. Youman's p4932

65. The definition of burst fracture of spine is:
a. Fracture of all the 3 columns
b. Fracture of posterior column
c. Fracture of anterior and middle column
d. Fracture of middle column with or without fracture of posterior column

Ref. Youman's p4992-4999

66. Chance fracture:
a. Is seen in seat-belt injuries and there is fracture in the axial plane of the vertebral body
b. Is seen in free-fall injuries and there is vertical fracture in the body
c. Is seen in motor vehicle accidents and the vertebral body is commuted
d. There is avulsion fracture of C_7 spinous process

Ref. Youman's p4992-4999

67. An elderly male has lower limb weakness. On MRI, the lesion is in extradural space of dorsal spine. Lesion is hyper in both T_1 and T_2 weighted sequences. There is heterogenous enhancement also. There is no bone or soft tissue involvement. The most likely diagnosis is:
a. Lymphoma
b. Metastasis
c. Lipomatosis
d. Angiolipoma

Ref. AJNR, 2014, Dec. 8

Answers

58. d.	**59.** a.	**60.** d.	**61.** d.	**62.** d.	**63.** a.	**64.** b.	**65.** d.	**66.** a.	**67.** d.

68. All the following statements about arachnoiditis are true, except:

a. Patient presents with radicular pain and weakness
b. Common variety occurs after lumbar disc surgery
c. The CSF may show increased protein and myelogram reveals a characteristic candle-guttering appearance
d. Administration of steroids is contraindicated

Ref. Adams, p1329-30

69. Which group correctly features the characteristic symptom with the toxin involved?

a. Ciguatera poisoning – perioral parasthesias, lathyrism – spastic paralysis, mushroom poisoning – areflexia flaccid paralysis
b. Lathyrism – spastic paralysis, mushroom poisoning – perioral parasthesias, Ciguatera poisoning – areflexic flaccid paralysis
c. Ciguatera poisoning – hot allodynia and symptoms recover with mannitol, Lathyrism – spastic paralysis, BOAA being the toxin, mushroom poisoning – Low serum CK
d. None of the above

Ref. Adams, p1275-1336

ANSWERS

68. d. **69.** a.

EXPLANATION

1. The Interval between odontoid tip and the basion remains constant when the CVJ is in the neutral position. A distance of greater than 3 mm in adults and 10 mm in infants has been suggested as abnormal but sensitivity and specificity of Dens-basion ratio has been found suboptimal. Power's ratio gives more precise diagnostic criterion. It is calculated as BC/OA ratio where BC is distance from basion to inner aspect of posterior atlantal arch (c) and OA is distance from opisthion (O) to inner aspect of anterior atlantal arch (A). The mean BC/OA ratio in normal subjects is 0.77 and value greater than 1 may indicate AOD.
2. Numerous measurements have been devised to radiographically quantitate atlanto-occipital subluxation. As per Dublin method: (a) Distance between posterior mandible and anterior atlas ≤13 mm, (b) Distance between posterior mandible and dens <20 mm.
3. OPLL is characterized by growth of posterior longitudinal ligament with development of ossification centers and eventual calcification and mature ectopic bone formation. Progressive hypertrophy and subsequent calcification of PLL within spinal canal confers a risk for spinal cord compression and neurologic compromise. It involves cervical spine (70–75% cases of OPLL) usually involves C5 level most, thoracic: 15–20% (usually T_4–T_6), lumbar: 10-15% (L_1–L_3). OPLL is a relatively common cause of cervical myelopathy in middle aged and elderly Japanese and is therefore believed to appear with higher frequency in Asian population. Posterior longitudinal ligament (PLL) is normally 1–2 mm thick, covers along dorsal aspect of vertebral bodies from axis (continuous with tectorial membrane) to sacrum. Has two layers, superficial and deep. OPLL has a strong hereditary component with autosomal dominant pattern of inheritance. OPLL occurs in 29% of siblings of patients in whom OPLL is diagnosed. An association between HLA haplotype and OPLL is usually seen. In OPLL patients, intrinsic growth factors may be integral in pathogenesis. Factors detected are: bone morphogenetic proteins (BMP-2), up-regulation of zinc finger protein-145, Down-regulation of MSX2 gene, transforming growth factor-B, ostocalcin, insulin like growth factor, parathyroid, platelet derived GF, retinoids, estrogen, interleukin-1. OPLL is also associated with high incidence of adult-onset obesity and impaired glucose tolerance.

   Clinical finding: Common in cervical spine (70%) middle aged and elderly (commonest 6th decade). Male: female ratio = 2:1 for cervical cases. Affect 2 to 4 levels. Patients may be asymptomatic. Symptomatic cases present as myelopathy or radiculopathy. Patients may have neck pain, paresthesias, radicular pain, motor weakness, hand discoordination, long tract signs (severe disease). Generally symptoms are insidious but even minor trauma (hyperextension) can lead to acute spinal cord injury.

   Diagnosis: Identified on lateral plain radiograph as longitudinal hyperdense area of calcification along dorsal margin of vertebral body. Based on these OPLL is divided into 4 subtypes: A-continuous, B-Segmental, C-Mixed and D-Localized. CT and MRI facilitate diagnosis with CT helpful for better lesion morphology. MRI demonstrating evidence of spinal cord signal changes indicating edema, gliosis or myelomalacia.

   Management: Conservative reserved for asymptomatic and those with radiographically small degree of stenosis. Surgical decompression is indicated for: Patients with myelopathic or radicular features like paresthesias, radicular pain, motor weakness, discoordination, gait disturbance, spasticity, bowel or bladder dysfunction. Anterior or posterior approach may be used. Anterior in: Young, with low surgical risk, short segment disease, canal compromise >60%, without previous surgery, patients with adequate bone density.

5. Regarding management of spinal cord injury, National Acute Spinal Cord injury study (NASCIS-2 and NASCIS-3) concluded that if treatment could be initiated within 6-hrs of injury, a 24-hour period of treatment with methyl prednisolone should be instituted. If the treatment is started between 6–8 hrs the loading dose is same but the duration of maintenance is 48 hrs and if the treatment couldn't be started within 8 hours of injury, steroids were of no benefit. Methyl prednisolone sodium succinate (MPSS) is given as an initial intravenous bolus of 30 mg/kg, administered over a period of 15 min., followed 45 minutes later by 5.4 mg/kg per hour infusion.
6. The Atlanto-Dental Interval (ADI) is the distance between anterior margin of dens and the closest point of anterior arch of C_1 on lateral cervical spine X-ray. Normal maximal ADI is in range of 2–4 mm.
   - **Adults:** Males ≤3 mm, Females ≤4 mm.
   - **Pediatrics:** (≤15 years), <5 mm.

7. Chamberlains line joins posterior margin of hard palate to posterior margin of foramen magnum (opisthion). At the maximum 3 mm of dens or half of dens can be above this line, more than this doubtful and 6 mm being definitely pathological.

8. Grisel's syndrome is non-traumatic atlantoaxial subluxation. It is a rare, dangerous complication after infectious processes or head and neck procedures. Hematogenous spread of infection to cervical spine with resulting edema and relaxation of ligamentous structures. Children with disorders that predispose them to ligamentous laxity such as Down's and Klippel-Feil syndromes are at increased risk of developing Grisel's syndrome. Most improve conservatively via traction and muscle relaxants. Few with higher grade subluxation require surgical fusion. Broad spectrum antibiotics are used.

10. Os odontoideum is a separate bone ossicle with smooth cortical borders separated from odontoid peg, occasionally fused with clivus. Mimics odontoid fracture. It has 2 anatomic types – (i) Orthotopic (ii) Dystopic. Most patients are neurologically intact and present with atlantoaxial instability which may be discovered incidentally. The fracture line in case of type-II odontoid fracture passes below the level of superior articular facet while as in os odontoideum it passes above.

11. Approximately 9 to 20% of all cervical fractures are dens fractures with most (65 to 74%) being type II. Anderson and D'Alonzo (1974) classification divides it into 3 types. ***Type I fracture:*** Avulsion fracture of tip of odontoid, which result from rotation and lateral flexion and injury to apical ligament. They are stable and usually managed conservatively. Fracture plane is cephalad to transverse ligament. Thin cut CT with sagittal and coronal reconstruction is optimal investigation, MRI and flexion-extension radiographs are useful if instability is an issue. ***Type II fracture:*** are most common and potentially most dangerous. Occur as a transverse fracture through the base of dens just superior to body of axis. About 15% also have neurologic injury. They are unstable and require some form of immobilization. ***Subtype III:*** Involves fracture at base of dens and body. Non-surgical management is: (1) rigid collar, (2) halo immobilization. Halo vest restricts cervical movement by 75% against 45% by collar. High risk of non-union seen in age >65 and displacement >6 mm.

Indications for surgery: (1) Irreducible or unstable fracture, (2) Significant neurologic deficit, (3) Previous non-union, (4) Delay in treatment, (5) Injuries that preclude halo-placement (skull, chest, facial injuries), (6) Patients with high risk of non-union (elderly, debilitated). Surgical management is (1) Anterior, (2) Posterior approach. Posterior approach involves use of C_1–C_2 fusion by wires, clamps or screws. Conventional wires and clamps cause loss of rotation at C_1–C_2 is >50%. Various bone and wire fusion techniques are Gallie, Brooks, Sonntag, Magerls. Anterior approach involves trans-odontoid screw fixation across the fracture. In anterior approach advantage is immediate stabilization and maintenance of rotation at C_1-C_2. Contraindication to trans-odontoid screw fixation is transverse ligament rupture, comminuted fracture and osteopenia (relative contraindication).

12. Nowadays trans-odontoid screw fixation is considered treatment of choice for type II odontoid fractures because of early stabilization and motion is also not restricted. Absolute contraindication of anterior approach is (1) Transverse ligament rupture (2) comminuted fracture. Fractures that slope obliquely and posteriorly are ideal for this procedure. Relative contraindications are: (1) Severe osteopenia and (2) Anterior obliquely sloping fractures.

13. The term "hangman's fracture" also known as traumatic spondylolisthesis of the axis was initially introduced by Schneider and Wood Jones after they exhumed 100 bodies from a mass grave in Egypt. These men were executed by judicial hanging in World War II. It is the second most common fracture of the C2 vertebra and accounts for 4–7 % of all cervical spine fractures and dislocations. Hangman's fracture is characterized by bilateral fracture through the pars interarticularis of C_2 with traumatic subluxation of C_2 on C_3. It results from hyperextension and distraction of cervical spine in judicial hanging when the knot is submental in location and in recent era motor vehicle accident is a commoner cause. The victim here lands on his forehead with resultant axial loading of spine. There is no distraction of the spinal segments which explains the absence of neurodeficits. Patients only complaint is pain and restricted neck movements. Treatment involves cervical traction, anterior C_2–C_3 discectomy and fusion with screw and plate. Alternatively transpedicular screw fixation is also a good option. Prognosis is excellent.

15. Burst fractures are largely the result of axial compression forces with flexion component. These injuries involve 2 columns, anterior and middle and retropulsion of bone into canal . Spinal cord injury is common. When posterior column also is involved the fracture qualifies as unstable burst fracture. Surgical treatment is anterior approach with corpectomy, cage/strut placement and anterior plate fixation.

17. For stabilization of cervical spine, weight of 5 lbs is used. Increase by 5–10 lb increments till desired alignment is attained. End points of traction: Don't exceed 10 lbs per vertebra level. Distraction of locked/perched facets achieved. If occipitocervical instability develops. If any disc space height exceeds 10 mm. Neurological deterioration clinically or on SSEP/MEP. Traction is contraindicated if MRI shows disc herniation.

18. "Rule of Spence" – "On AP or open-mouth odontoid X-ray, if the sum total overhang of both C_1 lateral masses on C_2 is ≥7 mm, the transverse ligament is probably disrupted.

20. Four basic goals for spinal stabilization:

1. Restoration of stability when it is compromised by trauma or degenerative changes.
2. Maintenance of alignment after correction.
3. Prevention of further alignment deformities.
4. Alleviation of chronic pain related to instability and pathological movement.

23. Elderly patients do not fare as well as younger patients, with or without surgery (only 41% over age 50 become ambulatory versus 97% for younger. Transient loss of all neurologic function (including segmental and polysynaptic reflexes and autonomic function) below level of spinal cord injury – flaccid paralysis and areflexia lasting varying periods (usually 1–2 weeks, occasionally several months and sometimes permanently qualifies as spinal shock.

25. In cervical spine injuries, traction is applied to:

1. Reduce fracture – dislocations
2. Maintain normal alignment.
3. Immobilize to prevent further cord injury.

Contraindications:

1. Atlantooccipital dislocation (occipitocervical dislocation)
2. Type IIA or III Hangman's fracture
3. Skull defect at anticipated pin site
4. Children less than 3 years of age

26. Avulsion of spinous process (usually C_7). Can also occur with whiplash injury, injuries that jerks arms upwards, neck hyperflexion, or direct blow to spinous process. This fracture is stable.

30. Many radiographic features of spondylodiscitis and tumor (metastatic and primary) are similar but tumors rarely involve the disc space, whereas most infections begin in or involve disc space.[Metastasis -disc space Maintained]

36. Treatment of atlantoaxial dislocation and C_2-odontoid fracture includes C_1–C_2 fusion via posterior approach using variety of bone and wire techniques. Various bone and wire fusion techniques described are Gallie (middle graft with a single wire) Brook's (bilateral sublaminar wires) and Sonntag (Interspinous) method, latest Magrel (transarticular C_1–C_2 fixation) and Harm's lateral mass C_1–C_2 fixation are becoming popular.

40. Compression fracture or wedge fracture result from flexion and axial loading. There is failure of anterior column but middle column is intact with no canal compromise or neural injury. Burst fracture involves two columns, anterior and middle with associated retropulsion of bone in canal. As per Denis's 3-column concept, disruption of all the three columns, anterior, middle and posterior leads to unstable fracture.

43. Lhermitte's sign (Lhermitte's phenomenon or barber chair phenomenon) was described in 1924. This sign is mostly described as an electric shock like condition by some patients of multiple sclerosis. This sensation occurs when the neck is moved in a wrong way or rather flexed. It can also travel down to the spine, arms, and legs, and sometimes the trunk. Neck flexion usually induces this sign while the reverse Lhermitte's phenomena is defined when symptoms are induced by neck extension. Reverse Lhermitte's phenomenon is said to be induced by extrinsic compression of the cervical cord and neck collar immobilization. Demyelination and hyperexcitability are the main pathophysiological reasons. It is caused by miscommunication between the nerves that have become demyelinated. Other causes for Lhermitte's sign include transverse myelitis, Behçet's disease, trauma, etc. Lhermitte's sign has also been associated with the intensity-modulated radiotherapy (IMRT) for head and neck cancer patients but the commonest association of this sign is with multiple sclerosis.

45. It occurs secondarily to a generalized bone disease such as osteomalacia, Paget's disease, hyperparathyroidism, rheumatoid arthritis, and osteogenesis imperfecta. Osteogenesis imperfecta is a clinically and genetically heterogeneous group of heritable disorders of connective tissue characterized by reduced bone mass (osteopenia) with associated bone fragility.

Basilar invagination: This is defined as when the tip of the dens projects more than 5 mm above a line joining the hard palate to the posterior lip of the foramen magnum (Chamberlain's line) or the tip of the dens is >7 mm above McGregor's line (the back of the hard palate to the lowest point of the occipital squama. It is usually congenital, when this happens secondary to the above bone diseases it qualifies as basilar impression.

52. A neurenteric cyst is a type of foregut duplication cyst, associated either with vertebral or central nervous system abnormalities. They are usually classified as spinal or intra-cranial.

The intraspinal cysts are usually extramedullary (80%) and ventral in location. They most commonly occur in the thoracic region (42%). They result from incomplete resorption of neurenteric canal.

53. The Currarino triad is an autosomal dominant genetic trait caused by a mutation in the HLXB9 homeobox gene featured by:

- Anorectal malformation or congenital anorectal stenosis
- Sacrococcygeal osseous defect
- Presacral mass

65. Burst fractures are a type of compression fracture which results in disruption of the anterior and middle columns (stable) or posterior columns also (unstable).

Imaging features are: burst vertebral body on axial CT, loss of posterior vertebral height on lateral views, retropulsed fragments in the spinal canal, vertical fracture through the posterior elements, interpedicular widening.

66. Chance fractures are flexion-distraction type injuries of the spine that extend to involve all three spinal columns. These are unstable injuries and have a high association with intra-abdominal injuries. They tend to occur from a flexion injury of the vertebral body and distraction type injury of the posterior element. Imaging: empty vertebral body sign: can be seen on an AP radiograph and results from the vertical separation of the posterior elements displacing the spinous processes or spinous process fracture fragments off the vertebral body on the AP projection, transverse fractures across the transverse processes, laminae, and articular processes, widening of the interpedicular distance: often suggests a burst component, widening of the facet joints .

69. Ciguatera is a foodborne illness caused by eating certain reef fish whose flesh is contaminated with a toxin made by dinoflagellates such as *Gambierdiscus toxicus*. Symptoms of ciguatera poisoning in humans include gastrointestinal and neurological effects viz. headaches, muscle aches, perioral paresthesia, numbness, ataxia, vertigo, and hallucinations, cold allodynia, which is a burning sensation on contact with cold. Neurological symptoms can persist and ciguatera poisoning is occasionally misdiagnosed as multiple sclerosis.

Lathyrism or neurolathyrism is a neurological disease of humans and domestic animals, caused by eating certain legumes of the genus *Lathyrus*. Symptoms include spastic paralysis of the lower limbs. The toxin responsible is known as β-*N*-oxalyl-amino-L-alanine, or BOAA).

Mushroom poisoning is usually the result of ingestion of wild mushrooms. Gastrointestinal symptoms predominate and neurotoxicity includes areflexic muscle paralysis.

5 CHAPTER

Miscellaneous

Nayil Khursheed, Arif Sarmast, Basharat Jan, Yagnesh Saija

IMPORTANT THEORY

PSEUDOTUMOR CEREBRI (PC)

Introduction

Modified Dandy's criteria. Signs and symptoms of increased ICP. Absence of focal deficits. Awake and alert patient. Normal CT scan/MRI. CSF pressure >20 cm H_2O in non-obese and >25 cm H_2O in obese. Obesity is the commonest factor associated with PC. Other conditions associated are Hematologic – anemia, polycythemia, thrombocytopenia. Medical/surgical – Otitis media, mastoiditis, sinus thrombophlebitis, head and neck surgery, pulmonary congestion. Drugs Steroid withdrawal. Oral contraceptives, tetracyclines, nitrofurantoin. sulfamethaxazole. Other factors associated are endocrine, metabolic and drug induced. Drugs commonly incriminated are: penicillin derivates, tetracyclines, steroids, indomethacin, phenytoin.

Pathophysiology

Loss of cerebral vasomotor tone. Increased water in brain, higher vasopressin in CSF as compared to serum. CSF absorption deficit is another theory.

Examination reveals papilledema. Mild weakness of lower limbs has also been reported. Imaging of the brain is normal. Opening pressure of CSF is raised. However, the CSF composition is normal. CT/MRI – Normal. Treatment is treatment of the cause, if the condition is idiopathic, a theco-peritoneal shunt usually helps. Medical treatment with acetazolamide usually is not fully effective. Patients with papilledema may benefit from optic nerve fenestration.

Common Conditions in Males

CP angle lipomas. Chordomas and chondrosarcoma. Pineal ependymomas. Syringomyelia. Dermoid. Epidermoids. Neurenteric cysts. Anterior encephaloceles. Arachnoid cysts. Spinal AVM.

Conditions in Which Sex Incidence is Equal

DACA aneurysm. Ependymoma. Adult age aneurysms. Neurosarcoidosis.

Common Conditions in Females

Intracranial aneurysms. Pseudotumor cerebri F:M – 8:1. Posterior encephaloceles. Sacrococcygeal teratoma. Meningiomas. Trigeminal neuralgia. Spondylolisthesis.

10 Percent Rule

10% cauda equina paragangliomas are malignant. 10% intracranial aneurysms are familial – most common being MCA. 10% of MCA aneurysms are giant aneurysms. 10% of A com aneurysms present with a catastrophic bleed and die within 24 hours. 10% chordomas are malignant.

20 Percent Rule

20% spinal ependymomas are malignant. 20% choroid plexus papillomas are calcified. 20% MCA aneurysms have visual field defects. 20% meningiomas are calcified. Hydrocephalus occurs in 20% of acute SAH.

Trigeminal Neuralgia

Treatment

1. Pharmacotherapy
2. *Destructive procedures*: Injection/avulsion
3. *Nondestructive procedures*: Decompression/compression

Destructive: Alcohol injection into peripheral portion of nerve, e.g. supra/infraorbital or V_2 or V_3, pain relief for about 1 year.

Disadvantages

Loss of sensations, weakness of mastication if V_3 gets the injection.

Alcohol injection into ganglion, other agents are hot water, phenol, wax, phenol in glycerol

Trigeminal branch avulsion – supraorbital/infraorbital, supratochlear, infratrochlear, lacrimal, inferior alveolar, mental, lingual.

Subtemporal retrogasserian neurotomy (Hartley et al): Extradural temporal approach to gasserian ganglion to facilitate intracranial neurotomy of 2nd and 3rd divisions.

Relief to pain 95–99%. Recurrence 5–20%. Mortality 2%.

Suboccipital retrogasserian neurotomy

Trigeminal tractotomy: Surgical division of descending part of 5th nerve in medulla, it has not gained widespread fame because of difficulty in dividing all of the descending trigeminocephalic tract and yet not injuring other tracts.

Nondestructive Procedures

Compression – Fogarty balloon – least risk of corneal anesthesia maximum risk of motor weakness.

Microvascular Decompression (MVD)

If no vessel is seen, division of caudal 2/3rd of sensory root at root entry zone (REZ).

Comparison of procedures

MVD and Fogarty compression – least risk of corneal anesthesia.

Glycerol rhizolysis – maximum recurrence.

RF lesioning – high chance of corneal anesthesia.

Fogarty balloon – maximum motor dysfunction.

MVD – least risk of facial numbness/parasthesias.

To conclude

V_1 pain – Forgaty balloon, MVD.

V_2, V_3 – RF lesioning, MVD.

If patient is >70 years, try to avoid surgery.

Percutaneous procedures-risks are of Dural AVM, maxillary artery fistula, carotid-cavernous fistula.

RF lesioning

Hartel's Technique

Needle is inserted 3 cm lateral to the angle of mouth. Needle direction – towards pupils – frontal view. Lateral view – towards a point on zygomatic arch 2.5 cms anterior to external auditory canal. The needle may erroneously pass into the superior orbital fissure, or it may hit carotid artery, optic nerve. Meningitis is a complication. If the carotid artery is hit that means the needle is too medial and inferior. 0.1–0.2V current for inducing a lesion is used. The lesion produced by the procedure is both current and time dependent. Patients with multiple sclerosis have 2 fold recurrence. Pain triggered from V2 division but projecting into 1st division needs treatment of 1st division. During RF patient should report loss of pain and not loss of touch.

Glycerol Rhizolysis

Anhydrous glycerol 99.9%, 0.7 ml is used. Pain relief – 90%. Recurrence – 30%.

Microvascular decompression (MVD)

Previous procedures are not a contraindication to MVD. However the success of MVD as a 2nd procedure is 43%, in such cases besides MVD partial division of sensory root is to be done. Intraoperative BERA is monitored. Preoperative EMG of temporalis and masseter is monitored.

Pain in V_1 distribution – offending vessel is caudal and vice versa. Offending vessels in decreasing order of frequency are- SCA-Vein-Unnamed artery-AICA-Vertebral artery-PICA. Permanent relief in 90% patients. Recurrence is 0.5% at 10 years.

Differential Diagnosis of Ring-enhancing Lesion

Some primary brain tumors, e.g. anaplastic astrocytoma. Metastasis. Granuloma. Abscess. Resolving hematoma. Infarct. Thrombosed aneurysm. Demyelination. Multiple sclerosis plaque

B/L Basal Ganglia Calcifications

Idiopathic. Fahrs disease (cerebrovascular ferrocalcinosis). Post infection (TB, Toxoplasma, cystecercosis, HIV). Carbon monoxide poisoning. Post chemoradiotherapy

B/L Basal Ganglia Hypodensity

Normal/perivascular spaces. Lacunar infarct. Toxic (CO, H_2S, Cyanide). Post infectious (Toxoplasmosis, AIDS, cryptococcsis). Venous infarct (Internal cerebral vein)

Sunderland's Classification of Nerve Injury

i. Loss of axonal conduction.
ii. Loss of continuity of axons with intact endoneurium.
iii. Transections of nerve fiber (axon and sheath) with intact perineurium.
iv. Loss of perineurium and fascicular continuity.
v. Loss of continuity of entire nerve trunk.

Seddon's Classification of Nerve Injury

- **Neurapraxia:** Physiological block
- **Axonotmesis:** Complete interruption of axon and myelin sheath with preservation of the connective tissue stroma of a peripheral nerve. The basement membrane, endoneurium, perineurium are normal. Complete distal wallerian degeneration occurs. There is loss of motor/sensory/autonomic functions.
- **Neurontmesis:** Complete anatomic severance and disruption of neural and connective tissue elements. No chance of spontaneous recovery.

Intraoperative Classification

i. Lesions in discontinuity
ii. Lesions in continuity
iii. Mixed

Tumors of Brachial Plexus

- Classification
  - Nerve sheath tumors
  - Non-nerve sheath tumors

A. Benign and Malignant

- Benign
  - Schwannoma
  - Neurofibroma
  - Neurothekeoma
- Malignant: neurofibrosarcoma
- **Benign:** Desmoid, lipoma, cavernoma, hemangioma, myositis ossificans, Malignant: Metastasis, Ewing's sarcoma, neuroblastoma
- S/S
  - Palpable mass
  - Pain – motor/sensory loss, Horners syndrome
  - Neurocutaneous markers
  - Tinel's sign
- **Schwannoma:** Commonest tumor, arise from schwannoma cells, restricted within the endoneurium, tumors are nontender, capsulated, age 30–40 years, sex ratio equal.
- **Neurofibroma:** May or may not be associated with NF-I. In NF-1, plexiform neurofibromas(bag of worms) arise from perineuronal cells, not capsulated, painful, usually >5 cm in size.
- **Neurothekeoma:** Common in females, it is basically a nerve-sheath myxoma
- Neurofibrosarcoma can be denovo or secondary to neurofibroma and constitute 50% of these tumors. If associated with NF-1, the time gap between a neurofibroma and its degeneration into neurofirosarcoma is less, than when neurofibrosarcoma occurs in the absence of NF-1
- **Desmoid:** Considered as low grade sarcoma, infiltrates nerves. Treatment is surgery followed by radiotherapy.

Surgical Approaches

a. Anterior supraclavicular – for roots, trunks
b. Anterior infraclavicular – for divisions, cords
c. Both – if tumor invades both 'a' and'b'
d. Posterior subscapular
e. Transaxillary
f. Thoracoscopic – if tumor extends into the thorax
g. Thoracotomy/sternotomy

Indications for Surgery in Brachial Plexus Tumor

1. Pain
2. Size >3 cm

3. Progressive increase in size
4. Cosmetic
5. Parasthesias/numbness
6. Suspicion of malignancy

Brain Abscess

- Otogenic/sinusitis – usually superficial and solitary
- Hematogenous–usually multiple, at gray-white junction and along MCA distribution
- Among metastatic – cardiogenic abscess is solitary
- 1/3rd of abscess – mixed organisms, especially common in otogenic abscess
- 1/3rd cultures are negative
- In neonates and infants –proteus, citrobacter are usually incriminated

Stages of Abscess Formation

1. Early cerebritis (1–3 days)-necrotic center, not demarcated from surrounding
2. Late cerebritis (4–9 days) mixed edema, necrotic center
3. Early encapsulation (10–13 days) – capsule develops less completely and develops late on the medial/ventricular side
4. Late capsule stage (>14 days) – is characterized by 5 histologic zones

D/D- Resolving hematoma, glioma, radiation necrosis, infarction

Acute Bacterial Meningitis

Cranial nerve dysfunction occurs in 10%. Cultures are positive in 50–70%. CSF flora -Gram-positive in 70–80% patients, Gram-negative in 50–70% patients. Seizures in 20%, 40% if age is <1 year. Post-operative meningitis seen in 0.5–0.7%. Ruptured meningocele - Gram-negative organisms. Dermal sinus -mixed organisms.

CAVERNOUS SINUS ANATOMY

Kawases triangle is bounded medially by V_3 and gasserian ganglion, laterally by GSPN and base by petrous apex

Contents – posterior surface of medial loop of carotid artery, petrous apex with Meckel's cave

Glassocks triangle – medially – GSPN, laterally – arcuate eminence, base – V_3

Contents – posterior and lateral loops of ICA, tensor tympani

Parkinsons triangle – medially – 4th cranial nerve, laterally – V_1, Base-anterior petroclinoid fold

Contents – medial loop, horizontal ICA, abducent nerve

Choroid Fissure

It is a C-shaped fissure. Choroid plexus is attached to it. The fissure extends between fornix medially and thalamus laterally. The plexus is attached to small projections on either side, on thalamic side these projections are called tenia choroidae, on fornix side these are called tenia fornics, except in temporal horn where these are called tenia fimbrae. While opening the choroidal fissure one should open near fornix or fimbra and not on the choroidal side, therefore less arteries encountered.

Cerebellar and Brainstem Fissures

These are:

Cerebellopontine and Cerebellomedullary

The former lies between lateral surface of pons and petrosal surface of cerebellum. This fissure is V-shaped, apex lies laterally. Fifth to 10th cranial nerves arise in this fissure. Fifth and 6th course above the middle cerebellar peduncle in the superior limb of the fissure and other cranial nerves arise below. Cerebellopontine fissure communicates inferiorly with cerebellomedullary fissure.

Foramen of Luschka lies at the level of lateral end of pontomedullary sulcus. It lies slightly inferior to 7th, 8th complex, i.e. at the level of junction of 9th nerve to brainstem and sits on 9th nerve rootlet.

Arterial relationship: AICA, branch of basilar, winds around pontomedullary sulcus and reaches the meatus and then enters the cerebellomedullary fissure and bifurcates terminally into superior and inferior divisions. At the area of pontomedullary sulcus, it has 3 segments, premeatal – from origin to the meatus, meatal – around the meatus, post meatal – from meatus till middle cerebellar peduncle. The AICA loop is seen in 50% near the internal auditory meatus and the loop usually travels below the 7th and 8th nerve complex.

Venous relationship: The main veins are pontomedullary vein, lateral medullary vein – these two join form vein of the middle cerebellar peduncle which extends and joins the vein of the cerebellopontine fissure to form petrosal vein (Dandy's vein) which drains into superior petrosal sinus.

Anatomy of Orbit

- Pear shaped – tapers posteriorly
- Medially – ethmoid, nasal, lacrimal, maxillary bones
- Laterally – Zygomatic and frontal bones anteriorly and greater wing of sphenoid posteriorly
- Roof – Anterior cranial fossa
- Floor – Roof of maxillary sinus
- Pierced by superior and inferior orbital fissure and optic canal, ethmoidal foramina, zygomaticofacial and intra-orbital foramina. Optic canal is 5–10 mm long, 5 mm wide, 5 mm high. Roof of optic canal is 2 mm thick. Canal lies between 2 struts of lesser wing, medial strut is thinner.
- Superior orbital fissure – 3, 4, cranial nerves, ophthalmic division of 5th, 6th nerve and superior ophthalmic vein pass through it.
- Inferior orbital fissure – maxillary division of 5th and inferior ophthalmic vein.
- Infraorbital canal – Infraorbital nerve
- Ethmoidal foramen – anterior and posterior ethmoidal arteries
- Zygomatico facial and zygomaticotemporal canals transmit vessels and branches of maxillary nerve to supply the temporal fossa.

Causes of Intermittent Myelopathy

- Spinal AVM
- Enterogenous cyst/arachnoid cyst
- Basial invagination
- Basilar ectasia
- AAD

Brainstem Syndromes

Mid-brain involvement

a. **Dorsolateral:** Ipsilateral Horners syndrome, ipsilateral cerebellar and contralateral spinothalamic tract involvement
b. **Paramedian (Benedicts syndrome):** Ipsilateral 3rd nerve and contralateral cerebellar signs, cerebellar sign is secondary to involvement of dentatorubral tract.
c. **Basal infarction (Webers):** Ipsilateral 3rd and contralateral hemiplegia

Pontine Involvement

a. Dorsolateral

- **Above mid pons:** Ipsilateral Horners, contralateral spinothalamic loss, facial sensation is– preserved
- **At mid-pons:** Ipsilateral Horners syndrome, contralateral spinothalamic, ipsilateral facial sensory loss, PPRF involvement ipsilateral gaze palsy
- **Lower pontine:** Ipsilateral Horners, contralateral spinothalamic, ipsilateral facial, PPRF, vestibulocochlear involvement.

At all levels, same degree of cerebellar involvement occurs:

a. Posterior column will be spared in dorsolateral involvement as medial lemnisci are too deep to get involved at this level.

b. **Paramedian:** Ipsilateral 6th and 7th nerve with conjugate gaze palsy with loss of posterior column on opposite side.

c. **Basal infarction:** Ipsilateral 6th nerve and 7th nerve (Millard-Gubler), contralateral -hemiplegia (incomplete), conjugate gaze – intact.

Medulla

Lateral medullary syndrome (dorsolateral):

Structures involved:

- 5th nerve spinal nucleus and tract
- Spinothalamic tract
- Descending autonomic nervous sys ANS
- Lower vestibular nuclei
- Any cerebellar peduncle
- 9, 10 CN (nucleus ambiguous)

Parinaud's Syndrome

Lid retraction (Colliers sign). Retraction of upward gaze. Light near dissociation. Convergence retraction nystagmus. Pseudoabducnes palsy – during horizontal eye movements, the abducting eye may move more slowly than the adducting eye, perhaps reflecting excess convergence tone.

Top of Basilar Syndrome

Infarction of midbrain, thalamus, portions of temporal and occipital lobes.

Internal Capsule

	Descending tracts	Ascending tracts
Anterior limb	Frontopontine	Anterior thalamic radiation
Genu	Corticonuclear	Anterior part of superior thalamic radiation
Posterior limb	Corticospinal Corticopontine Corticorubral	Superior thalamic radiation
Retrolentiform	Parieto and occipito-pontine, temporopontine	Posterior thalamic optic radiation
Sublentiform	Temporopontine	Auditory radiation

Blood Supply of Internal Capsule

Anterior limb	Ventromedial	Heubners artery
	Dorsolateral	Perforators of MCA
Genu	Dorsal part	Lateral striate branches of MCA
	Ventromedial	Perforators of ACA, ICA, anterior choroidal artery
Post limb	Dorsal part	Lateral striate branches of MCA
	Rostral	Perforators of ICA, ACA and anterior choroidal artery
Retrolenticular		Capsular branches of anterior choroidal artery

Parietal Lobe Disorders

Unilateral involvement	Abolition of optokinetic nystagmus (OKN)
	Loss of cortical sensations
	Mild hemiparesis
	Homonymous hemianopia
Dominant	Ideomotor/ideational apraxia
	Gerstmann syndrome
	Alexia
Nondominant	Anosognosia
	Constructional/dressing apraxia
	Environmental agnosia
	Tendency to keep eyes closed
Bilateral involvement	Balints syndrome

Occipital Lobe

Unilateral involvement	Homonymous hemianopia unformed hallucinations
Left occipital lobe	Alexia
	Simultagnosia
Right occipital lobe	Loss of topographic memory
	Metamorphopsia and hallucinations are common with right occipital lobe involvement than with left
Bilateral involvement	Cortical blindness
	Prosopagnosia
	Antons syndrome
	Balint's syndrome
	Loss of perception of color

Disconnection Syndromes

- **Acute:** occurs after total callosotomy – mutism, apraxia, hemi-anopia, left hemineglect, increased focal motor seizures, urge incontinence.
- Posterior (sensory) disconnection syndrome – After splenial sectioning:
  Tactile transfer deficits – in which objects placed in left hand cannot be named
  Visual transfer deficits – objects projected tachistoscopically to right field cannot be named
- Split brain syndrome – occurs after total or near total callositomy in 3–5% patients.
  Language impairment – speech initiation is difficult
  Alien hand
  Impaired attention – memory sequencing in which patient is unable to pursue multiple tasks simultaneously.

Seizure Classification

1. Partial
   a. Simple
   b. Complex
   c. Partial with secondary generalization
2. Generalized
   a. Tonic
   b. Clonic
   c. Tonic-clonic
   d. Myoclonic
   e. Atonic
   f. Absence
3. Unclassified

Dysarthria

- **Spastic paralysis:** b, p, d alphabets are impaired
- **Facial paralysis:** m, w, b, p
- **Tongue paralysis:** l, d, n, s, t, x, z (linguals)
- **Palatal paralysis:** Produces nasal speech b and d becomes m and n respectively. Speech worsens when head is bent forwards.

Classification of Cortical Aphasias

Fluency	Comprehension	Repetition	Type of aphasia
Fluent	Good	Good	Anomic
		Bad	Conduction
	Good	Good	Transcortical sensory
		Bad	Wernickes
Nonfluent	Good	Good	Transcortical motor
		Bad	Brocas
	Bad	Good	Mixed transcortical
		Bad	Global

Subcortical aphasia:

- Anomic in thalamic lesions and global in basal ganglia lesions.

Paraphasias:

- Semantic (verbal) – Cat for dog
- Phonemic (literal) – breen for green

Echolalia – temporoparietal lesion

Pure word deafness – middle or superior temporal gyrus

Alexia

Without agraphia (pure word blindness) – lesion is in left occipital lobe and splenium and right hemianopia is associated.

With agraphia – lesion is in left angular gyrus, associated with hemianopia, and Gerstmans syndrome.

Apraxias

Apraxias: Ideomotor. Ideational. Constructional. Dressing.

Ideomotor: Patient is able to carry out work spontaneously, but not to command

Ideational: Fragmented motor takes are carried out on command, but full task cannot be done. Lesion – left supramarginal gyrus (SMG).

If lesion is in left supramarginal gyrus – apraxia is bilateral. If between connections from SMG and left motor cortex – apraxia is on right side. If between SMG and corpus callosum – apraxia is on left side. Constructional and dressing apraxia – non-dominant angular gyrus

Thus lesion in:

- Left angular gyrus – Gerstman's syndrome
- Right angular gyrus – Constructional and dressing apraxia
- Left supramarginal gyrus – Ideomotor/ideational apraxia
- Left angular gyrus – Alexia with agraphia

Respiration

Respiratory center – from mid-pons to medulla, supracortical control is by forebrain. Disconnection of brainstem center from forebrain – Cheyne Stoke's breathing.

Central neurogenic breathing – lesion in pontine tegmentum anterior to aqueduct.

Kussmaul breathing – deep regular breathing – metabolic acidosis.

Apneustic breathing – deep inspiratory gasps, lesion in dorsolateral pons.

Ataxic breathing – irregular in rate and rhythm – medullary lesion.

Cluster breathing – medullary damage, periodic breathing which is irregular in frequency and amplitude with variable pauses between clusters of breaths.

Nystagmus

Pendular-it is always central

Jerk- can be central or peripheral

Points to be checked in nystagmus

Is the nystagmus congenital. Direction of the fast component. Binocular/unilocular. Null zone/fatiguability. Effect of OKN/change in head position. Conjugate/dissociated. Torsional/vertical component. Is it alternating spontaneously. Is it present in primary position or on change of gaze (gaze evoked). Does convergence dampen it. Associated movements – e.g. palatal myoclonus. Is there a lateral component, i.e. increase in nystagmus after covering one eye. Family history of nystagmus.

Alexanders law – vestibular nystagmus is maximum in the direction of fast component.

Plexopathy

Neoplastic plexopathy of brachial plexus	Radiation plexopathy
Lower trunk commonly involved	Upper trunk involved
Pain is a feature	Dysesthesias present
No myokimia	myokimia is present

Thoracic Outlet Syndrome

Auscultate the proximal and distal brachial artery and check for bruit, while keeping the upper limb extended at elbow, abducted at shoulder and externally rotated (Adson's test). Elevate the upper limb alternately clench and release, if there is numbness parasthesias, pallor of hand it is suggestive of Thoracic outlet syndrome (Ross test).

Speech

Apraxia of speech is misarticulation of phonemes for different words at different times. Dysarthria – misarticulation of specific words. Aphasia has to be differentiated from disorder of thought. In the latter the content of speech is altered, but linguistic structure is maintained. Anomic aphasia can be seen in memory losses also. Rule of thumb is that if a patient is able to copy, write, type and the content of the language are normal – there is no aphasia. A fluent paraphasic speech can be seen in psychosis, delirium, dementia, encephalopathy. In psychosis, delirium, encephalopathy – other features like drowsiness, agitation, hallucinations, memory disturbances will be seen, moreover, the content of speech will be abnormal, but linguistic structure is maintained.

In dementia and fluent aphasia – difference is slightly difficult, though in dementia, memory disturbances and visuo-spatial impairment will be seen.

Opercular syndrome – lesion in both perisylvian cortices. Patient has sensory disturbance in one hand and ipsilateral corner of mouth, able to follow commands of limbs, but not of cranial nerves, occurs in patients with multiple strokes.

Medial Temporal Lobe Epilepsy (TLE)

40% of TLE patients have febrile seizures. TLE is caused by medial temporal sclerosis (MTS), tumors/AVM, etc. MTS occurs early in life. In MTS there is loss of neurons. Paradoxial TLE is defined as TLE with negative MRI. Unfavorable outcome after surgery is seen in- Normal pre-operative MRI, bilateral temporal EEG changes, no pathology seen in the surgical specimen on HPE, disabiling seizure during Ist year of surgery.

Medial Temporal Sclerosis

Grade I: High signal of Hippocampus + Amygdala + atrophy of these structures and temporal lobe

Grade II: As above, but no atrophy of temporal lobe

Grade III: Only high signal, no atrophy

Grade IV: Only atrophy of Hippocampus + Amygdala, no signal changes.

Vagal Nerve Stimulation

Indications – Intractable seizures, extratemporal seizures.

Contraindications – Bilateral vagotomies, extratemporal epilepsy, cardiorespiratory disease, acid peptic disorder, dysautonomia.

Generalized seizures respond better than partial seizures. Effect on seizure control is cumulative. 40% decrease in seizures at 36-months. In L.G. syndrome, 20% patients have 50% reduction in seizures and 50% had 20% decrease in seizures. Usually the left vagus is stimulated because chances of bradycardia are more with right vagal stimulation.

S/E – Bradycardia, shortness of breath, hoarseness of voice.

Multiple Subpial Transection

Indications

1. Seizure focus in eloquent area
2. Landau Klifner syndrome
3. Epilepsia partialis continua
4. Rasmussens encephalitis. Best seizure control rate is for (1), next for (2).

Hemispherectomy

It is indicated in patients with Sturge-Weber syndrome, Rasmussens encephalitis, cerebral infantile hemiplegia.

Callostomy

It is indicated in atonic seizures, tonic seizure, tonic-clonic seizure, infantile hemiplegia, forme-fruste hemiplegia, Rasmussens encephalitis, migrational disorders, HHH syndrome.

Natural Course of Epilepsy

70% have medically controlled seizures within 2 years of AED, 30% have uncontrolled.

After temporal lobectomy–70% get controlled at 2 years.

Extratemporal resection – outcome rate: seizure freedom – 22%, improvement – 73%, Failure – 27%.

Hemispherectomy: 67% seizure freedom, 21% improvement, 12% failure.

Callosotomy- Atonic-seizure cure rate-80%, GTC: 50–75%, partial: 30–40%.

Engels grading of postoperative seizure control:

Grade I: Free of disabling seizure

Grade II: Rare disabiling seizure

Grade III: Worthwhile improvement

Grade IV: No worthwhile improvement.

TRANSCRANIAL DOPPLER

Transcranial Doppler (TCD) ultrasonography was introduced in 1982 by Aaslid and colleagues as a non-invasive technique for monitoring blood flow velocity (FV) in the basal cerebral arteries. TCD is based on the use of a range-gated, pulsed-doppler ultrasonic beam of 2 MHz frequency. The ultrasonic beam crosses the intact skull at points known as 'windows' and is reflected back from the moving erythrocytes in its path. The difference between the transmitted signal and the received signal is called the Doppler shift, and can be expressed by the formula;

Doppler shift = 2*V*Ft*cosu/C

where V is the velocity of the reflector (red cells), Ft is the transmitted frequency C is the speed of sound in soft tissue, and cosu is the correction factor based on the angle of insonation (u).

In TCD, Ft (2 MHz) and C (1540 m/s) remain constant; therefore, frequency shift depends mainly on the blood FV and the angle of insonation of the TCD probe. Within a vessel, different erythrocytes move at different speeds. The Doppler signal obtained from blood flowing in vessels is therefore, a mixture of different frequency components. Time is represented on the horizontal scale, frequency shift (velocity) on the vertical scale, and signal intensity as the relative brightness or color.

Either transcranial spectral Doppler sonography, Power M-mode doppler sonography, or transcranial color-coded duplex sonography (TCCS) should be performed with the patient supine. A TCD examination should be performed with a real-time imaging scanner with Doppler capability using a 1 to 5 MHz transducer. Doppler images and/or data are obtained at 2 to 5 mm intervals with a 3 to 6 mm gate. Color or spectral doppler ultrasound should be used to locate the intracranial vessels. Duplex ultrasound is preferred over nonimaging doppler methods for more precise localization and insonation within the targeted vessels when imaging through the fontanelles. The superior sagittal sinus can be evaluated through an open sagittal suture. With TCD, four 'windows' (temporal, orbital, foramen magnum and submandibular) can be used for insonation different cerebral arteries.

1. The temporal window is defined as an area 2 cm above the line drawn from the tragus to the lateral canthus of the eye. On gray-scale images, the hypoechoic heart-shaped cerebral peduncles and echogenic star shaped basilar cistern are the reference landmarks for the circle of Willis. Flow in the MCA is directed toward the transducer and ACA should be away from the transducer. PCA is found located immediately anterior to the heart shaped cerebral peduncles.
2. The foramen magnum can be used to study the vertebral and basilar arteries. Patient should be turned to one side and the neck flexed so that the chin touches the chest. The transducer is placed over the upper neck at the base of the skull and angled cephalad through the foramen magnum towards the nose.

3. The transorbital view can be used in patients with suspected carotid stenosis or occlusion. It helps in examination of the ophthalmic arteries and carotid siphons.
4. The submandibular approach can be used to sample the distal ICA in the neck to calculate mean flow velocity ratios between the MCA and ICA, the so-called hemispheric or Lindegaard index in patients with subarachnoid hemorrhage and signs of vasospasm.

The middle cerebral artery (MCA) is the most commonly insonated because of the ease of access through the temporal window and the quality of the signal and MCA carries 50–60% of the ipsilateral carotid artery blood flow, thus can be taken to represent blood flow to the hemisphere. Having identified the vessel, the examiner should attempt to follow the vessel toward the bifurcation of the internal carotid artery (ICA) into the MCA and anterior cerebral artery. This provides greater confidence that the vessel is indeed the MCA. The depth of insonation is then reduced back to 45–55 mm following the positive deflection of the MCA FV waveform. The point of maximum deflection is taken for measurements. Insonation of the MCA can be further confirmed by the ability to follow the signal for at least 10 mm, and reduction in FV with compression of the ipsilateral carotid artery. From the FV waveform, systolic, diastolic and time-averaged mean values can be calculated. The values for mean MCA FV in healthy adults range from 35 to 90 cm/s under normal physiological conditions. This variability, despite constant cerebral blood flow (CBF), is mainly the reflection of variability in the diameter of the MCA or the angle of insonation. Also, there is a considerable degree of variation both between subjects and within subjects measured at different times. MCA FV varies cyclically by around 10%. Side to side variation has been assessed and difference of more than 14% should be considered abnormal. Day to day variation should be less than 10 cm/s in 95% of individuals. Inter-observer variability has been reported as around 7.5% on the same day, and around 13% on different days. At birth, MCA FV is approximately 24 cm/s increasing to 100 cm/s at 4–6 year. Thereafter, it decreases steadily to about 40 cm/s in the seventh decade. MCA FV is affected by subject arousal, exercise, menstrual cycle, pregnancy, hematocrit and these factors should be taken into consideration when changes in MCA FV are assessed.

Indications of TCD

1. Detection and follow-up of stenosis or occlusion in a major intracranial artery in the circle of Willis and vertebrobasilar system, including monitoring of thrombolytic therapy for acute stroke patients.
2. Detection of cerebral vasculopathy.
3. Detection and monitoring of vasospasm in patients with spontaneous or traumatic subarachnoid hemorrhage.
4. Evaluation of collateral pathways of intracranial blood flow, including after intervention.
5. Detection of circulating cerebral microemboli.
6. Assessment of dural venous sinus patency.
7. Assessment of cerebral vasomotor reactivity.
8. As an adjunct in the confirmation of the clinical diagnosis of brain death.
9. Intraoperative and periprocedural monitoring to detect cerebral embolization, thrombosis, hypoperfusion, and hyperperfusion.
10. Assessment of arteriovenous malformations.
11. Detection and follow-up of intracranial aneurysms.
12. Evaluation of positional vertigo or syncope.

Tubercular Meningitis

Studies in bacterial meningitis have shown that CSF concentrations of tumor-necrosis-factor [TNF]- correlate with disease severity. TNF- concentrations in TBM are lower than they are in bacterial meningitis. Adenosine deaminase is produced by lymphocytes and monocytes. Its detection in CSF has been reported with variable success, with sensitivities and specificities as high as 99% being suggested. A trial comparing concentrations of adenosine deaminase in the CSF found increased concentrations in 30% of those with pyogenic meningitis, and almost universally raised concentrations in TBM and neurobrucellosis. The advent of DNA amplification techniques such as PCR has turned attention away from serological techniques. In paucibacillary TB the concept of amplifying specific genetic material to detectable levels is attractive. Use of PCR in the diagnosis of TBM is promising, but still poorly defined. Sensitivities vary from 33 to 90%, specificities from 88 to 100%.

Three general processes produce the subsequent neurological pathology: adhesion formation, an obliterative vasculitis, and an encephalitis or myelitis. Adhesions result from a dense basal meningeal exudate that develops after inoculation of bacilli into the subarachnoid space. The exudate contains lymphocytes, plasma cells, and macrophages, with increasing quantities of fibrin. Blockage, through adhesion formation, of the basal subarachnoid cisterns can result in obstruction of the CSF and hydrocephalus. Adhesions around the interpeduncular fossa and related structures can compromise cranial nerves, particularly II, IV, and VI, and the internal carotid artery. An obliterative vasculitis of both large and small vessels can result in infarction and stroke syndromes.

[J Neurol Neurosurg Psychiatry 2000;68:289–299].

Bacterial Meningitis

Cognitive impairment is found in 32% of patients and this proportion is similar for survivors of pneumococcal and meningococcal meningitis. Survivors of pneumococcal meningitis performed worse on memory tasks and tended to be cognitively slower than survivors of meningococcal meningitis. The frequency of cognitive impairment and the numbers of abnormal test results for patients with and without adjunctive dexamethasone were similar. Male gender and cranial nerve palsy at discharge are risk factors for cognitive impairment.

[J Neurol Neurosurg Psychiatry 2007;78:1092–1096].

False Localizing Signs in Neurology and Neurosurgery

False localizing neurological signs reflect dysfunction distant from the site of the pathology. Hence challenging the traditional clinico-anatomical correlation paradigm on which neurological examination is based.

False localizing signs occur in two contexts:

1. As a consequence of raised ICP, which is symptomatic of intracranial pathology (tumor, hematoma, abscess).
2. Idiopathic (idiopathic intracranial hypertension [IIH]) and with spinal cord lesions. Associated lesions may be intra- or extraparenchymal.

Cortical Functions

Signs traditionally thought to be of cortical origin, such as aphasia and inattention, may sometimes occur with exclusively subcortical pathology; conversely exclusively cortical lesions may results in dysarthria. Hemi-neglect is much commoner with right rather than left parietal lobe lesions. False localizing ipsilateral hemi-neglect has been reported in patients with posterior fossa tumors like meningioma causing left pontine compression, despite normal imaging of cerebral hemispheres.

Cranial Nerves

Oculomotor Nerve

Unilateral fixed dilated pupil (Hutchinson's pupil) may occur with an ipsilateral lesion such as an intracerebral hemorrhage, due to transtentorial herniation of the brain compressing the oculomotor nerve against the free edge of the tentorium. Because of the fascicular organization of the fibers within the oculomotor nerve, the externally placed pupillomotor fibers are most vulnerable. Very occasionally, fixed pupil may occur contralateral, and hence false localizing, to cranial pathology. The exact mechanism for this clinical observation is not known. The mechanism for this third nerve palsy has traditionally been ascribed to extrinsic compression of the third nerve on the margin of the tentorium. An alternative explanation, possibly relevant to false localizing third nerve palsy, is that raised ICP causes kinking of the nerve over the clivus, just posterior to the clinoid. Another suggestion is that a central mechanism might be responsible. Supratentorial pressure causing the brainstem to buckle as it descends because of caudal tethering of the neuraxis at the first dentate ligament ("dynamic axial brainstem distortion"). Divisional third nerve palsy is usually associated with lesions at the superior orbital fissure or anterior cavernous sinus, where the superior division of the oculomotor nerve passes to the superior rectus and levator palpabrae, and the inferior division to the medial and inferior recti and inferior oblique muscles. Divisional third nerve palsies may sometimes occur with more proximal lesions, presumably as a consequence of the topographic arrangement of the fascicles within the nerve, for example with intrinsic brainstem disease (e.g. stroke) or with pathology in the subarachnoid space where the nerve rootlets emerge from the brainstem (e.g. malignant infiltration).

Trochlear Nerve

False localizing fourth nerve palsies, causing diplopia on downward and inward gaze, have occasionally been described in the context of IIH. Trochlear nerve palsy might be overlooked in cases in which other cranial nerves are affected (sixth, third) because the signs are subtle.

Trigeminal Nerve

Trigeminal nerve hypofunction (trigeminal sensory neuropathy) or hyperfunction (trigeminal neuralgia) may on occasion be false-localizing, for example in association with IIH or with contralateral pathology, often a tumor.

For example, trigeminal neuralgia has been associated with a contralateral chronic calcified subdural hematoma, which caused rotational displacement of the pons, with resolution after removal of the hematoma. As with the idiopathic condition, there has been debate about the pathophysiology of trigeminal neuralgia associated with contralateral tumors. Some favor vascular compression of the nerve root as the proximate cause of paroxysmal ephaptic transmission, whereas others implicate angulations and distortion of the nerve root entry/exit zone as a consequence of displacement of brain tissue caused by an expanding mass lesion in the posterior fossa.

Abducent Nerve

Sixth nerve palsies are the most common false-localizing sign of raised ICP. Stretching of the nerve in its long intracranial course or compression against the petrous ligament or ridge of the petrous temporal bone have been suggested as the mechanism for false-localizing sixth nerve palsy.

Facial Nerve

Lower motor neuron type facial weakness has been described in the context of IIH sometimes occurring bilaterally to cause facial diplegia usually with concurrent sixth nerve palsy or palsies. Hemifacial spasm has rarely been described with contralateral posterior fossa lesions.

Vestibulocochlear Nerve

Hearing loss has on occasion been reported as a complication of IIH.

Multiple Lower Cranial Nerve Involvement

Concurrent false-localizing involvement of multiple cranial nerves has been noted on occasion, for example, trigeminal, abducens and facial nerves with a contralateral acoustic neuroma and trigeminal, glossopharyngeal and vagus nerves with a contralateral laterally-placed posterior fossa meningioma.

Motor System

Kernohan's Notch Syndrome: False-localizing Hemiparesis

A supratentorial lesion, such as acute subdural hematoma, may cause transtentorial herniation of the temporal lobe, with compression of the ipsilateral cerebral peduncle against the tentorial edge; since this is above the pyramidal decussation, a contralateral hemiparesis results. Occasionally, however, the hemiparesis may be ipsilateral to the lesion, and hence false-localizing; this occurs when the contralateral cerebral peduncle is compressed by the free edge of the tentorium. This is the Kernohan-Woltman notch phenomenon, or Kernohan's notch syndrome. There may be concurrent homolateral third nerve palsy, ipsilateral to the causative lesion.

Brainstem Compression: False-localizing Diaphragm Paralysis

Hemi-diaphragmatic paralysis with ipsilateral brainstem (medullary) compression by an aberrant vertebral artery has been described, in the absence of pathology localized to the C3–C5 segments of the spinal cord where phrenic motor neurons originate, hence it is a false-localizing sign.

Foramen Magnum/Upper Cervical Cord

Paresthesia in the hands with intrinsic hand muscle wasting and distal upper limb areflexia, with or without long tract signs, suggestive of a lower cervical myelopathy may occur with lesions at the foramen magnum or upper cervical cord ('remote atrophy').

Lower Cervical/Upper Thoracic Cord

Compressive lower cervical or upper thoracic myelopathy may produce spastic paraplegia with a mid-thoracic sensory level (or 'girdle sensation'). For example, in one case a spastic paraplegia with a sensory level at T_{10} was associated with cervical compression from a herniated disc at C5/C6.

Radiculopathy

False-localizing radiculopathy may occur in the context of IIH and cerebral venous sinus thrombosis, manifesting as acral paresthesias, backache and radicular pain, and less often with motor deficits which on occasion may be sufficiently extensive to mimic Guillain-Barré syndrome (flaccid-areflexic quadriplegia). The postulated mechanism for such radiculopathy is mechanical root compression due to elevated cerebrospinal fluid (CSF) pressure.

Cerebellar Syndrome

Frontocerebellar pathway damage, for example, as a result of infarction in the territory of the anterior cerebral artery, may result in incoordination of the contralateral limbs, mimicking cerebellar dysfunction. Suboccipital exploration to search for cerebellar tumors based on these clinical findings was known to occur before the advent of brain imaging.

Pseudo-internuclear Ophthalmoplegia

To describe internuclear ophthalmoplegia, usually indicative of medial longitudinal fasciculus dysfunction, in patients with myasthenia gravis this 'pseudo internuclear ophthalmoplegia' has also been observed in dermatomyositis.

Pseudoathetosis

Pseudoathetosis or abnormal writhing movements usually of the fingers, caused by a failure of joint position sense (proprioception). They indicate disruption of the proprioceptive pathway, from peripheral nerve to parietal cortex. It may be mistaken for choreoathetosis. However, these abnormal movements are relatively constant irrespective of whether the eyes are open or closed and occur in the absence of proprioceptive loss.

Pseudosyringomyelia

Pseudosyringomyelia" has been used to describe a selective loss of pain and temperature sensation with relative preservation of vibration and position sense seen in amyloid polyneuropathy and Tangier disease,(a small fiber sensory neuropathy), in the absence of any spinal cord pathology, and hence false localizing.

Most importantly, since false localizing signs may be indicative of serious, even life threatening, pathology within neural pathways, awareness of them and the situations in which they occur, will facilitate appropriate and timely investigation and management.

CNS CYSTICERCOSIS

Viable cysticerci in brain parenchyma measure approximately 10 mm. These cysts tend to lodge in the cerebral cortex or the basal ganglia because of the high vascular supply in these areas. Subarachnoid cysticerci may be located within cortical sulci or in the CSF cisterns at the base of the brain. After a long period of infection some cysticerci lose their scolices and grow to reach 50-mm or more, which more frequently occurs in cysts located in the subarachnoid cisterns, because their growth is not limited by the effect of pressure within the brain parenchyma. After entering the CNS, cysticerci are viable and induce slight inflammatory changes in the surrounding tissues. At this stage, called the vesicular stage, parasites have a transparent membrane, clear vesicular fluid, and larva or scolex. They may remain for decades in this stage or, as the result of a complex immunological attack from the host, may begin a degenerative process that may lead to the death of the parasite and its further transformation into an inert nodule. After cysticidal treatment or successful immune response, the first sign of involution of cysticerci is the colloidal stage, in which the transparent vesicular fluid is replaced by a viscous and turbid fluid, readily identifiable by MR imaging studies and the scolex dies. Colloidal cysticerci are surrounded by a thick collagen capsule, and the surrounding brain parenchyma shows an intense astrocytic gliosis associated with microglial proliferation, diffuse edema, neuronal degenerative changes, and perivascular cuffing of lymphocytes. Thereafter, the wall of the cyst thickens and the scolex is transformed into coarse mineralized granules; this stage, in which the cysticercus is not longer viable, is called the granular nodular stage. Finally, in the calcified stage the parasite remnants appear as a mineralized (calcified) nodule. When parasites enter into the granular and calcified stages, the edema subsides but the astrocytic changes in the vicinity of the lesions are conspicuous. The exact duration of each of these stages in the natural history of the infection has not been established, because considerable differences exist among individuals, particularly in relation to the intensity of the endogenous immune response. Albendazole is another strong cysticidal drug, initially tested at doses of 15 mg/kg/day for 1-month period. It was later found, however, that at similar doses the length of therapy could be shortened to 1-week without lessening the drug efficacy. Albendazole destroys 75 to 90% of parenchymal brain cysts and has been shown to be superior to praziquantel in several comparative trials. Another advantage of albendazole over praziquantel is that the former also destroys subarachnoid and ventricular cysts because of its better penetration in CSF, as well as the fact that it can be administered jointly with corticosteroid agents for anti-inflammatory therapy.

Intraventricular NCC

The presence of cysts inside the cerebral ventricular system, occurs in approximately 30% of patients with NCC. Intraventricular cysts are firmly encapsulated. They may circulate freely throughout the CSF pathways or become attached to theependyma anywhere in the ventricles, but their predilection is for the occipital horn of the lateral and fourth ventricles. Intraventricular cysts may be single or multiple, and frequently coexist with multiple parenchymal and subarachnoid cysts. Seizures subsequently develop in many patients with intraventricular cysts because of the concomitant parenchymal cysts. Approximately 30% of all patients with NCC develop hydrocephalus due to CSF obstruction by intraventricular or subarachnoid lesion. The larvae prefer well perfused parenchymal sites; the ventricles become populated with cysts when the parenchyma is filled. A cyst in the fourth ventricle, however, tends to be solitary, without accompanying parenchymal cysts.

Intraventricular cysts have a more aggressive behavior than their parenchymal counterparts. Symptoms associated with the parenchymal lesions largely result from the host's inflammatory response to the dead or dying larva; irritation and edema of the brain and epileptic seizures may develop.

Intraventricular cysts may become symptomatic at the time of implantation secondary to obstruction of CSF flow, with consequent hydrocephalus and the symptoms and signs of increased ICP. When involution begins, the inflammatory reaction around a dead or dying cyst produces ependymitis, scarring, obstruction, and ventriculitis.

Neuroimaging Studies. For several reasons CT scanning may fail to demonstrate small cysts that do not de- form the ventricles: 1) they share the same density as CSF; 2) the cyst wall and the scolex are not visible; and 3) the cyst does not show contrast enhancement. A large intraventricular cyst may be seen on CT scans, even without hydrocephalus, if it deforms the ventricle and the cyst is outlined by the normal ventricular cavity. A cyst de- forming or enlarging the fourth ventricle is usually well visualized on CT scans if narrow (3 or 5 mm) slices are obtained. Edema of the adjacent tissues is frequently present if the cyst is in the inflammatory stage. Computerized tomography scanning may also reveal calcified inactive parenchymal lesions.

Magnetic resonance imaging is the most important neuroimaging study, revealing intraventricular cysts in approximately 80% of cases. A viable active intraventricular cyst appears as a spherical lesion of 10 to 20 mm in diameter on T_1-weighted and fluid-attenuated inversion- recovery imaging. The scolex is frequently demonstrated as a mural nodule having the hyperintensity of fat. A cystic lesion with a scolex is one of the absolute diagnostic criteria. The cyst wall appears as a thin hyperintensity between the darkness of the cyst content and the CSF. On T_2-weighted imaging, the cyst contents are isointense with the surrounding tissues, and the scolex is hyperintense. The differential diagnosis of IVNCC includes toxoplasmosis, fungal and bacterial meningitis, hydrocephalic sequelae of tubercular meningitis, echinococcosis, intraventricular neoplasms, and non-infectious granulomatous chronic meningitis.

Neurosurg. Focus 2002;12:1-7

TOPICAL HEMOSTATS IN NEUROSURGERY

Hemostasis

Hemostasis comes from the coordinated activation of platelets and plasma clotting factors to form a platelet fibrin clot. Two processes, primary and secondary hemostasis is done by collagen for the intrinsic pathway, and the extrinsic pathway is activated by the release of tissue factors from the damaged zone. Coagulation begins almost instantly after an injury to the blood vessel has damaged the endothelium lining the vessel. Exposure of blood to the space under the endothelium initiates two processes: changes in platelets, and the exposure of subendothelial tissue factor to plasma Factor-VII, which ultimately leads to fibrin formation. Platelets immediately form a plug at the site of injury; this is called primary hemostasis. Secondary hemostasis occurs simultaneously: Additional coagulation factors or clotting factors beyond Factor-VII, respond in a complex cascade to form fibrin strands, which strengthen the platelet plug.

The two converge and enter the common pathway which begins with the conversion of Factor X to Xa, the conversion of prothrombin to thrombin, which is integral in clot stabilization via fibrin. This common pathway is facilitated by Factor V.

First Attempts

Until the early 1950, neurosurgeons used as topical hemostatic agents fresh chicken breast which was delivered to the operation theatre just before the beginning of the operation. Electrocoagulation device was not very good, and they often had to apply the chicken flesh on the brain during ten minutes while washing the field with warm serum, and removed it before closing the dura. Fresh muscle harvested from the temporal site or the thigh is still commonly used for extradural dural hemostasis and may be left in situ.

Topical Hemostats

Surgicel, Surgical Fibrillar, Gelfoam, Microfibrillar collagen (Avitene), Thrombin, Bone wax, Ostene, Fibrin glue, Floseal, Hydrogen peroxide (3%).

Surgicel

Surgicel is an oxidized cellulose polymer (the functional unit is poly- anhydroglucuronic acid) formed by dissolving pure α-cellulose (plant derived) in an alkaline solution. It is then regenerated into continuous fiber, knitted into gauze, and oxidized. Introduced in 1940s. Manufactured by Johnson and Johnson's Ethicon subsidiary. Applied dry, absorbs within 4 to 8 weeks. It forms a brownish or black gelatinous mass in contact with blood.

Surgicel is composed of solid fibers with irregular contours on cross-section.

Acts as a physical matrix to which platelets can adhere which, in turn, aids in clot formation. Additional pressure of the mass also contributes to the hemostatic process. Relatively bacteriostatic because of its relatively low pH, it deactivates and denatures some of the bacterial proteins thus making them more susceptible to antibiotics. Needs to be applied dry.

Gelatin Sponge (Gelfoam/Surgifoam)

Introduced in the 1940s for neurosurgical procedures. It is a water-insoluble, off-white, non-elastic, porous, pliable. Derived from purified pork skin gelatin. Absorbs approximately 45 times its weight in blood and can expand to approximately 200% of its initial volume. It may be cut without fraying. Absorbed in approximately four to six weeks. Not to be used in combination with blood salvage equipments as their fibers can pass through the 40 mm filters of salvage systems. Can be used dry or saline soaked, better when excess saline is removed

Surgicel Fibrillar

Oxidized regenerated cellulose (1969). Layers can be peeled off in desired amounts. It conforms to irregular surfaces, even hard-to-reach areas. Surgical visualisation is improved by ability to cauterise directly through it. Fully absorbed within 14 days. 33% faster hemostasis vs SURGICEL. Proven bactericidal properties.

[Oxidized regenerated cellulose as a cause of paraplegia after thoracotomy: case report and review of the literature. (Spinal Cord. 2005 Jul;43(7):445-7.]

Microfibrillar Collagen (Avitene)

This substance (Avitene) was introduced in 1970. Microfibrillar applied collagen products come from the purification of bovine collagen, followed by microcrystallization. It is presented as a powder, and is more effective than gelatin based hemostasis, since it is able to activate the clotting cascade. Binds tightly to blood surfaces. Causes minimal swelling especially when compared to Gelfoam. In addition to being collagen and causing contact activation, it does somehow directly activate platelets with subsequent aggregation. May reduce the number of free platelets in normal individuals. Loses effectiveness in thrombocytopenia (<10,000). It is absorbed in 3-months and needs to be applied dry.

Thrombin (Thrombostat/Thrombinar)

Thrombin is marketed as bovine (Thrombin-JMI, King Pharmaceuticals, Bristol, TN), human pooled plasma (Evithrom, J and J), and recombinant (Recothrom, Zymogenetics, Seattle, WA). Thrombin directly activates fibrinogen and converts it into fibrin monomers. Can be used directly or combined with gelatin sponge. Produced from bovine prothrombin hence antigenic. If injected into large vessels can lead to thrombosis and complications.

A phase 3, randomized, double-blind comparative study of the efficacy and safety of topical recombinant human thrombin and bovine thrombin in surgical hemostasis

(Chapman WC, Singla N, Genyk Y, McNeil JW, Renkens KL Jr, Reynolds TC, Murphy A, Weaver FA. J Am Coll Surg 2007;205:256-65).

The three commercially available thrombins are functionally equivalent in terms of efficacy with 95% or greater of patients achieving hemostasis within 10-minutes of application and approximately two-thirds of patients achieving hemostasis within 3-minutes. The human antibodies to bovine FII and FV have been linked to coagulopathy and potentially fatal complications.

(Sarfati MR, Dilorenzo DJ, Kraiss LW, Galt SW. Severe coagulopathy following Intraoperative use of topical thrombin. Ann Vasc Surg 2004;18:349-51.)

Bone Wax

Pioneered by Sir Victor Horsley (1892).

Horsley's wax: bees wax, 7 parts; **almond oil**, 1 part; **salicylic acid**, 1 part.

Modern wax: 88% refined beeswax and 12% isopropyl palmitate (softening agent). Effective in controlling bleeding from bone. Once smeared across the bleeding edge, immediate hemostasis occurs.

Complications

1. Bone wax inhibits osteogenesis.
2. Increases infection rates (the number of bacteria needed to produce osteomyelitis is reduced by a factor of 10^4 (10,000).
3. Remains as a foreign body for many years.

Ostene

Sterile mixture of water-soluble alkylene oxide copolymers. Inert artificial material feels and works like wax. Does not increase infection rates, does not interfere with bone healing, and is non-inflammatory.

Fibrin Glue (Tisseel/Crosseal)

Commercially available/autologous.

2 components:

a. Fibrinogen, factor 13, fibronectin, *aprotinin*, plasminogen, cryoprecipitate
b. Thrombin and calcium.

When combined, the fibrinogen is activated by thrombin and converted into fibrin monomer which form an adhesive glue at the tissues applied. The fibrin monomer interacts with the patient's own factor VIII and calcium to convert the final product into a fibrin polymer that allows for platelets activation and aggregation with subsequent hemostasis. Aprotinin inhibits premature fibrin degradation. Supply a source of fibrinogen to the site of injury and do not need active bleeding or blood-derived fibrinogen to polymerize. They are presented with a dual chamber syringe that allows for the combination of the thrombin and fibrinogen when the plunger is depressed. They also can be used in spray. Many commercial products are now on the market: Tisseel (Baxter), Evicel formerly called Crosseal (Johnson and Johnson. Tisseel is now bovine free.

Other Uses

To reinforce dural closure and prevent CSF leak.

In anastomosis of nerves and nerve grafts.

(Micro neural anastomosis with **fibrin glue**: an experimental study. Suri A, Mehta VS, Sarkar C. Neurology India 2002).

Fixation of bone fragments to repair skull defects.

Flowables

Human plasma thrombin with bovine gelatin matrix. **(Floseal)**

Create a granular hemostat that employs both active and mechanical components to achieve hemostasis. It is applied as a paste to which is recommended that gentle pressure be applied with a moist saline sponge for 2-minutes to achieve hemostasis.

Hemostatic matrix sealant in neurosurgery: a clinical and imaging study. (Roberto Gazzeri and Marcelo Galarza and Massimiliano Neroni and Alex Alfieri and Marco Giordano).

Acta Neurochir (2011) 153:148–155. Effective hemostasis, defined as cessation of bleeding, was achieved no later than 3 min after topical agent application in all patients except in 11 cases out of 214 cases it was used.

The role of Flo Seal in reducing epidural fibrosis in a rat laminectomy model.

(Dogulu F, Durdag E, Cemil B, Kurt G, Ozgun G Neurol Neurochir Pol. 2009 Jul-Aug;43(4):346-51).

Application of Flo Seal at a laminectomy site may be useful to decrease adhesion at the interface between the dura mater and epidural fibrosis.

Hydrogen Peroxide

It has been used for decades as a hemostatic agent, 3% solution is used in neurosurgery.

Mechanism: Exact mechanism is not known, presumed to be because of mechanical air locking of the small vessels because of oxygen released from H_2O_2, and is also credited to create a disruption of the blood-barrier and an aggregation of the platelets and neutrophils leading to thrombus formation. Recent evidence suggest significant tissue damage in surrounding functional brain.

(Hydrogen peroxide–induced stroke: elucidation of the mechanism in vivo J Neurosurg 110:94–100, 2009)

CNS Cryptococcosis

In patients with AIDS, cryptococcosis (Cryptococcus neoformans) is the third most common CNS infection, with only HIV encephalopathy and toxoplasmosis being more common. Cryptococcus proliferates in the subarachnoid spaces and spreads into the perivascular spaces, dilating them. The confluence of dilated perivascular spaces leads to the formation of gelatinous pseudocysts, usually in the basal ganglia and dentate nuclei regions. Clinical Presentation: Most patients present with symptoms or signs of subacute meningitis or meningoencephalitis, with fever, malaise, nausea, vomiting, lethargy, and altered mental status.

Key Diagnostic Features*:* Classic MR findings are clusters of small hyperintense T_2-weighted lesions in the basal ganglia showing subtle peripheral enhancement, representing the dilated perivascular spaces. In cases with larger pseudocysts, high T_2-FLAIR signal can be seen as the gelatinous material has different relaxation times than

CSF, and therefore will not be suppressed. In the absence of parenchymal lesions, communicating hydrocephalus (subacute to chronic cases) may raise suspicion.

In patients with AIDS and a CD4 count below 200 cells/mm^3, meningeal enhancement, cryptococcomas, and choroid plexitis or gelatinous pseudocysts are a rare finding probably due to 1) the patient's inability to mount an immune response to the organisms, and 2) the organism's thick mucoid capsule that isolates it from the patient's inflammatory cells. The diagnosis should be confirmed with the patient's serum or CSF agglutination test for cryptoccocal polysaccharide antigen, Indian ink stain of CSF and CSF cultures.

DDx: Other opportunistic infections (e.g., toxoplasmosis), although these lesions are parenchymal rather than located in the subarachnoid space, and also elicit a more pronounced inflammatory reaction.

(AJNR, case of the week 2015; June 25)

Uremic Encephalopathy

Uremic complications of CNS may result from either multiple metabolic derangements associated with dialysis for treatment of end-stage renal disease due to the rapid removal of urea during hemodialysis in patients with chronic uremia.

Clinical Presentation: Altered mental status, headache, nausea and vomiting, myoclonus, tremor, and focal or generalized seizures.

MRI demonstrates bilateral symmetrical swollen lentiform nuclei with a hyperintense T_2/FLAIR signal rim delineating the boundaries of the putamen [Lentiform fork sign]. The lateral arm of the fork corresponds to the edematous external capsule. The "stem" of the fork is formed by the fusion of edematous external and internal capsules. The medial arm splits in two, the internal and external medullary laminae, which divide the lentiform nucleus into three components (the putamen, globus pallidus externus and globus pallidus internus). Associated diffuse cerebral edema can also be seen. Restricted diffusion is not one of the classic described findings but might represent a more advanced stage with irreversible neuronal damage.

Fork sign can be seen in other conditions that result in metabolic acidosis, including methanol or ethylene-glycol toxicity, and acidopathies such as propionic acidemia, pyruvate dehydrogenase deficiency, nonketotic hyperglycinemia, and hydroxyglutaric aciduria.

(AJNR, case of the week 2015; June 8)

Acute Cerebellitis

Acute cerebellitis is a rare inflammatory syndrome characterized by cerebellar dysfunction. It usually occurs as a primary infectious, post-infectious or post- vaccination disorder, and mostly presents in early childhood.

Clinical Presentation: Trunk and limbs ataxia, fever, abnormal eye movements, dysarthria, headache, nausea, vomiting and decreased level of consciousness. The condition is self-limited to fatal, depending on the amount of cerebellar swelling.

Diagnostic Features: Bilateral hemispheric cerebellar swelling with cortical and white matter T_2-hyperintensities; leptomeningeal enhancement may be present. Less frequent features are obstructive hydrocephalus, unilateral involvement, normal T_2-signal.

CSF: Elevated protein and leukocytes, with lymphocytic predominance, normal glucose, anti- HSV, EBV, VZV, mumps, rubella, Lyme disease.

DD-Lhermitte-Duclos disease, Vasculitis, Drug intoxication (e.g., heroin inhalation, or "chasing the dragon")

Treatment: Steroids, Aciclovir, decompressive craniectomy if necessary

(AJNR, case of the week 2015; June 4)

Chronic Lymphocytic Inflammation with Pontine Perivascular Enhancement Responsive to Steroids (CLIPPERS)

Pathogenesis: unknown

Clinical Presentation: Dysarthria, ataxia and diplopia. Usually responds to treatment with steroids.

Pathology: Perivascular spaces infiltrated with lymphocytes

Key Diagnostic Features: Numerous patchy FLAIR signal hyperintensities, typically at the pontocerebellar junction. Minimal enhancement. Can sometimes extend cephalad to involve the midbrain, basal ganglia, and the periventricular white matter. Occasionally involves the spinal cord. No restricted diffusion. Imaging findings reversible upon treatment with steroids. Diagnosis on imaging is largely one of exclusion.

DDx: Lymphoma, Histiocytosis, Encephalitis, Vasculitis, Sarcoidosis.

Rx: Corticosteroids, if no response to immunosuppressive therapy.

(AJNR, case of the week 2015; May 11)

Radiculopial Artery Aneurysm Rupture

Isolated spinal artery aneurysms are rare. Such aneurysms can be seen arising from the anterior, posterior spinal arteries or branches and collaterals, including the radiculopial and radiculomedullary arteries.

A recent review of the literature found descriptions of spinal artery aneurysms in 43 patients, 60.5% of which have other underlying vascular pathologies such as arterial dissection, aortic coarctation, vasculitis, fibromuscular dysplasia, infection, pseudoxanthoma elasticum, and connective tissue disorder. The average age at diagnosis was 46-years. **Unlike cerebral artery aneurysms, spinal artery aneurysms seldom occur at branching points, and are not usually associated with atherosclerotic disease.**

Clinical Presentation: Acute headache, meningismus, severe back pain (related to the blood in the spinal canal and not the arterial dissection), and focal cord ischemia and/or compression.

Key Diagnostic Features: SAH with disproportionate amount of blood in the spinal canal, foramen magnum and posterior fossa. Epidural-subdural spinal hematomas may be present. In any patient presenting with a SAH and symptoms related to the spinal cord, a spinal artery aneurysm has to be considered as one of the potential sources of hemorrhage. Focal clot within the spinal canal may point to the location of the aneurysm. A perimedullary focal enhancement can be seen representing blood and contrast stasis in the pseudoaneurysm. Localized spinal angiogram is necessary to confirm the diagnosis.

Rx: If the aneurysm is located in the dorsal surface of the cord, surgery may be performed. Conservative management is an option, specially in patients who are poor surgical candidates or when the aneurysm is located on the ventral surface of the cord. Endovascular treatment is usually not recommended.

(AJNR, case of the week 2015; April 23)

POEMS Syndrome

POEMS syndrome is a poorly understood entity characterized by polyneuropathy, organomegaly, endocrinopathy, M-protein (monoclonal plasma cell proliferative disorder), and skin changes. Etiology not established, likely secondary to imbalance of inflammatory cytokines.

Clinical Presentation: Symmetrical and ascending peripheral neuropathy most common manifestation, pulmonary manifestations (PAH, restrictive lung disease), endocrinopathy (most commonly gonadal axis). Skin changes include scleroderma, hyperpigmentation, hemangioma/telangiectasia.

Key Diagnostic Features: Radiographic findings of POEMS syndrome are nonspecific. Almost always associated with sclerotic bone lesions. Organomegaly (hepatomegaly, splenomegaly) may be noted. Lymphadenopathy (including Castleman's disease) is a common feature.

DD: Lymphoma, Osteoblastic metastatic disease, Multiple myeloma

Rx: Multisystem disease, no standardized therapy. Radiation may be utilized in a solitary bone lesion. High-dose chemotherapy with autologous stem cell support.

Mitochondrial Encephalopathy Lactic Acidosis Stroke-like Episodes (MELAS)

MELAS is characterized by stroke-like events that are acute in onset, often transient.

Generally presents between the ages of 3-months and 40 years. Seizures, nausea/vomiting, headaches, and hearing loss are common symptoms. Linked to mutations in mitochondrial DNA inherited from the mother.

Key Diagnostic Features: Hyperintense T_2-lesions, predominately in the gray and subcortical white matter in the temporal, parietal, and occipital lobes. Frontal lobes are not commonly involved. Lesions generally spare the deep white matter and may cross vascular boundaries. Basal ganglia calcification is often seen (better appreciated on CT – interval progression of calcification is suggestive of MELAS). Follow-up MRI studies may show lesion resolution, sometimes with interval appearance of new lesions.

DDx: Ischemic stroke, Kearns-Sayre syndrome, Leigh syndrome, Pearson syndrome

Rx: Aimed at increasing the production of ATP. Coenzyme-Q10 has been helpful to some patients. Other therapies include carnitine, riboflavin, ascorbic acid, and L-arginine.

(AJNR, case of the week 2015; March 2)

Infantile Krabbe Disease (KD)

KD, also known as "globoid" cells leukodystrophy. Autosomal recessive disorder involving chromosome 14 (14q31), caused by a deficiency of galactocerebroside beta-galactosidase (GALC) that leads to accumulation of cytotoxic metabolite psychosine, resulting in demyelination due to apoptosis of myelin-forming cells.

Clinical Presentation varies with patient age. Infantile, late infantile, juvenile, and adult forms are recognized. The infantile form is the most common and manifests as hyperirritability, increased muscle tone, and fever. Disease progression is characterized by cognitive decline, myoclonus, opisthotonus, and nystagmus. Typically, KD is rapidly progressive and fatal.

CT performed during the initial stage may demonstrate symmetric high-attenuation foci in the thalami, caudate nuclei, corona radiata, posterior limbs of the internal capsule, and brainstem. The centrum semiovale, periventricular white matter, and deep gray matter demonstrate high signal intensity at T_2WI.

Gaucher disease, Niemann-Pick disease (NPD), GM-1 gangliosidosis, metachromatic leukodystrophy (MLD), status marmolatus, and cerebral palsy form a list of differential diagnosis.

Rx: Umbilical cord blood transplantation is the only available treatment, and is only effective before symptoms develop.

(AJNR, 2001;22:1782-5)

Adrenomyeloneuropathy

Adrenomyeloneuropathy (AMN) is an adult variant of X-linked adrenoleukodystrophy, characterized by ABCD1 gene mutation, that results in impaired peroxisome function with accumulation of very long chain fatty acids (VLCFA) and demyelination.

Patients present with progressive spastic paraparesis beginning in distal lower extremities with hyperreflexia, impaired vibration sense, and sphincter dysfunction. Patients can also have adrenal insufficiency.

Key Diagnostic Features: MR findings: Spinal cord atrophy, mostly at thoracic level. Cerebral demyelination is confined to white matter tracts, or diffuse depending on subtype. Most common finding is increased T_2-signal (demyelination) along corticospinal tracts, and less commonly along the spinothalamic tract and audiovisual pathways.

Laboratory confirmation: Laboratory confirmation: Genetic analysis for ABCD1 gene mutation; increased VLCFA's within CSF and plasma

DDx: Amyotrophic lateral sclerosis

Rx: Steroid replacement *(AJNR, case of the week 2014; Feb 6)*

MULTIPLE CHOICE QUESTIONS

1. **Weber's syndrome is:**
   a. 3rd cranial nerve palsy with opposite side weakness of limbs
   b. 6th and 7th cranial nerve palsy
   c. 6th and 7th cranial nerve palsy with opposite side weakness of limbs
   d. Ipsilateral anesthesia of face and contralateral anesthesia of limbs

   Ref. Greenberg, 4th/e, p811

2. **Dolls eye response is seen in:**
   a. Stuporous patients
   b. Brain dead patients
   c. Normal individuals
   d. Hypothermic patients

   Ref. Greenberg, 4th/e, p558

3. **The target site for treatment of tremors is:**
   a. Midbrain
   b. Thalamus
   c. Internal capsule
   d. None of the above

   Ref. Thieme, 1st/e, p216-8

4. **All the procedures are done for trigeminal neuralgia relief except:**
   a. Microvascular decompression
   b. Radiofrequency ablation
   c. Glycerol rhizotomy
   d. 5th nerve stimulation

   Ref. Thieme, 1st/e, p79-97

5. **The commonest cause of bilateral trigeminal neuralgia is:**
   a. Diabetes
   b. Multiple sclerosis
   c. Bilateral 5th nerve schwannomas
   d. None of the above

   Ref. Greenberg, 4th/e, p14

6. **The commonest symptom in diabetic autonomic neuropathy is:**
   a. Stress incontinence
   b. Retrograde ejaculation
   c. Impotence
   d. Dumping syndrome

   Ref. Greenberg, 4th/e, p436

7. **Which lobar pathology is responsible for geographical apraxia?**
   a. Left temporal
   b. Right parietal
   c. Left parietal
   d. Right temporal

   Ref. Adams, 7th/e, p486

8. **Gerstman's syndrome is caused by lesion in:**
   a. Right angular gyrus
   b. Left angular gyrus
   c. Left supramarginal gyrus
   d. Right paracentral lobule

   Ref. Bickerstaff, 6th/e, p272

9. **Lesion in the left angular gyrus will cause:**
   a. Bimanual astereognosis
   b. Gerstman's syndrome
   c. 'a' and 'b'
   d. Word deafness

   Ref. Bickerstaff, 6th/e, p272, Adams, p487

10. **Loss of topographic memory is caused by lesion in the:**
    a. Right occipital lobe
    b. Left occipital lobe
    c. Left temporal lobe
    d. Right temporal lobe

    Ref. Adams, 7th/e, p493

ANSWERS

1. a.	**2.** c.	**3.** b.	**4.** d.	**5.** b.	**6.** c.	**7.** b.	**8.** b.	**9.** c.	**10.** a.

11. Bilateral lesions in the occipital lobes will cause all the following except:
a. Cortical blindness
b. Anton's syndrome
c. Prosopagnosia
d. Anomia
Ref. Adams, 7th/e, p493

12. All the following statements about Broca's aphasia are correct except:
a. It occurs when the lesion involves dormant (left) posterior inferior frontal gyrus
b. Comprehension is preserved
c. Writing to dictation is possible
d. Words are mis-spelt
Ref. Adams, 7th/e, p505-8

13. All the following statements about conduction aphasia are true except:
a. It occurs when the motor or sensory speech areas get disconnected
b. Repetition is severely impaired
c. Speech output is normal or reduced
d. Comprehension is impaired
Ref. Adams, 7th/e, p510

14. Tactile agnosia is caused by lesions in the:
a. Contralateral angular gyrus
b. Contralateral supramarginal gyrus
c. Ipsilateral angular gyrus
d. Ipsilateral para central lobule
Ref. Adams, 7th/e, p487

15. Alexia without agraphia occurs because:
a. Left inferior parietal lobule is disconnected from all the visual input
b. Right inferior parietal lobule is disconnected from the visual input
c. Left occipital lobe is disconnected from right temporal lobe
d. Right temporal lobe is disconnected from right superior parietal lobule
Ref. Adams, 7th/e, p511

16. Posterior cerebral artery embolus on right side will cause:
a. Left homonymous hemianopia
b. Right homonymous hemianopia
c. Total blindness
d. Left superior temporal quadrantnopia
Ref. Adams, 7th/e, p493

17. Which of the following is not a cause of raised ICP without localization?
a. Frontal polar lesions
b. Temporal polar lesions
c. Pseudotumor cerebri
d. Bilateral falcine meningioma
Ref. Greenberg, 4th/e, p259

18. Dementia is most commonly caused by lesion in:
a. Frontal lobe b. Temporal lobe
c. Perisylvian area d. Parietal lobe
Ref. Adams, 7th/e, p431-5

19. The term walnut brain is seen in:
a. Alzheimer's disease
b. Multi-infarct dementia
c. Pick's disease
d. None of the above
Ref. www.medical-dictionary.thefreedictionary.com

20. In which of the following conditions, sella is usually normal?
a. Acromegaly
b. Prolactimomas
c. Non-functioning pituitary adenomas
d. None of the above
Ref. Youmans, 5th/e, p1169-96

21. Which formula/rule helps to differentiate true leucocytosis from a traumatic spinal tap?
a. Rule of Spence b. Steel's rule
c. Fishman's formula d. None of the above
Ref. Greenberg, 4th/e, p99

Answers

11. d. **12.** c. **13.** d. **14.** b. **15.** a. **16.** a. **17.** d. **18.** a. **19.** c. **20.** d.
21. c.

22. All the following statements about microvascular decompression for 5th cranial neuralgia are true except:

a. Previous procedures for trigeminal neuralgia are a contraindication for the procedure

b. Preoperative EMG of temporalis and masseter muscles is monitored

c. The commonest vessel involved in compression of the 5th cranial nerve is the superior cerebellar artery

d. The success of second MVD is less than the first

Ref. Thieme, 1st/e, p79-97

23. Which of the following entities is classified by Suwanwela and Suwanwela classification?

a. Tuberous sclerosis b. Syringomyelia

c. Spina bifida d. Encephaloceles

Ref. Greenberg, 4th/e, p71

24. All the following receptors have been found in meningiomas except:

a. Estrogen and progesterone receptors

b. Androgen receptors

c. Glucocorticoid receptors

d. D-2 dopamine receptors

Ref. Al-Mefty, p273-8

25. All the following are features of retrocochlear deafness except:

a. The air-bone gap gets widened

b. Tone decay

c. Speech discrimination is poor

d. None of the above

Ref. Greenberg, 4th/e, p264-5

26. A patient in whom pseudotumor cerebri is suspected will have the following features except:

a. Raised ICP symptoms

b. Normal CSF composition

c. Associated with vitamin A toxicity

d. Hydrocephalus on MRI

Ref. Youmans, 5th/e, p1419-1424

27. All the following lesions can have intracranial extension except:

a. Nasal polyp

b. Juvenile angiofibroma

c. Esthesioneuroblastoma

d. Nasal encephalocele

Ref. Youmans, 5th/e, p1311-5

28. In all the following conditions, patients usually present with cough headaches except:

a. Chiari malformation

b. Arachnoid cysts

c. Craniostenosis

d. Pseudotumor cerebri

Ref. Youmans, 5th/e, p1419-24, 3289-99, 3347-59

29. Chassaignai's tubercle is seen on:

a. Transverse process of C_6

b. Spinous process of C_7

c. Articular process of C_5

d. Anterior arch of atlas

Ref. Greenberg, 4th/e, p421

30. Match the following:

a. Kocher's point 1) 3 cm above and posterior to helix

b. Dandy's point 2) 6 cm above and 4 cm lateral to inion

c. Frazier's point 3) 3 cm above and 2 cm lateral to inion

d. Keen's point 4) Precoronal in midpupillary line

Ref. Greenberg, 4th/e, p406-708

31. Tubercular meningitis can cause:

a. Communicating hydrocephalus

b. Noncommunicating hydrocephalus

c. both 'a' and 'b'

d. None of the above

Ref. Neurosurgery Quarterly 2011;21(4): 267-71

ANSWERS

22. a.	**23.** d.	**24.** d.	**25.** a.	**26.** d.	**27.** a.	**28.** c.	**29.** a.	**30.** a.	**31.** c.

32. The ventral horn of spinal cord is motor and dorsal horn is sensory, it is known as:

a. Rule of Spence
b. Rule of Steel
c. Rule of Bell and Magendie
d. None of the above

Ref. www.medical-dictionary.thefreedictionary.com

33. If all the pregnant mothers take adequate folate during periconceptual period, the incidence of spina bifida will decrease by:

a. 30%
b. 60%
c. 70%
d. 100%

Ref. Youmans, 5th/e, p3257

34. In which of the following tumors malignant transformation has not been reported?

a. Colloid cyst
b. Pilocytic astrocytoma
c. Lhermitte-Duclos disease
d. Epidermoid cyst

Ref. Greenberg, 4th/e, p289, Youmans, p3687-9

35. A 65-year-old female with known chronic renal disease is getting a session of hemodialysis, during the procedure she started with altered sensorium–the possibilities could be:

a. Dialysis-dementia syndrome
b. Subdural hematoma
c. Hypertensive encephalopathy
d. All the above

Ref. Neurology India 2004;52:475-7

36. The following statement about audiometry in a patient of vestibular schwannoma is true:

a. Low tone decay
b. Air-bone gap
c. Impaired speech discrimination
d. None of the above

Ref. Greenberg, 4th/e, p264-5

37. Phalens test is done in:

a. Median nerve entrapment
b. Ulnar nerve entrapment
c. Occipital nerve entrapment
d. Anterior interosseous neuropathy

Ref. Greenberg, 4th/e, p445

38. All the following conditions are the differential diagnoses of ulnar nerve entrapment except:

a. Syrinx
b. Intramedullary tumor
c. Amyotrophic lateral sclerosis
d. Pancoasts tumor compressing the upper trunk of brachial plexus

Ref. Greenberg, 4th/e, p449-50

39. The following statements about Erb's paralysis are true except:

a. There is paralysis of pronation of forearm
b. There is paralysis of extensors of elbow
c. There is paralysis of lateral rotators of shoulder
d. All the above

Ref. Greenberg, 4th/e, p440

40. Which of the following statements about neoplastic plexopathy of brachial plexus is true?

a. Lower trunk is commonly involved
b. Pain is a feature
c. Myokimia is absent d. All are true

Ref. Adams, p1427-30

41. All the following are common in pediatric age group except:

a. Diastatic fractures b. 1 Pond fractures
c. CSF rhinorrhea d. Growing skull fractures

Ref. Youmans, 5th/e, p3473, 3480

42. Calcification at which of the following sites is not a cause of worry:

a. Temporal lobe in an adult
b. Pineal gland in a 2-year child
c. Choroid plexus in an elderly
d. Hypothalamus in an adult

Ref. Youmans, 5th/e, p3603-11, p3595-9

ANSWERS

32. c. **33.** c. **34.** a. **35.** d. **36.** c. **37.** a. **38.** d. **39.** d. **40.** d. **41.** c. **42.** c.

43. The commonest cause of facial nerve palsy is:

a. Acoustic neuroma
b. Bell's palsy
c. Facial nerve schwannoma
d. CP angle epidermoid

Ref. Greenberg, 4th/e, p128

44. All the following are derived from neural crest except:

a. Adrenal medulla
b. Autonomic ganglia
c. Ventral root ganglia
d. Carotid body

Ref. Developmental Biology, 6th ed, Gilbert SF, Sunderland: Sinauei Associates 2000

45. All the following can cause hemifacial spasms, except:

a. Aberrant vessel loop
b. Aneurysm from anterio inferior cerebellar artery
c. Vestibular schwannoma
d. Astrocytoma of motor strip

Ref. Patten, 2nd/e, p74-5

46. All the following statements are true about sellar arachnoid cysts except:

a. Never occur in infancy
b. Are extradural in location
c. Are not associated with a subarachnoid cistern
d. Are always noncommunicating arachnoid cyst

Ref. Youmans, 5th/e, p3294-5

47. All the following statements about CNS tuberculosis are true except:

a. About 50% of tuberculomas have history of TB in the past
b. About 10% of TBM have opticochiasmatic arachnoiditis
c. TBM has mortality of 50%
d. About 40% have pulmonary TB

Ref. Neurosurgery Quarterly 2011, 21:4; 267-71

48. Which of the following antiepileptics is an enzyme inducer?

a. Carbamazepine
b. Valproic acid
c. Lamotrigine
d. None of the above

Ref. Youmans, 5th/e, p2470

49. In which of the following conditions pituitary stalk is not thickened?

a. Syphilis
b. Sarcoidosis
c. Lymphocytic hypophysitis
d. Cushing's disease

Ref. Pediatric Neurology 2011;44(6):463-6

50. Infundibuli are most commonly encountered at the origin of which of the following arteries:

a. Basilar artery
b. Anterior choroidal artery
c. Posterior communicating artery
d. Superior cerebellar artery

Ref. Rhoton, p87-9

51. All the following statements about Horner's syndrome are true except:

a. Miosis is present
b. There is pseudoenophthalmos
c. Anhidrosis is present
d. Ciliospinal reflex is present

Ref. Adams, 7th/e, p566-7

52. Downbeat nystagmus is usually seen in:

a. CV junction anomalies
b. Vestibular neuronitis
c. Viral labrynthitis
d. Drug induced

Ref. Adams, 7th/e, p291

53. Injury to greater superficial petrosal nerve will lead to:

a. Impaired caloric test
b. Impaired Schimer's test
c. Impaired audiometry
d. None of the above

Ref. Greenberg, 4th/e, p128

Answers

43. b. **44.** c. **45.** d. **46.** d. **47.** c. **48.** a. **49.** d. **50.** c. **51.** d. **52.** a. **53.** b.

54. In traumatic head injury causing blindness, the most vulnerable segment of optic nerve is:
a. Intracanalicular
b. Intraorbital
c. Intraocular
d. Intracranial
Ref. Youmans, 5th/e, p3468

55. All the following structures form the medial wall of the orbit except:
a. Ethmoid
b. Lacrimal bone
c. Sphenoid bone
d. Palatine bone
Ref. Schmidek and Sweet, 4th/e, p200

56. Which of the following triangles is named as Kawase's triangle?
a. Posterolateral middle fossa triangle
b. Posteromedial middle fossa triangle
c. Inferolateral paraclival triangle
d. Inferomedial paraclival triangle
Ref. Schmidek and Sweet, 4th/e, p959

57. In which of the following conditions is there increasing evidence that it is related to polymorphism in apolipoprotein E4?
a. Hyperlipoproteinemias
b. Atherosclerosis
c. Alzheimer's disease
d. Macular degeneration
Ref. Adams, 7th/e, p1116

58. Which osmotic agent has additional properties of inhibiting apoptosis?
a. Mannitol
b. Glycerol
c. Urea
d. None of the above
Ref. Journal of Neurosurgery 2011;114:545-8

59. Which of the following osmotic agents has a reflection coefficient?
a. Mannitol
b. Hypertonic saline
c. Urea
d. Glycerol
Ref. Neurosurgery Focus 2007;22(5):E-12

60. The following drug is best for treating vasogenic edema:
a. Steroids
b. Acetazolamide
c. Frusemide
d. Mannitol
Ref. Youmans, 5th/e, p801-2

61. Which osmotic agent went into disrepute because of its allergic reactions?
a. Glycerol
b. Albumin
c. Urea
d. Hypertonic saline
Ref. Neurosurgery focus 2007;22(5):E-12

62. A 15-year-girl was operated for glioblastoma multiforme. She received adjuvant therapy also. In her postoperative period she was put on diphenyl-hydantoin to control her seizures. Six months later, her baseline investigations revealed Hb levels of 3.8g%, with low white cell and platelet count. The cause of this could be:
a. Bone marrow metastasis from GBM
b. Development of renal failure with chemotherapy
c. Di-phenylhydantoin toxicity
d. None of the above
Ref. Greenberg, 4th/e, p676

63. The most accurate test to differentiate between 'SIADH' and cerebral salt wasting (CSW) is:
a. Serum osmolality
b. Serum ADH levels
c. Body weight
d. Central venous pressure measurement
Ref. Greenberg, 4th/e, p482

ANSWERS

54. a. **55.** d. **56.** b. **57.** c. **58.** a. **59.** b. **60.** a. **61.** b. **62.** c. **63.** b.

64. In management of aneurysmal SAH, the hematocrit of the patient shall be between 30 and 35, to achieve such a goal hemoglobin levels should be:

a. 10 g%
b. 15 g%
c. 20 g%
d. None of the above

Ref. Youmans, 5th/e, p1822

65. Which of the following statements is false?

a. There is inverse relation between viscosity of blood and hematocrit
b. If the hematocrit is low, the oxygen carrying capacity of blood is reduced
c. The mean arterial pressure while managing aneurysmal rupture should be 120–150 mm Hg
d. For unclipped aneurysms, hypertension is not aimed and only hemodilution and hypervolemia are the goal

Ref. Youmans, 5th/e, p1813-5

66. A 45-year-male reports with 5 days' history of rapidly progressive hemiparesis. Imaging reveals an enhancing mass. Biopsy of the lesion revealed perivascular lymphocytes which were predominantly T-cell type. Bielschowsky stains showed preservation of axons and myelin stain showed loss of myelin. The most probable diagnosis is:

a. CNS lymphoma
b. Multiple sclerosis
c. Tubercular encephalitis
d. Acute demyelinating encephalomyelitis

Ref. Robbins and Cotran, p1310-1

67. Which of the following varieties of lipomyelomeningioceles is a surgical challenge?

a. Caudal lipomyelomeningocele
b. Transitional lipomyelomeningocele
c. Dorsal lipomyelomeningocele
d. All the above

Ref. Thieme 1st/e, p208

68. A 10-year-old boy on imaging shows tonsillar descent of 6 mm and cervical cord syrinx. The next best step in his management shall be a:

a. Foramen magnum decompression
b. Lumbosacral MRI to look for tethered cord syndrome
c. Syrinogo-subarachnoid shunt
d. Foramen magnum decompression and a syringo-subarachnoid shunt

Ref. Greenberg, 4th/e, p92-3

69. A 35-year-old male develops progressive quadriparesis. MRI spine reveals a cervical cord syrinx. He gives past history of tubercular meningitis. The best treatment of syrinx is:

a. Syringosubarachnoid shunt
b. Syringopleural shunt
c. Foramen magnum decompression only
d. Foramen magnum decompression with release of arachnoid adhesions

Ref. Greenberg, 4th/e, p228

70. Which of the following advantages is best known about prenatal repair of spina-bifida as compared to postnatal repair?

a. Incidence of infection is less
b. Incidence of secondary tethering is less
c. Incidence of shunt dependence is less
d. None of the above

Ref. Thieme, 1st/e, p193-208

71. The incidence of secondary tethoring syndrome in repair of spina-bifida is reduced by:

a. Application of hyaluronic acid topically at the end of surgery
b. Application of lasser beam at the surgical site
c. Application of cryoprobe
d. None of the above

Ref. Thieme, 1st/e, p193-208

ANSWERS

64. a. **65.** a. **66.** b. **67.** b. **68.** b. **69.** b. **70.** c. **71.** a.

72. A teenager reports with neck swelling in the posterior triangle of neck for 3-weeks duration. On examination, she is noted to have upper motor neuron (UMN) signs in all the four limbs. Her MRI is most likely to reveal:

a. Lipoma of neck with intradural extension
b. Dumbell neurofibroma
c. Osteoma from C_2 vertebra
d. Meningioma

Ref. Child's Nervous System 2011;27(9): 1503-6

73. A 6 months old child is noticed to have pus discharge from a puncture wound near the occiput. Contrast MRI done shows cerebellar abscess communicating via a track to the exterior. The most likely diagnosis is:

a. Infected dermoid with cerebellar abscess
b. Spontaneous cerebellar abscess
c. Cerebellar abscess secondary to CSOM
d. Infected pilocytic astrocytoma

Ref. Pediatric Neurology, 2011;45(3):197-9

74. A 45-year-old male with an artificial pacemaker complains of neurogenic intermittent claudication of 6-months duration. He was advised myelogram which showed serpiginous filling defects in the conus-cauda region. The most likely diagnosis is:

a. AVM
b. Redundant cauda equina syndrome
c. Both 'a' and 'b'
d. None of the above

Ref. Greenberg, 4th/e, p225

75. Which of the following is/are the theories to explain slit ventricle syndrome?

a. Reduced compliance of brain
b. Craniocerebral disproportion
c. Venous hypertension
d. All the above

Ref. Thieme, 1st/e, p51-5

76. Which of the following is/are the procedures to deal with slit ventricle syndrome?

a. Subtemporal decompression
b. Change the shunt valve
c. Change the lower end
d. Endoscopic third ventriculostomy

Ref. Thieme, 1st/e, p51-5

77. All the following statements regarding frusemide are correct, except:

a. Frusemide decreases CSF production
b. Frusemide increases free water excretion
c. Frusemide induces hypo-osmolarity
d. Administered along with mannitol, it causes more sustained reduction in ICP

Ref. Neurosurgery Focus 2007;22(5):E-12

78. Which of the following scales is most commonly used for assessing the neurocognitive outcome in adults?

a. Vineland maturity scale
b. Wechsler intelligence scale
c. Malins scale
d. Binet-Kamat scale

Ref. Youmans, 5th/e, p5288

79. All the following regarding Pagets disease are true:

a. Both inner and outer tables are affected and there is widening of diploe
b. There are both lytic and blastic lesions
c. Radiology shows a cotton wool skull which consists of focal sclerosis within previous areas of osteoporosis circumscripta
d. There is no chance of transformation into giant cell tumor

Ref. Osborn, Section 4, p38-9

80. Nerve injuries secondary to injections:

a. Should be repaired as early as possible
b. Should be repaired if recovery does not take place within 3–4 months
c. Should never be repaired
d. None of the above

Ref. Youmans, 5th/e, p3974-5

ANSWERS

72. b. **73.** a. **74.** c. **75.** d. **76.** d. **77.** c. **78.** b. **79.** d. **80.** b.

81. All the following about Guillain-Barre syndrome are true, except:

a. It is an axonal polyneuropathy

b. Parasthesias, numbness and ascending weakness are the classical features

c. Usually the disease is preceded by a viral respiratory or gastrointestinal disease

d. CSF protein is elevated

Ref. Adams, 7th/e, p1380-3

82. All the following statements about radiosurgery are correct, except:

a. In LINAC, X-rays are generated by Compton scattering and in Gamma knife these are generated by Bremsstrahlung

b. Cobalt-60 is the source of radiation in Gamma knife

c. LINAC delivers its maximum dose deeper than Gamma knife

d. Gamma knife radiosurgery cannot be delivered to the spinal tumors in general while as such locations are amenable to LINAC

Ref. Schmidek and Sweet, 4th/e, p657-9

83. Which of the following tumors is amenable for intracavitary brachytherapy?

a. Solid craniopharyngioma

b. Cystic low grade glioma

c. Solid high grade glioma

d. None of the above

Ref. Schmdek and Sweet, 4th/e, p707-9

84. Which of the following statements regarding post-traumatic facial nerve palsy is correct?

a. It is common with longitudinal fractures of the petrous temporal bone and pregeniculate segment is commonly involved

b. It is common with transverse fractures of the temporal bone and pregeniculate segment is commonly involved

c. It is common with longitudinal fractures of the temporal bone and postgeniculate segment is commonly involved

d. None of the above

Ref. Youmans, 5th/e, p5273-5

85. Which of the following neurocognitive tests assesses the executive functions?

a. California verbal learning test

b. Stroop color and word test

c. Benton visual retention test

d. None of the above

Ref. Youmans, 5th/e, p5288-9

86. The best statistical test to detect sensitivity and specificity is:

a. Bland-Altman nomogram

b. Box-Whisker plot

c. Chi-square test

d. ROC analysis

Ref. www.medcal.com

87. For the definitions of non-traumatic persistent and permanent vegetative states, the time interval should be at least:

a. 1 and 3 months respectively

b. 1 and 12 months respectively

c. 3 and 6 months respectively

d. 3 and 12 months respectively

Ref. Youmans, 5th/e, p284

88. All the following statements regarding CNS germinoma are true except:

a. There is mild heterogenous enhancement

b. CSF seedlings may be diagnosed by contrast MRI which reveals a sugar coated appearance

c. Diffusion weighted MRI shows restricted diffusion

d. Pineal region is the most favorite site for CNS germinoma

Ref. Osborn, Neoplasms and Tumor like lesions, p133

89. The average amount of cerebral blood at a given time is approximately:

a. 20 ml

b. 30 ml

c. 50 ml

d. 70 ml

Ref. Youmans, 5th/e, p1488-90

ANSWERS

81. a. **82.** a. **83.** b. **84.** b. **85.** b. **86.** d. **87.** a. **88.** a. **89.** c.

90. All the following surgical approaches are for clipping of Basilar top aneurysms, except:
a. Pterional craniotomy via extended lateral corridor (PAVEL)
b. Pterional approach
c. Sub-temporal approach
d. Retrosigmoid suboccipital approach

Ref. Youmans, 5th/e, p2041-53

91. Spinal stenosis and myelopathy is seen in all the following conditions, except:
a. Mucopolyssacharidosis
b. Achondroplasia
c. Autosomal polycystic kidney disease
d. Hurler's syndrome

Ref. Greenberg, 4th/e, p207

92. The criteria for spinal canal stenosis is a Pavlov ratio of:
a. Less than 1 b. Less than 1.5
c. Less than 2 d. Less than 2.5

Ref. Clinics in Orthopedic surgery 2009;1(1): 6-10

93. An acromegalic patient can have features of intermittent claudication because of:
a. Direct effect of GH on muscles of the limb
b. Spinal canal stenosis
c. Axonal degeneration because of direct effect of GH
d. None of the above

Ref. Schmidek and Sweet, 4th/e, p439

94. All the following are risk factors for aneurysm formation and rupture, except:
a. Hypertension
b. Smoking
c. Familial history
d. Radiation exposure

Ref. Neurosurgery Clinics, p485-93

95. In which of the following causes of myelopathy, seizures also are seen?
a. Adrenoleukodystrophy
b. Lathyrism
c. Amyotrophic lateral sclerosis
d. Radiation induced myelopathy

Ref. Adams, 7th/e, p1034-5

96. All the following about spinal epidural abscess are correct, except:
a. The commonest organism isolated is Staphylococcus aureus
b. Cervical spine is the commonest location
c. Posterior location of the abscess is commoner
d. Treatment lies in urgent surgical decompression and antibiotic therapy

Ref. Greenberg, 4th/e, p644-6

97. Which of the following is/are true about steroid induced osteoporosis?
a. Steroids increase the activity of osteoclasts and decrease the activity of osteoblasts
b. Steroids decrease the absorption of calcium from gut
c. Steroids suppress testosterone
d. All the above

Ref. Youmans, 5th/e, p4235

98. All the following are true about Paget's disease of bone, except:
a. Both osteogenesis and bone resorption are accelerated
b. Only osteogenesis is accelerated and hence bone is thickened
c. There is increased secretion of hydroxyl-proline in urine
d. Mithramycin is one of the drugs for treatment

Ref. Youmans, 5th/e, p1399-400

99. A female patient complains of back pain and pain in the posterior aspect of thigh. Pain is worse in the morning and evenings. On examination, surprisingly she has no neuro-deficits. The most likely diagnosis is:
a. Myofascial syndrome
b. Neuropathic syndrome
c. Inflammatory syndrome
d. Hysteria

Ref. Youmans, 5th/e, p4330

ANSWERS

90. d. **91.** c. **92.** a. **93.** b. **94.** d. **95.** a. **96.** b. **97.** d. **98.** b. **99.** a.

100. The most common site of metastasis from hemangiopericytoma is:

a. Lung
b. Bone
c. Liver
d. Kidney

Ref. Youmans, 5th/e, p1137

101. Following statement describes the Adie pupil correctly:

a. Unilateral dilated pupil with response to near focus and no or minimal response to light
b. Unilateral constricted pupil with response to near focus and no or minimal response to light
c. Unilateral dilated pupil with response to light better than response to near focus
d. Unilateral constricted pupil with response to light better than response to near focus

Ref. Adams, 7th/e, p297

102. In which of the following conditions are the classical findings of vertigo fluctuating sensoneural deafness, tinnitus or poor speech discrimination noted?

a. Cerebellopontine angle arachnoid cyst
b. Meniere's disease
c. Vestibular schwannoma
d. Benign paroxysmal positional vertigo

Ref. Greenberg, 4th/e, p124

103. Swelling of the nasal mass on jugular venous compression to differentiate nasal polyp from encephalocele is known as:

a. Hitselberg sign
b. Furstenberg sign
c. Lemon sign
d. None of the above

Ref. Greenberg, 4th/e, p961

104. Cobweb fibrin clot in cerebrospinal fluid is usually seen in:

a. SAH
b. TBM
c. Pyogenic meningitis
d. Viral meningoencephalitis

Ref. Neurosurgery Quarterly 2011;21(4): 267-71

105. Endoscopic third ventriculostomy, a communication, is made from:

a. Third ventricle and 4th ventricle, bypassing the tumor
b. Lateral ventricles and 3rd ventricle
c. Third ventricle and prepontine cistern
d. Third ventricle and cisterna magna

Ref. Greenberg, 4th/e, p411

106. The postoperative surgical outcome in epilepsy is determined by:

a. Glasgow coma scale
b. Glasgow outcome scale
c. Engel's score
d. Modified Rankin scale

Ref. Medically Refractory Epilepsy, 1st/e, p25

107. All the following are true about temporal lobe epilepsy except:

a. Aura is a common phenomenon
b. Gets induced by hyperventilation
c. Responds well to carbamazepine
d. Mesial temporal sclerosis may be the underlying cause

Ref. Handbook of Epilepsy, p42-4

108. Which of the cranial nerve stimulation helps to control epilepsy?

a. II
b. VII
c. IX
d. X

Ref. Youmans, 5th/e, p2643-6

109. All the following procedures are done to control epilepsy except:

a. Amygdalohippocampectomy
b. Multiple subpial transections
c. Hemispherectomy
d. Deep brain stimulation

Ref. Youmans, 5th/e, p2565-72

ANSWERS

100. b. **101.** a. **102.** b. **103.** b. **104.** b. **105.** c. **106.** c. **107.** b. **108.** d. **109.** d.

110. The commonest MRI finding in complex partial seizures is:

a. Middle cerebral arteryaneurysm projecting into the temporal lobe
b. Hippocampal sclerosis
c. Tumors
d. Cavernomas

Ref. Handbook of Epilepsy, p43

111. All the following statements about complex partial seizures are true except:

a. In temporal lobe CPS aura is present, in extratemporal CPS it is absent
b. Automatism in temporal CPS is simple and stereotyped and in extratemporal CPS it is complex
c. Duration of a seizure in temporal lobe is very brief and in extratemporal, it lasts for 3–5 minutes
d. Seizure frequency in temporal CPS is 2–5/month and in extratemporal CPS it is 5–20/day

Ref. Handbook of Epilepsy, p42-4

112. All the following statements about complex partial seizure and absence seizures are true except:

a. CPS occurs at any age while as absence seizure usually occurs at 4–12 years
b. Duration of a seizure in CPS is about 3–5 minutes and in absence seizures, it is 5–10 minutes
c. Hyperventilation has no effect on CPS and it induces seizures in absence seizures
d. Interictal EEG in CPS shows focal spike and in absence seizure it is normal

Ref. Handbook of Epilepsy, p31-6, 42-4

113. The definition of intractable epilepsy is:

a. One seizure per month for a period of 5 years
b. One seizure per month for a period of 2 years
c. Two or more seizures per month for a period of 5 years
d. Two or more seizures per month for a period of 2 years

Ref. Medically Refractory Epilepsy, 1st/e, p2

114. Following are the candidates for anterior temporal lobectomy except:

a. Complex febrile seizures during childhood
b. Typical CPS of temporal semiology
c. MRI showing hippocampal sclerosis
d. Primary generalized epilepsy

Ref. Medically Refractory Epilepsy, 1st/e, p187-95

115. All the following statements about pseudoseizures are true except:

a. Prolactin levels are raised during the activity
b. Cyanosis during the ictus is unusual
c. Eyes are in closed position during the ictus
d. Duration of the episode is larger, usually minutes

Ref. Greenberg, 4th/e, p666

116. All the following statements about frontal lobe CPS are true except:

a. Usually occur when patient is awake
b. The episodes are brief
c. Semiology is stereotyped
d. Thrashing of legs during the episodes is common

Ref. Handbook of Epilepsy, p44-5

117. All the following changes on MRI suggest mesial temporal sclerosis except:

a. Atrophy of temporal horn of lateral ventricle
b. Atrophy of ipsilateral fornix
c. Blurred gray/white matter interface of temporal lobe
d. Atrophy of hippocampus/amygdala

Ref. Medically Refractory Epilepsy, 1st/e, p130-1

118. In all the following syndromes, seizure is a prominent feature except:

a. West syndrome
b. Lennox-Gastaut syndrome
c. Gorlin's syndrome
d. Landau-Kleffner syndrome

Ref. Handbook of Epilepsy, p93, p96-8

ANSWERS

110. b. **111.** c. **112.** b. **113.** d. **114.** d. **115.** a. **116.** a. **117.** a. **118.** c.

119. The most common cause of temporal complex partial seizure is:

a. Ganglioglioma
b. Dysembryoplastic neuroepithelial tumor (DNET)
c. Tuberculoma
d. Mesial temporal sclerosis

Ref. Handbook of Epilepsy, p43

120. All the following are features of acute disconnection syndrome except:

a. Mutism
b. Apraxia
c. Right hemineglect
d. Urge incontinence

Ref. Adams, 7th/e, p494-5

121. All the following are features of herpes encephalitis, except:

a. In children it is caused by HSV-1 and in adults by HSV-2
b. Medial temporal lobe and gyrus rectus are predominantly involved
c. There is evidence of restricted diffusion on DWI
d. MRS reveals increased choline peaks

Ref. Greenberg, 4th/e, p627-8

122. The term 'Nasal glioma' is:

a. Grade II astrocytoma in nose
b. Herniation of normal brain into the nose through a defect in the cribriform plate
c. Is a misnomer for inflamed nasal polyp
d. Is basically a neuroglial heterotopia

Ref. Greenberg, 4th/e, p961

123. Which of the following statements is/are true about cerebellar action tremors?

a. These are worsened by fatigue
b. These get improved by eye closure
c. Alcohol tends to worsen the tremors
d. All are correct

Ref. Movement Disorders, p453-4

124. All the following statements about vision are correct, except:

a. Papilledema does not cause loss of vision
b. Snell's chart is used for testing both near and distant visions
c. The common causes of visual deterioration lie in the eye itself
d. 'b' and 'c'

Ref. Bickerstaff, 6th/e, p38-49

125. Regarding the assessment of visual fields by direct confrontation method all the following are correctly mentioned, except:

a. The fields have to be checked in both eyes one by one and then simultaneously in both the eyes to differentiate between visual inattention from visual field defect
b. The object should be moved from field of vision towards the blind area because it is easier to detect disappearances than appearances of objects
c. The examiner and the patient should face each other at same height and when examiner covers the left eye the patient shall cover the right eye
d. None of the above

Ref. Bickerstaff, 6th/e, p38-50

126. The commonest cranial nerve involved in tubercular meningitis after optic nerve involvement is:

a. Oculomotor nerve
b. Trochlear nerve
c. Olfactory nerve
d. Vestibulocochlear nerve

Ref. Zuger A, Lowy FD. Tuberculosis. In: Scheld WM, Whitley RJ, Durack T, eds. Infections of the Central Nervous System. 2nd ed. Philadelphia: Lippincott-Raven;1997:417-43

127. The worried appearance in Parkinsonism plus syndromes is because of contraction of:

a. Frontalis
b. Procerus
c. Orbicularis oris
d. Masseter

Ref. Movement Disorders, p235

128. Which lobar involvement causes applause sign?

a. Frontal lobe
b. Temporal lobe
c. Parietal lobe
d. Occipital lobe

Ref. Movement Disorder, p236

Miscellaneous (MCQs)

ANSWERS

119. d. **120.** c. **121.** a. **122.** d. **123.** d. **124.** b. **125.** b. **126.** a. **127.** b. **128.** a.

129. Which type of gait is seen in Parkinsons disease?

a. Festinant
b. Marche a petit pas
c. Freezing
d. All the above

Ref. Movement Disorders, p79-85

130. A heavy meal of oral glucose shall reduce blood pressure in:

a. Parkinsons disease
b. Multisystem atrophy
c. Maple syrup urine disease
d. Diencephalic epilepsy

Ref. Movement Disorders, p243

131. In all the conditions ubiquitin gets accumulated in brain except:

a. Alzheimers disease
b. Picks disease
c. Creutzfeldt-Jacobs disease
d. Frontotemporal dementia

Ref. Movement Disorders, p239

132. All the following statements about peripheral vertigo are true except:

a. It always has a 5–10 second latent period
b. It rapidly fatigues and does not recur on repeated movement
c. Vomiting is usual
d. It is usually self-limited

Ref. Movement Disorders, p319-21

133. The commonest organisms incriminated in mycotic aneurysms is:

a. Streptococcus
b. Staphylococcus
c. Pseudomonas
d. Klebsiella

Ref. Neurosurgery Clinics, p579

134. All the following statements are true regarding type of resection in craniopharyngioma except:

a. Seizures are common in radical excision
b. Long-term morbidity is common in radial excision
c. Immediate postoperative morbidity and mortality is common in radial resection
d. Radical excision is good for small tumors without involvement of the hypothalamus

Ref. Youmans, 5th/e, p1217-8

135. Other than folate deficiency which elementary deficiency is supposed to have a role in neural tube defects:

a. Molybedenum
b. Zirconium
c. Calcium

Ref. Youmans, 5th/e, p3217

136. A 2-month-old baby presents with seizures. MRI reveals hyperintense signals on both T_1-W and T_2-W images involving both the medial temporal lobes and cerebellum. He also has a nevus in the back. The most likely diagnosis is:

a. Intracranial metastasis from melanoma
b. Congenital nevus with subarachnoid bleed
c. Neurocutaneous melanosis
d. Ataxia telangectasia

Ref. AJNR 1995;16:603-6

137. A 40-year-adult female reports with an on and off headache. MRI shows bilateral subdural hygromas with tonsillar descent. Sulci are wide. Her CT myelogram shows a small dural rent in the lumbar area. This patient will respond best to:

a. Epidural blood patch
b. Burr hole drainage of subdural hygromas
c. Subduro-peritoneal shunts
d. Subpial resection of cerebellar tonsils

Ref. Greenberg, 4th/e, p9

138. A middle-aged male reports with abnormal body movements. MRI shows signal intensity changes in bilateral caudate head giving rise to a giant Panda appearance. His ophthalmologic examination will reveal:

a. Loss of red reflex
b. KF ring
c. Papilledema
d. Primary optic atrophy

Ref. Movement Disorders, p590-1

ANSWERS

129. d. **130.** b. **131.** c. **132.** c. **133.** a. **134.** b. **135.** b. **136.** c. **137.** a. **138.** b.

139. Out of the following causes of nonepileptic seizures, which one responds to antiseizure medication:

a. Episodic movement disorder
b. Syncope
c. Parasomnias
d. Transient global amnesia

Ref. Handbook of Epilepsy, p133-135

140. Normal descent of tonsils below foramen magnum is up to:

a. 3 mm
b. 5 mm
c. 7 mm
d. 8 mm

Ref. Youmans, 5th/e, p3347

141. Which of the following is usually not a feature of Chiari?

a. Herniation of brainstem and 4th ventricle through foramen magnum
b. Hydrocephalus
c. Neck pain
d. None of the above

Ref. Youmans, 5th/e, p3347-50

142. Which of the following Chiari malformations is usually incompatible with life?

a. Chiari 1
b. Chiari 1.5
c. Chiari 2
d. Chiari 3

Ref. Greenberg, 4th/e, p79

143. In which of the following conditions, probst bundles are seen?

a. Dandy Walker malformation
b. Agenesis of corpus callosum
c. Holoprosencephaly
d. Spinal dysraphism

Ref. Greenberg, 4th/e, p84

144. In tethered cord syndrome, the filum is:

a. < 2 mm thick
b. > 2 mm thick
c. > 5 mm thick
d. > 6 mm thick

Ref. Greenberg, 4th/e, p93

145. All the mentioned features distinguish filum terminale from nerve roots intraoperatively except:

a. Filum terminale has ligamentous-like strands
b. Filum terminale is thicker than the nerve roots
c. Filum has whiter appearance
d. Filum has vessels on its surface

Ref. Schmidek and Sweet, 4th/e, p1898

146. The prevalence of neural tube defects is highest in:

a. American-Africans
b. American whites
c. Hispanics
d. Asians

Ref. Youmans, 5th/e, p3217

147. The current definition of folate deficiency is:

a. Erythrocyte folate level less than 140 ng/ml
b. Erythrocyte folate levels <250 ng/ml
c. Serum folate level of <5 ng/ml
d. Serum folate level of <4 ng/ml

Ref. Youmans, 5th/e, p3218

148. All the following regarding neural tube defects (NTD's) are true except:

a. Obesity is not a risk factor for NTD's
b. The amniotic fluid alpha-fetoprotein (AFP) and acetyl-cholinesterase (ACh E) have high accuracy of diagnosing it
c. Folate deficiency is a high-risk factor
d. None of the above

Ref. Youmans, 5th/e, p3218-9

149. Lemon sign on cranial USG is:

a. Scalloping of frontal bones
b. Scalloping of parietal bones
c. Herniation of cerebellum below the foramen magnums
d. Loculation of CSF within the 4th ventricle

Ref. Youmans, 5th/e, p3349

ANSWERS

139. a. **140.** b. **141.** a. **142.** d. **143.** b. **144.** b. **145.** d. **146.** c. **147.** a. **148.** a. **149.** a.

150. The most common complication after myelomeningocele repair is:

a. Superficial wound dehiscence
b. Hydrocephalus
c. Respiratory difficulty
d. Sphincter disturbance

Ref. Schmidek and Sweet, 4th/e, p1904

151. At term, the normally developing spinal cord ends at:

a. L_1 vertebral level
b. L_2 vertebral level
c. L_3 vertebral level
d. L_4 vertebral level

Ref. Youmans, 5th/e, p3236

152. The tuft of hair at the back is usually associated with:

a. Diplomyelia
b. Diastematomyelia
c. Rachischisis
d. Meningocele-manque

Ref. Greenberg, 4th/e, p94

153. Split cord malformations are how many times more common in females than males:

a. Twice
b. Thrice
c. Four times
d. Six times

Ref. Youmans, 5th/e, p3268

154. The triad of Dandy-Walker syndrome is, dilatation of 4th ventricle, agenesis of vermis and

a. Herniation of tonsil
b. Supratentorial hydrocephalus
c. Platybasia
d. Meningocele

Ref. Youmans, 5th/e, p3285-6

155. Which of the following cystic lesions causes bobbing movements of the head?

a. Sylvian fissure arachnoid cysts
b. Suprasellar arachnoid cysts
c. Cysts of the frontal lobe
d. Pontine cysts

Ref. Youmans, 5th/e, p3294

156. All the following about primary vein of Galen aneurysm are true except:

a. It is dilatation of vein of Galen secondary to parenchymal AVM's
b. Can result in cardiac failure
c. Can result in hydrocephalus
d. Can result in spasticity of the limbs

Ref. Youmans, 5th/e, p3434

157. All the following statements about arachnoid cysts are correct except:

a. These cysts occur both in children and adults
b. All the subtypes of arachnoid cysts are commoner in males
c. The arachnoid cyst wall may sometimes contain bits of choroids plexus
d. The symptomatic cysts are best treated by endoscopic procedures

Ref. Youmans, 5th/e, p3289-96

158. A child with anal atresia, renal anomalies and absent sacrum fits best into the diagnosis of:

a. Anorectal malformation
b. VATER group of anomalies
c. Caudal regression syndrome
d. Scimitar sacrum

Ref. Youmans, 5th/e, p4317

159. The apparent viscosity of blood falls as vessel diameter reduces. This effect is known as:

a. Cushing effect
b. Fahraeu's effect
c. Fogging effect
d. None of the above

Ref. Youmans, 5th/e, p1468

160. Which of the following statements about CSF formation is/are true?

a. Formation of CSF occurs by ultrafiltration of plasma
b. Formation is by active transport of sodium and bicarbonate
c. Formation rate is about 0.35 ml/min
d. All are true

Ref. Greenberg, 4th/e, p98

ANSWERS

150. a. **151.** c. **152.** b. **153.** b. **154.** b. **155.** b. **156.** a. **157.** b. **158.** c. **159.** b. **160.** d.

161. All the following are true about normal pressure hydrocephalus except:
a. About 60% of cases have no known etiology
b. NPH is seen following head injury, subarachnoid bleed
c. ICP monitoring reveals increasing number of 'A' waves
d. Dementia, gait apraxia and urinary incontinence are the cardinal symptoms of this entity

Ref. Greenberg, 4th/e, p592-3

162. All the following statements about normal pressure hydrocephalus (NPH) are true except:
a. Prognosis for dementia is better for patients with NPH of known etiology
b. Cerebral blood flow is low in patients with NPH
c. After CSF diversion, the cerebral blood flow improves in all the patients
d. Prognosis for dementia is better for patients with small sulci

Ref. Greenberg, 4th/e, p592-5

163. Neurofibrillary tangles are seen in all the following conditions except:
a. Pick's disease
b. Post head injury
c. Alzheimer's disease
d. Progressive supranuclear palsy

Ref. Greenberg, 4th/e, p3

164. Which of the following cranial nerves give rise to schwannomas?
a. Oculomotor b. Trochlear
c. Trigeminal d. All the above

Ref. Youmans, 5th/e, p1147-64, p1344-6

165. The commonest site of meningioma is:
a. Skull base b. Convexity
c. Sphenoid ridge d. Intraventricular

Ref. Youmans, 5th/e, p1111

166. All the following conditions are associated with pseudotumor cerebri except:
a. Hypervitaminosis
b. Addison's disease
c. Malnutrition
d. Pregnancy

Ref. Youmans, 5th/e, p1419-26

167. The cerebral metabolic rate of oxygen in human brain is:
a. 2.3 mg/100 g of brain/minute
b. 3.3 mg/100 g of brain/minute
c. 4.3 mg/100 g of brain/minute
d. 5.5 mg/100 g of brain/minute

Ref. Youmans, 5th/e, p5048

168. The normal value of pressure-volume-index (PVI) is:
a. 5–10 ml b. 10–15 ml
c. 25–30 ml d. 35–50 ml

Ref. Youmans, 5th/e, p5054

169. With a bolus of intravenous mannitol, the following changes occur:
a. Cerebral blood volume (CBV) decreases and cerebral blood flow (CBF) increases
b. CBV increases and CBF decreases
c. CBV decreases and CBF increases
d. None of the above

Ref. Youmans, 5th/e, p5058

170. Definition of absolute hyperemia in case of traumatic brain injury is:
a. Cerebral blood flow > 35 ml/100 g of brain/minute
b. CBF >55 ml/100 g of brain/minute
c. CBF >75 ml/100 g of brain/minute
d. CBF >100 ml/100 g of brain/minute

Ref. Youmans, 5th/e, p5051

171. Which of the following conditions is/are bad prognostic factors in a head injury patient?
a. Systolic BP of 70 mm Hg
b. PaO_2 of 50 mm Hg
c. Pyrexia
d. All the above

Ref. Youmans, 5th/e, p5113-5

ANSWERS

161. c. **162.** c. **163.** a. **164.** d. **165.** b. **166.** c. **167.** b. **168.** c. **169.** a. **170.** b. **171.** a.

172. After 6th cranial nerve, which is the most common cranial nerve to get involved in head injury:

a. Oculomotor nerve b. Facial nerve
c. Vestibulocochlear d. Vagus nerve

Ref. Facta Universitatis, Medicine and Biology series 2003;10(3):145-7

173. After head injury, perilymph fistula exists via

a. Round window b. Oval window
c. a and b d. Utricle

Ref. Youmans, 5th/e, p2904

174. Injury to fornix during resection of 3rd ventricular colloid cyst causes:

a. Seizures b. Memory impairment
c. Hemialexia d. Mutism

Ref. Schmidek and Sweet, 4th/e, p856

175. The 5th wave in brainstem evoked audiometry is produced by:

a. Cochlear nucleus b. Olivary nucleus
c. Lateral lemniscus d. Inferior colliculus

Ref. Youmans, 5th/e, p335

176. The following skeletal deformities of camptocormia, head ptosis, striatal toe are seen in:

a. Parkinson's disease b. Multiple sclerosis
c. Steroid toxicity d. Nemaline myopathy

Ref. Movement Disorder, p83

177. Which of the following charts is used to test near vision?

a. Snell's chart b. Jager's chart
c. Hess's chart d. None of the above

Ref. Bickerstaff, 6th/e, p38-9

178. Which of the following statements about ptosis caused by oculomotor nerve lesion or due to sympathetic output lesion is correct?

a. In ptosis caused by third nerve lesion the pupil also is dilated but in the latter, size of the pupil is unaffected
b. In ptosis caused by third nerve lesion or sympathetic nerve lesion even a voluntary attempt cannot correct ptosis
c. In the former the forehead shall show permanent wrinkling while in the latter it is not seen
d. None of the above

Ref. Patten, 2nd/e, p12-3

179. Which of the following statements about Horners syndrome is correct?

a. It is a caused by lesion in the superior cervical ganglion
b. It can also be seen during migraine
c. Cocaine does not dilate the pupil in Horners syndrome
d. All the above are correct

Ref. Patten, 2nd/e, p12-3

180. All the following statements about optokinetic nystagmus are true, except:

a. It is a normal physiologic response
b. The response is absent in temporal lobe lesions
c. It is absent in brainstem lesions also
d. It can detect vision in patients who feign blindness

Ref. Patten, 2nd/e, p21

181. The weakness in the muscles secondary to pyramidal tract lesions occur mostly in:

a. Abductors and extensors of the upper limbs and flexors of the lower limb
b. Adductors and extensors of the upper limbs and flexors of the lower limbs
c. Abductors and extensors of upper limbs and extensors of the lower limbs
d. Adductors and flexors of the upper limbs and flexors of the lower limbs

Ref. Bickerstaff, 6th/e, p146

182. The cerebral metabolic rate of glucose and oxygen are:

a. 25–30 μmol/100g/min and 150–160 μmol/100g/min respectively
b. 40–50 μmol/100g/min and 250–350 μmol/100g/min respectively
c. 50–70 μmol/100g/min and 350–400 μmol/100g/min respectively
d. None of the above

Ref. Youman's p1479

ANSWERS

172. b. **173.** c. **174.** b. **175.** d. **176.** a. **177.** b. **178.** c. **179.** d. **180.** b. **181.** a. **182.** a.

183. The cerebral blood flow below which there is electrocerebral silence is:

a. 10 ml/100 g/min b. 18 ml/100 g/min
c. 25 ml/100 g/min d. 33 ml/100 g/min

Ref. Youman's p1515

184. During awake craniotomy speech area is stimulated by a current of 5 mA and motor area is stimulated by a current of:

a. 10 mA b. 20 mA
c. 5 mA d. 2.5 mA

Ref. JNS 2013;118:243-49

185. Which agent has recently shown presence as a very good anticonvulsant especially for medically refractory epilepsy like Dravet syndrome?

a. Marijuana b. Clobazam
c. Valproic acid d. Levetiracetam

Ref. Neurosurgery 2015;76(4):357-61

186. The average lag time between neural injury and electrophysiological alert during somatosensory evoked potential monitoring is:

a. 2 min b. 5 min
c. 10 min d. 15 min

Ref. Neurosurgery Focus 2012;33(5):E10

187. Which of the following statements regarding type of suture involved and characteristic headshape is a mismatch?

a. Sagittal suture – scapohcephaly
b. Bicoronal – anterior plagiocephaly
c. Metopic – trigonocephaly
d. Sagittal plus metopic – scaphocephaly

Ref. Youman's p3305

188. All the following are causes of secondary craniostenosis except:

a. Hyperthyroidism b. Hyperparathyroidism
c. Thalassemia d. Polycythemia vera

Ref. AJR 1970;109, 2, 277

189. In which of the following postoperative conditions hypertrophic-olivary-degeneration is seen?

a. Endoscopic third ventriculostomy
b. Basilar top aneurysm clipping
c. Brainstem cavernoma
d. None of the above

Ref. Neurosurgery 2013;72(4):573-89

190. The triangle of Guillain-Mollaret triangle is formed by:

a. Fastigial nucleus, inferior olivary nucleus, substantia nigra
b. Dentate nucleus, red nucleus, inferior olivary nucleus
c. Inferior olivary nucleus, red nucleus, posteromedial nucleus of thalamus
d. Ventromedial nucleus of thalamus, caudate nucleus, dentate nucleus

Ref. AJNR 2014;35:792-802

191. Hypertrophic olivary degeneration is seen in all the following conditions except:

a. Trauma b. Tumors
c. Demyelination
d. Rapid correlation of hyponatremia

Ref. Neurosurgery 2013;72(4):573-89

192. Which four criteria depict idiopathic intracranial hypertension?

a. Raised ICP, papilledema, normal CSF, abnormal CT brain
b. Raised ICP, papilledema, abnormal CSF, normal CT brain
c. Raised ICP, papilledema, normal CSF, normal CT brain
d. Raised ICP, optic atrophy, abnormal CSF, normal CT brain

Ref. Neurosurgery 2004;54(3):538-52

193. All the following statement are true about infantile Krabbe disease except:

a. Also known as globoid cells leukodystrophy
b. Autosomal dominant disorder involving chromosome-14
c. The toxic metabolite is psychosine
d. There is apoptosis of myelin-forming cells

Ref. AJNR, Feb. 13, 2014

ANSWERS

183. b. **184.** a. **185.** a. **186.** d. **187.** b. **188.** b. **189.** c. **190.** b. **191.** d. **192.** c. **193.** b.

194. All the following statements about adrenomyeloneuropathy are correct except:

a. It is an adult variant of x-linked adrenoleukodystrophy
b. There is ABCD-1 gene mutation
c. There is depletion of very long chain fatty acids and demyelination
d. Spinal cord is atrophic

Ref. AJNR, Feb. 6, 2014

195. All the following statements regarding Meckel cave meningoceles are correct except:

a. These develop secondary to congenital or acquired herniation of posterolateral wall of Meckel's cave into petrous apex
b. Most commonly present as CSF leak
c. Imaging reveals expansion of the petrous apex
d. Non-enhancing on PET scan

Ref. AJNR, Jan. 30, 2014

196. All the following statements about paraneoplastic polyneuropathy are correct except:

a. It is a form of predominantly distal, symmetrical sensory or sensorimotor polyneuropathy
b. Anti-HV antibody is usually associated with small cell cancer of the lung
c. Cerebellar degeneration also can occur as part of paraneoplastic syndrome
d. The overall prognosis however is good

Ref. Adams, p1392-93

197. All the following statements about malignant hyperthermia are correct, except:

a. It occurs after halothane anesthesia
b. Masseter spasm is the first indication of this entity
c. All the muscles except masseter become lax
d. Intravenous dantrolene is life saving

Ref. Adams, p1563

198. Which of the anti-neoplastic agents causes progressive symmetrical neuropathy:

a. Procarbazine b. Vincristine
c. L-asparaginase d. 5-FU

Ref. Adams, p1283-84

199. All the following statements about lead encephalopathy are true except:

a. CSF pressure is high
b. Glucose levels in CSF are low
c. Protein levels are increased
d. None of the above

Ref. Adams, p1277

200. In which group of vitamin deficiencies, cerebellar ataxia is a common sign?

a. Thiamin, cobalamin, nicotinamide
b. Thiamin, pyridotine, folate
c. Cobalamin, nicotinamide, folate
d. Biotin, folate, nicotinamide

Ref. Adams, p1219

201. Which of the following substances is typified by the features of snorting, craving, beading of cerebral vessels, rhabdomyolysis, liver dysfunction?

a. Amphetamine b. Cocaine
c. Marijuana d. Lithium

Ref. Adams, p1269

202. All the following statements about Pick's disease are true except:

a. Cerebral degeneration involves only gray matter
b. There is atrophy of bilateral hippocampi
c. There may be ballooning of cortical neurons
d. The disease mostly involves frontal and temporal lobes

Ref. Adams, p1118

203. All the following statements about progressive supranuclear palsy are correct except:

a. It usually occurs in 6th decade
b. Patients develop supranuclear ophthalmoplegia, pseudobulbar palsy and axial dystonia
c. Patients also have a peculiar wide-eyed unblinking stare imparting an expression of perpetual surprise
d. Patient always lies in a stooped posture

Ref. Adams, p1139

ANSWERS

194. c. **195.** b. **196.** d. **197.** c. **198.** b. **199.** b. **200.** a. **201.** b. **202.** a. **203.** d.

204. All the following statements about Friedreich ataxia are true except:
a. It is a progressive spinocerebellar ataxia
b. It is supposed to be secondary to gene mutation on chromosome-6
c. The protein involved in this disorder is frataxin
d. Many of the patients die of cardiac arrhythmia
Ref. Adams, p1145

205. The anatomical substrates involved in Wallenberg's syndrome are following except:
a. Vestibular nuclei
b. Spinothalamic tract
c. Descending sympathetic tract
d. 2, 4, 6th cranial nerves
Ref. Adams, p844

206. All the following statements regarding punch-drunk syndrome are true except:
a. It is the cumulative effect of repeated cerebral injuries observed in boxers
b. Patients develop forgetfulness, slowness in thinking
c. Levy bodies are seen on autopsy
d. Purkinje's cells are lost and granular cell layer is thinned
Ref. Adams, p944-45

207. All the following statements about Shagreen patch are true except:
a. Shagreen patches are seen in tuberous sclerosis
b. These patches are mostly seen on thoracic region
c. It is a plaque of subepidermal fibrosis
d. It has an orange-peel appearance
Ref. Adams, p1071

208. In osmotic demyelination syndrome, the lesions occur in the following sites grouped together; which of the groups includes an erroneous site of involvement:
a. Pons, thalamus, subthalamic nuclei, internal capsule
b. Thalamus, internal capsule, lateral geniculate body
c. Midbrain, pons, muscle, deep layers of cerebral cortex
d. Muscle, pons, cerebellar nuclei, amygdaloid nuclei
Ref. Adams, p1193

209. The first symptom in Wilson's disease usually is:
a. Muscular rigidity
b. Tremor of the outstretched hands
c. Ataxia
d. Dementia
Ref. Adams, p1196

210. The classic triad of Wernicke-Korsakoff syndrome includes which of the following:
a. Ataxia, disturbed mentation, seizures
b. Ophthalmoplegia, ataxia, seizures
c. Disturbed mentation, seizures, ophthalmoplegia
d. Ophthalmoplegia, ataxia, disturbed mentation
Ref. Adams, p1207

211. All the following statements regarding amyotrophic lateral sclerosis are correct except:
a. Men are affected more frequently than women
b. The dorsal interosseous space becomes hallowed giving rise to the 'Cadaveric' or 'skeletal' hand
c. Sphincter control is lost early in the cause of the disease
d. Coarse fasciculations are usually evident in the weakened muscle
Ref. Adams, p1152-53

212. All the following statements regarding retinitis pigmentosa are correct except:
a. The disease affects only the pigment epithelium of the retina
b. Males are affected more commonly than females
c. Inheritance is more often autosomal recessive
d. As a result of gene abnormality of chromosome-3, the amount of opsin and rhodopsin is reduced
Ref. Adams, p1165

ANSWERS

204. b. **205.** d. **206.** c. **207.** b. **208.** d. **209.** b. **210.** d. **211.** c. **212.** a.

213. Following statements about deafness are true except:

a. Sensorineural deafness is characterized by a partial loss of perception of high pitched sounds
b. The features of cochlear type of hearing loss are recruitment and diplacusis
c. Since each cochlear nucleus is connected to both temporal lobes, hence lesion of a temporal lobe unlikely causes deafness
d. In sensorineural deafness, Rinne's test is negative in the affected ear

Ref. Adams, p306

214. Following statements about tinnitus are true except:

a. Tonal and non-tonal tinnitus refer to objective and subjective tinnitus
b. The tonal type is commoner than non-tonal tinnitus
c. Pseudotumor cerebri causes pulsatile tinnitus
d. Tinnitus in middle ear disease becomes severe at night

Ref. Adams, p308

215. All the following statements about seizures are correct except:

a. Fencer posture (tonic elevation and extension of the contralateral arm) is seen in temporal lobe lesions
b. This posture is seen in medial frontal lobe lesions
c. In visual seizures red is the most frequently reported color followed by blue
d. Postictal aphasia has a localizing value

Ref. Adams, p337-8

216. Which of the following statements about tussive and valsalva syncope are true?

a. The affected individuals are usually heavy-set males
b. The mechanism is that coughing increases ICP
c. Weight lifters black out is also attributable to it
d. All are true

Ref. Adams, p395

217. All the following statements about nocturnal epilepsy are true except:

a. These often occur in adults
b. Deprivation of sleep may induce seizure on the other hand
c. Seizures occur mainly in the stage-4 of NREM sleep
d. EEG recordings during sleep are most helpful to diagnose this disorder

Ref. Adams, p418-19

218. All the following statements regarding bacterial meningitis are true except:

a. Pneumococcal, H. influenza and meningococcal forms are the common pathogens
b. These pathogens are all inhabitants of nasopharynx
c. Onset of meningococcal is rapid and may be associated with rash or purpura
d. The spinal pressure is consistently low and raises the possibly that the patient is suffering from severe meningitis

Ref. Adams, p739-40

219. The phenomenon of gait disorder in frontal lobe disorder is called as:

a. Magnetic feet
b. Slipping clutch
c. Gait ignition failure
d. All the above

Ref. Adam, p128

220. Following statements about astasia-abasia are true except:

a. Patients tough unable to stand or walk display normal use of lower limbs while in bed
b. They usually have a normal neurological examination
c. It is nearly always a hysterical condition
d. It cannot be mimicked by vermian lesions

Ref. Adams, p131

ANSWERS

213. d. **214.** a. **215.** a. **216.** d. **217.** a. **218.** d. **219.** d. **220.** d.

221. Following statements are true about migraine except:

a. Crash migraine may lead a clinician think of subarachnoid bleed
b. The headache is always hemicranial
c. It may be accompanied by neurological deficit
d. Some elderly patients may have no or less headache but only neurologic abnormality (aura without migraine)

Ref. Adams, p183

222. Following statements about basilar migraine are true except:

a. Patients may have vertigo, staggering and incoordination of the limbs
b. Dysesthesia and tingling in both hands may be present
c. Headache is typically bitemporal
d. Symptoms last for 10-30 minutes usually

Ref. Adams, p183

223. Reproduction of pain along sciatic nerve distribution on coughing, or compressing both jugular veins is:

a. Neri sign
b. Naffziger sign
c. Bragard sign
d. Sicard sign

Ref. Adams, p214

224. The following statements about myofascial pain syndrome are true except:

a. The pain is localized to certain patients in skeletal muscles
b. Ill defined tender nodules can be felt in the muscle tissue
c. Most of the patients are sedentary women
d. Relief is given by excision of the tender nodules

Ref. Adams, p231

225. Following statements about pendular nystagmus are true except:

a. Pendular nystagmus is more common than jerk
b. Pendular nystagmus occurs in albinos
c. It is always binocular and in one plane
d. Spasmus nutans is a type of pendular nystagmus and is accompanied by head nodding

Ref. Adams, p290

ANSWERS

221. b. **222.** c. **223.** b. **224.** d. **225.** a.

EXPLANATION

1. Cr. N. III palsy with contralateral hemiparesis (no sensory loss). Third nerve palsies from parenchymal lesions may be relatively pupil sparing. Usually due to occlusion of interpeduncular branch of basilar artery: -central midbrain infarction, disrupting cerebral peduncle and issuing fibers of CN III. May also be due to aneurysm of basilar bifurcation or BA·SCA junction.

2. Also called as oculocephalic response or reflex, provides similar information as oculovestibular reflex but poses a greater risk to the spinal cord if cervical spine is injured. In an awake patient the eyes will either move with the head or if the movement is slow enough and the patient is fixating on an object there will be a contraversive conjugate eye movement. In a comatose patient with an intact brainstem and cranial nerves there will also be contraversive conjugate eye movement (a positive dolls eye response). In brain dead patients it is absent.

3. When the medications fail to control the tremor, surgery should be considered. Stereotactic ablation of the ventral intermediate nucleus (Vim) of the thalamus used to be the preferred surgical procedure for control of essential tremor (ET), but has become obsolete with the advent of deep brain stimulation (DBS) of the thalamus. Thalamic DBS involves the placement of an electrode in the Vim nucleus. This electrode is connected to a wire, which is tunneled under the skin and attached to an implantable pulse generator located in the subcutaneous tissue overlying the pectoralis muscle. This pulse generator can then be switched on or off and programmed using a portable computer. The clinical effect of DBS is identical to that of ablation, but DBS holds an advantage over ablation in that turning the stimulator off can reverse its effects. Thalamic stimulation can also be performed bilaterally with fewer side effects than thalamotomy.

4. Over time, the drugs used for the treatment of trigeminal neuralgia (TN) often lose effectiveness. For patients in whom medical therapy has failed, surgery is a viable and effective option. Around 25–50% of patients eventually stop responding to drug therapy and require some form of alternative treatment. Three operative strategies now prevail: percutaneous procedures, gamma knife surgery (GSK), and microvascular decompression (MVD). Ninety percent of patients are pain-free immediately or soon after any of the operations, although the relief is much more long-lasting with microvascular decompression. Percutaneous surgeries make sense for older patients with medically unresponsive trigeminal neuralgia. Younger patients and those expected to do well under general anesthesia should first consider microvascular decompression—presently, this is the most cost-effective surgery although it is also more invasive.

Pain-free intervals after percutaneous procedures (percutaneous retrogasserian glycerol rhizotomy [PRGR] and percutaneous balloon microcompression [PBM]) last 1.5–2 years, 3–4 years after another (percutaneous radiofrequency trigeminal gangliolysis [PRTG]), and 15 years commonly after microvascular decompression. Those in whom the first percutaneous procedure fails may undergo a repeat procedure, which usually provides relief. More recently, however, posterior fossa exploration has frequently revealed some structural cause for neuralgia (despite normal findings on computed tomography [CT] scans, magnetic resonance images [MRI], or arteriograms), such as an anomalous artery or vein impinging on the trigeminal nerve root. In such cases, simple decompression and separation of the anomalous vessel from the nerve root produces lasting relief of symptoms. In elderly patients with limited life expectancy, radiofrequency rhizotomy is sometimes preferred, as it is easy to perform, has few complications, and provides symptomatic relief for a considerable period.

5. 2% of patients with multiple sclerosis have trigeminal neuralgia whereas 18% of patients with bilateral trigeminal neuralgia have multiple sclerosis.

8. Gerstmann syndrome is characterized by four primary symptoms:

1. **Dysgraphia/agraphia:** deficiency in the ability to write
2. **Dyscalculia/acalculia:** difficulty in learning or comprehending mathematics
3. **Finger agnosia:** inability to distinguish the fingers on the hand
4. Left-right disorientation

This disorder is often associated with brain lesions in the dominant (usually left) hemisphere including the angular gyrus near the temporal and parietal lobe junction. The angular gyrus is generally involved in translating visual patterns of letter and words into meaningful information, such as is done while reading. In adults, the syndrome may occur after stroke or in association with damage to the parietal lobe. In addition to exhibiting the above symptoms, many adults also experience aphasia, which is a difficulty in expressing oneself when speaking, in understanding speech, or in reading and writing.

There are few reports of the syndrome, sometimes called developmental Gerstmann syndrome, in children. The cause is not known. Generally, children with the disorder exhibit poor handwriting and spelling skills, and difficulty with math functions, including adding, subtracting, multiplying, and dividing. An inability to differentiate right from left and to discriminate among individual fingers may also be apparent. In addition to the four primary symptoms, many children also suffer from constructional apraxia, an inability to copy simple drawings.

9. Lesions causing damage to the angular gyrus can give rise to a constellation of symptoms. The classic symptoms include Gerstmann's tetrad and behavioral manifestations such as depression, poor memory, frustration and belligerence. The angular gyrus, located in the left temporal lobe, is part of the language system of the brain, which also includes Broca's area and Wernicke's area; damage to the angular gyrus gives rise to alexia and agraphia. Even if the angular gyrus is spared, it can still be isolated by lesions immediately subcortical to it or by lesions involving the mesial part of the occipital cortex and the splenium of the corpus callosum, which will result in alexia and agraphia. Left angular gyrus is dominant for stereognosis bimanually.

10. Topographic memory involves the ability to orient oneself in space, to recognize and follow an itinerary, or to recognize familiar places. Getting lost when traveling alone is an example of the failure of topographic memory. Although loss of topographic memory is considered a parietal lobe syndrome, right medial temporoparietal lesions will be most common and may be in the territory of posterior cerebral artery. It can occur with unilateral stroke in either hemisphere.

11. Anton's syndrome is a condition where the patient is unaware of being blind and denies the problem even when it is pointed out to him. On the contrary, in cortical blindness patient is aware of his blindness and does not deny it. In both, bilateral lesions of the occipital lobes are seen. The ability to recognize visually presented objects and words depends on the integrity not only of the visual pathways and primary visual area of the cerebral cortex (area 17 of Brodmann) but also of those cortical areas that lie just anterior to area 17 that is areas 18 and 19 of the occipital lobe and area 39 - the angular gyrus of the dominant hemisphere (visual association areas). Bilateral infarction in the distal PCAs produces cortical blindness (blindness with preserved pupillary light reaction). The patient is often unaware of the blindness or may even deny it (Anton's syndrome). Tiny islands of vision may persist, and the patient may report that vision fluctuates as images are captured in the preserved portions. Rarely, only peripheral vision is lost and central vision is spared, resulting in 'gunbarrel' vision. Although cerebrovascular disease is the most common cause, surgery, particularly cardiac surgery and cerebral angiography are also major causes. The mode of recovery from cortical blindness can be phased through visual agnosia and partially impaired perceptual function to full recovery. Even with recovery, the patient may complain of visual fatigue (asthenopia) and difficulties in fixation and fusion.

Prosopagnosia (Greek: "prosopon" – "face", "agnosia" – "not knowing"), also called face blindness, is a cognitive disorder of face perception where the ability to recognize familiar faces, including your own face (self-recognition), is impaired, while other aspects of visual processing (e.g., object discrimination) and intellectual functioning (e.g., decision making) remain intact. The term originally referred to a condition following acute brain damage (acquired prosopagnosia), but a congenital or developmental form of the disorder also exists, which may affect up to 2.5% of the population. The specific brain area usually associated with prosopagnosia is the fusiform gyrus, which activates specifically in response to faces. Prosopagnosia can be caused by lesions in various parts of the inferior occipital areas (occipital face area), fusiform gyrus (fusiform face area), and the anterior temporal cortex.

12. Expressive aphasia (non-fluent aphasia) is characterized by the loss of the ability to produce language (spoken or written). It is one subset of a larger family of disorders known collectively as aphasia. Expressive aphasia differs from dysarthria, which is typified by a patient's inability to properly move the muscles of the tongue and mouth to produce speech. Expressive aphasia also differs from apraxia of speech which is a motor disorder characterized by an inability to create and sequence motor plans for speech. Comprehension is typically only mildly to moderately impaired in expressive aphasia. This contrasts with receptive aphasia, which is distinguished by a patient's inability to comprehend language or speak with appropriately meaningful words. Expressive aphasia is also known as Broca's aphasia in clinical neuropsychology and agrammatic aphasia in cognitive neuropsychology and is caused by acquired damage to the anterior regions of the brain, including (but not limited to) the left posterior inferior frontal gyrus or inferior frontal operculum, also described as Broca's area (Brodmann area 44 and Brodmann area 45) Expressive aphasia is also a symptom of some migraine attacks.

Sufferers of this form of aphasia exhibit the common problem of agrammatism. For them, speech is difficult to initiate, non-fluent, labored, and halting. Writing is difficult, as well. Intonation and stress patterns are deficient. Language is reduced to disjointed words, and sentence construction is poor, omitting function words and inflections (bound morphemes). While, in general, word comprehension is preserved, meaning interpretation dependent on syntax and phrase structure is substantially impaired. This can be demonstrated by using phrases with unusual structures.

13. Conduction aphasia, also called associative aphasia, is a relatively rare form of aphasia. An acquired language disorder, it is characterized by intact auditory comprehension, fluent (yet paraphasic) speech production, but poor speech repetition. They are fully capable of understanding what they are hearing, but show significant difficulty in repeating phrases, particularly as the phrases increase in length and complexity and as they stumble over words they are attempting to pronounce. Patients will display frequent errors during spontaneous speech, such as substituting or transposing sounds. They will also be aware of their errors, and will show significant difficulty correcting them. Typical lesion location for conduction aphasia is on the supramarginal gyrus of the parietal lobe, posterior to the primary sensory cortex and just above Wernicke's area. The classical explanation for conduction aphasia is that of a disconnection between the brain areas responsible for speech comprehension (Wernicke's area) and speech production (Broca's area), due specifically to damage to the arcuate fasciculus, a deep white matter tract. Recent research has challenged this notion on the basis that patients with conduction aphasia more often have lesions in the supramarginal gyrus or deep parietal matter. However, conduction aphasia remains a controversial topic from the understanding of its neurologic foundations.

Conduction aphasics will show relatively well-preserved auditory comprehension, which may even be completely functional. Spontaneous speech production will be fluent and generally grammatically and syntactically correct. Intonation and articulation will also be preserved. Speech will often contain paraphasic errors: phonemes and syllables will be dropped or transposed (e.g., "snowball" → "snowall", "television" → "vellitision", "ninety-five percent" → "ninety-twenty percent"). The hallmark deficit of this disorder, however, is in repetition. Patients will show a marked inability to repeat words or sentences when prompted by an examiner. When prompted to repeat words, patients will be unable to do so, and produce many paraphasic errors. Oral reading can also be poor. Patients recognize their paraphasias and errors and will try to correct them, with multiple attempts often necessary for success. Error sequences frequently share one or more similarly located phonemes but differ in at least one aspect that makes the substituted morpheme(s) semantically distinct.

Symptoms of conduction aphasia, as with other aphasias, can be transient, lasting only several hours or a few days. As aphasias and other language disorders are frequently due to stroke, their symptoms can change and evolve over time, or simply disappear. This is due to healing in the brain after inflammation or hemorrhage, which leads to decreased local impairment. Furthermore, plastic changes in the brain may lead to the recruitment of new pathways to restore lost function. However, chronic conduction aphasia is possible, without transformation to other aphasias.

14. Although much has been written on the subject of tactile agnosia since the time of the classical description by Dejerine, "syndrome sensitif cortical", some authors have pointed out that the underlying failure in tactile agnosia is mainly impaired perception of microgeometrical properties (such as textures) of objects due to lesions in the primary sensory cortex (SI) and that macrogeometrical properties (such as shape and size) are recognized in the secondary somatosensory area (SII) and the posterior parietal cortex in a parallel processing fashion. The site of lesion is in contralateral supramarginal gyrus. It is possible that left sided agnosia in a right handed person may also be caused by a lesion of the corpus callosum.

15. Alexia is defined as loss of reading ability in a previously literate person due to an acquired brain lesion. Alexia without agraphia (pure alexia) results from a lesion in the left occipital lobe and adjacent splenium (posterior corpus callosum) that disconnects visual input from language areas, first described by Dejerine. The most common pathological process is usually an infarction in the territory of the posterior cerebral artery (PCA) due to occlusion by thrombi or emboli, although PCA compression during tentorial herniation and space occupying lesion may also cause this syndrome.

In the classic syndrome of pure alexia without agraphia, patients can write but cannot read their own writing; speech, auditory comprehension, and repetition are normal. Naming deficit, especially for colors, may be present. Associated defiits include a right hemianopia and frequently, a deficit of short-term memory. The classic syndrome of pure alexia without agraphia is caused by lesion in left occipital cortex and posterior sector of the corpus callosum- (the splenium), thus interrupting the flow of visual input into the language network. There is usually a right hemianopia, but the core language network remains unaffected. Pure alexia may or may not be associated with color naming and visual object agnosia.

16. Major PCA stroke syndromes

The major posterior cerebral artery (PCA) stroke syndromes (many of which occur concomitantly) include the following:

- Paramedian thalamic infarction
- Visual field loss
- Visual agnosia
- Balint syndrome
- Prosopagnosia
- Palinopsia, micropsia, and macropsia
- Disorders of reading
- Disorders of color vision
- Memory impairment
- Motor dysfunction

Visual field loss

Unilateral infarction produces homonymous hemianopia. Sparing of the macula is encountered frequently in infarction of the occipital lobes due to PCA occlusion. Macular sparing may be caused by collateral vascular supply to the macular region or by the very large macular representation in the occipital cortex; additionally, bilateral representation of macular vision has been suspected.

Bilateral infarctions of the occipital lobes produce varying degrees of cortical blindness depending on the extent of the lesion. Patients often exhibit Anton syndrome, a state in which they fervently believe they can see when they cannot. Patients may describe objects that they have not seen previously in exquisite detail, completely in error and oblivious to that error. Another intriguing phenomenon is blind sight. Although cortically blind, patients can respond to movement or sudden lightening or darkening of their environment.

Infarction of the lateral geniculate nucleus may produce hemianopia, quadrantanopia, or sectoranopia. The vascular supply is dual; the anterior choroidal artery supplies the anterior hilum and anterolateral areas, and the posterior choroidal artery supplies the rest. Occlusion of the posterior choroidal artery may produce a distinct syndrome of hemianopia, hemidysesthesia, and memory disturbance due to infarction of the lateral geniculate, fornix, dorsomedial thalamic nucleus, and posterior pulvinar.

19. A term referring to a brain with narrowed gyri and widened sulci which is seen in extreme frontal and temporal lobe atrophy, with relative sparing of the posterior brain. The finding is characteristic of Pick's disease and has been fancifully likened to the appearance of a walnut; asatrophy evolves, compensatory ventricular enlargement—ex vacuo hydrocephalus—occurs

21. When many RBCs and WBCs are present in the CSF due to a traumatic tap, It may be important to tell if the WBC are elevated or if they are present in the same ratio as in the peripheral blood. In non-anemic patients, there should be 1–2 WBCs for every 1000 RBC. (as a correction subtract 1 WBC for every 700 RBCs). In the presence of anemia or peripheral leukocytosis use Fishman s formula.

$WBC_{CSF\ ORIGINAL} = WBC_{CSF} - WBC_{Blood} \times RBC_{CSF}/RBC_{Blood}$

22. Microvascular decompression in trigeminal neuralgia is an effective treatment method. The favorable long-term impact of MVD in TN ranges from 69%. The general morbidity, such as hearing loss, and sensory disorders in the trigeminal distribution varies between 0.2 and 4.5%. The aim of the operation is to remove the suspected compression of the nerve by a loop of an artery (sometimes a vein) near the brain stem, usually superior cerebellar artery (SCA). Usually the arachnoid surrounds the facial and vestibulocochlear nerve; these cranial nerves should not be detached. The whole area around the trigeminal nerve is then inspected. Usually at the front of the nerve an artery loop is to be found—the SCA. This is mobilized and positioned in a new place and separated from trigeminal nerve by Teflon. This is done so that there is minimal or no contact with the nerve.

As a complication hearing loss or reduced hearing may occur (usually transient), for example, because the cranial nerve VIII has been compromised by the release of the trigeminal nerve decompression. Other risks are bleeding and infection. Bleeding in this vital structures area means of course a serious complication. Cerebral spinal fluid leakage is also one of the possible complications. There are a number of factors which are strongly correlated with a good outcome of TN after MVD. These factors include age, gender, and the type of compression. Venous compression correlates with a worse outcome. Previous procedures done for TN are not a contraindication for MVD, instead these are the patients who benefit from MVD.

24. Expression of a number of steroid hormone and growth factor receptors is characteristic of meningiomas. Analysis of receptors for progesterone, estrogen, androgen and platelet derived growth factor (PDGF) in human meningioma tissue specimens have given positive results.

25. **Retrocochlear lesion:** VIII nerve dysfunction (typical with vestibular schwannoma), as opposed to cochlear lesions (dysfunction of the hearing end organ). Progressive unilateral or asymmetric sensorineural hearing loss of high tones occurs in >95% of VS. High frequency hearing loss is also the most common hearing loss with age or noise exposure but is usually symmetrical. An unexplained hearing difference from one ear to the other of> 10–15 dB on PTA is suspicious and should be investigated further.

26. Idiopathic Intracranial hypertension (IIH); also called as pseudotumor cerebri, also called as benign intracranial hypertension (plus numerous other obsolete terms) is a heterogeneous.

Group of conditions characterized by intracranial pressure with no evidence of intracranial mass, hydrocephalus, infection or hypertensive encephalopathy. Some but not all authors exclude patients with intracranial hypertension in the presence of dural sinus thrombosis. IIH is thus a diagnosis of exclusion. It has a juvenile form and an adult form.

29. Chassaignaie's tubercle... (anterior tubercle of transverse process of C6) also called as carotid tubercle (the most prominent in C spine) usually at the level of cricoid cartilage, approximately 1.5–2 inches above the clavicle.

30.
1. **Frazier's burr hole:** placed prophylactically before posterior fossa craniotomy for emergency ventrilculostomy in event of post-operative swelling. Location: 3–4 cm from midline, 6–7 cm above inion.
2. **Keen's point (posterior parietal):** (placement in trigone) 2.5–3 cm posterior and 2.5–3 cm superior to pinna.
3. **Dandy's point:** 2 cm from midline and 3 cm above inion (maybe more damaging to visual pathways than Frazier's point).
4. **Kocher's point:** places catheter in frontal horn. The right side is commonly used. Commonly employed for ICP monitors
   a. **Entry site:** 2–3 cm from midline which is approximately the mid pupillary line in forward gaze 1 cm anterior to coronal suture (to avoid motor strip)
   b. **Trajectory:** direct catheter perpendicular to surface of brain which can be approximated By aiming in coronal plane towards medial canthus of ipsilateral eye in AP plane towards external auditory meatus.
   c. **Insertion length:** advance catheter with stylet till CSF is obtained (should be <5–6 cm this may be 3–4 cm with markedly dilated ventricles). Advance catheter without stylet 1 cm deeper.

31. In TBM, a thick gelatinous exudate develops around the basal cisterns, the sylvian fissure and the brainstem. As this may cause obstruction to the outflow from the fourth ventricle or indeed from the cerebral aqueduct, hydrocephalus frequently develops in these children, and this further exacerbates the clinical condition by raising the intracranial pressure (ICP). The brain itself shows edema, perivascular infiltration with lymphocytes and mononuclear cells, and a microglial reaction. Indeed, a vasculitic-like syndrome may result, where inflammatory changes may be seen in the vessel wall, and the lumen of these vessels may be narrowed or even occluded by formation of the thrombi, and this may result in small areas of infarction. In the majority of patients, the location of the infarctions is in the distribution of the medial striate and thalamoperforating arteries. Rarely, hemorrhagic transformation of these infarcts may occur. It may not be out of place to point out that the ventriculomegaly that occurs in these patients is not always due to obstructive hydrocephalus, and hence associated with high ICP, but may be due to brain "softening". Some amount of non-obstructive hydrocephalus is present as well.

33. Neural tube defects (NTDs) remain an important yet potentially preventable cause of neonatal mortality. Dietary change and selective termination of affected pregnancies has resulted in severe NTDs rarely being seen in high-income countries. Periconceptional folic acid supplementation has a large effect on the occurrence of NTDs (70% reduction).

36. Pure Tone Audiogram (PTA) may be useful as a first step screening test. Air conduction assesses the entire system, bone conduction assesses from the cochlea and proximally. PTA assesses the functionality of hearing (to help in treatment decision making) and acts as a baseline for future comparision. The single numerical score is an average of the threshold for frequencies across the audio spectrum.

Speech Discrimination: maintained in conductive hearing loss, moderately impaired in cochlear hearing loss, poorest in retrocochlear lesion. A score of 4% suggests retrocochlear lesion. Rollover phenomenon decreased speech discrimination of >20% at high sound intensity is typical of retrocochlear lesion.

37. **Phalen's test:** 30–60 secs of complete wrist flexion exaggerates or reproduces pain or tingling. Positive in 80% of cases of cases of carpal tunnel syndrome.

38. Ulnar nerve entrapment differential diagnosis include:

- Alcohol (Ethanol) Related Neuropathy
- Amyotrophic Lateral Sclerosis
- Brachial Plexus Abnormalities
- Cervical Disc Disease
- Cervical Spondylosis
- Epicondylitis
- Pancoast tumor involving the lower trunk of brachial plexus
- Thoracic Outlet Syndrome
- Traumatic Peripheral Nerve Lesions

39. **Erb's palsy:** Upper brachial plexus injury (C5-7) e.g from forceful separation of humeral head from shoulder commonly due to difficult parturition or motorcycle accident. Paralysis of deltoid, biceps, rhomboids, brachioradialis, supra and infraspinatus and occasionally supinator.

Motor: Arm hangs at side internally rotated and extended at elbow (tip position). Hand motion is unaffected.

40. Neoplastic brachial plexopathy (NBP) is an uncommon diagnosis in most physiatrists' offices, but the condition can mimic symptoms of many common upper limb neuropathies. Approximately 10% of all peripheral nerve lesions involve some type of brachial plexus lesion. Neoplastic invasion of the brachial plexus is an uncommon, though not rare, cause of plexopathy.

Lesions of the brachial plexus occur most often secondary to neoplasms that reach the plexus by direct extension (Pancoast syndrome) or, more commonly, by metastasis through lymphatics from the axilla. Pain in the shoulder, radiating down the limb, may be observed, as well as pain in the medial forearm and hand with lower trunk innervation (C8-T1 roots) in some series. The most common pathophysiology revealed on electrodiagnostic tests is axonal loss. Peripheral pain mechanisms may include lowering of the nociceptor threshold by prostaglandins and other noxious chemical substances and persistent nociceptor stimulation. Compression or infiltration of the nerves of the plexus by a tumor may produce neuralgia and inflammation.

Some historical findings suggestive of NBP include the following:

- Onset of limb pain less than 6 months following radiation
- Rapid progression
- Horner syndrome (in two thirds of patients with Pancoast syndrome)
- Severe pain is predominant
- Other metastases
- Focal mass or neoplasm on biopsy

The most reliable feature of NBP (in 80% of patients) is early severe unrelenting pain. Fewer than 20% of radiation induced brachial plexopathy (RBP) patients present with pain, and approximately 33% have minimal or no pain throughout the course of the disease. Two thirds of patients with RBP show severe neurologic deficit progression over several years, while in one third of patients progression spontaneously ceases after 1–3 years. More common findings in RBP include the following:

- Slowly progressive course, duration greater than 4-years
- Predominant parasthesias
- Involvement of the upper trunk or C5–C6 portions of the plexus
- Conduction block on supraclavicular stimulation
- Myokymia on needle examination

42. Choroid plexus: the most common site for physiological calcification (in lateral ventricles where it is usually bilateral and symmetric; rare in 3rd & 4th ventricles. Increases in frequency and extent with age (prevalence: 75% by 5th decade), rare under 3 year. Involvement in the temporal horn is often associated with neurofibromatosis. Normal intracranial calcifications can be defined as age-related physiologic and neurodegenerative calcifications that are unaccompanied by any evidence of disease and have no demonstrable pathological cause.

The most common sites include:

- Pineal gland
  - Seen in 2/3 of the adult population and increases with age.
  - Calcification over 1 cm in diameter or under 9 years of age may be suggestive of a neoplasm.
- Habenula
  - It has a central role in the regulation of the limbic system and is often calcified with a curvilinear pattern A few millimeters anterior to the pineal body in 15% of the adult population.
- Choroid plexus
  - A very common finding, usually in the atrial portions of the lateral ventricles.
  - Calcification in the third or fourth ventricle or in patients less than 9 years of age is uncommon.
- Basal ganglia calcification
  - Are usually idiopathic incidental findings that have an incidence of ~1% (range 0.3–1.5%) and increases with age.
  - Usually demonstrate a faint punctuate or a coarse conglomerated symmetrical calcification pattern.
  - Falx, dura mater or tentorium cerebelli- occur in ~10% of the elderly population.
  - Dural and tentorial calcifications are usually seen in a laminar pattern and can occur anywhere within the cranium.
- Petroclinoid ligaments
  - Common age-related degeneration sites and usually have laminar or mildly nodular patterns.
- Superior sagittal sinus
  - Common age-related degeneration sites and usually have laminar or mildly nodular patterns.

43. Bell's palsy is the commonest cause of facial nerve palsy

Cause of facial nerve palsy

Etiologies producing primary facial nerve palsy include:

1. Bell's palsy
2. Herpes zoster
3. Trauma; basal skull fractures
4. Birth:

A. Congenital

1. Bilateral facial nerve palsy (facial diplegia) of Mobius syndrome, unique in that is it affects upper face more than lower face.
2. Congenital facial diplegia may be part of facioscapulohumeral or myotonic muscular dystrophy".

B. Traumatic

5. **Otitis media:** with acute otitis media, facial palsy usually improves with antibiotics; with chronic suppurative otitis, surgical intervention is required.
6. Central facial paralysis and nuclear facial paralysis;
7. **Neoplasm:** usually cause. Hearing loss and (unlike Bell's palsy) and slowly progressive facial paralysis
8. Neurosarcoidosis
9. Diabetes
10. Lyme disease
11. Guillain-Barré syndrome
12. Occasionally seen in Klippel-Feil syndrome

44. Neural crest cells are a transient, multipotent, migratory cell population unique to vertebrates that gives rise to a diverse cell lineage including melanocytes, craniofacial cartilage and bone, smooth muscle, peripheral and enteric neurons and glia.

After gastrulation, neural crest cells are specified at the border of the neural plate and the non-neural ectoderm. During neurulation, the borders of the neural plate, also known as the neural folds, converge at the dorsal midline to form the neural tube. Subsequently, neural crest cells from the roof plate of the neural tube undergo an epithelial to mesenchymal transition, delaminating from the neuroepithelium and migrating through the periphery where they differentiate into varied cell types. The structural derivatives of neural crest include:

Mesoectoderm odontoblasts, dental papillae, the chondrocranium (nasal capsule, Meckel's cartilage, scleral ossicles, quadrate, articular, hyoid and columella), tracheal and laryngeal cartilage, the dermatocranium (membranous bones), dorsal fins and the turtle plastron (lower vertebrates), pericytes and smooth muscle of branchial arteries and veins, tendons of ocular and masticatory muscles, connective tissue of head and neck glands (pituitary, salivary, lacrymal, thymus, thyroid), Endocrine cells: chromaffin cells of the adrenal medulla, parafollicular cells of the thyroid, glomus cells type I/II. Peripheral nervous system: Sensory neurons and glia of the dorsal root ganglia, cephalic ganglia (VII and in part, V, IX, and X), some Merkel cells in the whisker, Satellite glial cells of all autonomic and sensory ganglia, schwann cells of all peripheral nerves, melanocytes and iris pigment cells.

MOTEL PASS

Melanocytes, Odontoblasts, Tracheal cartilage, Enterochromaffin cells, Laryngeal cartilage Parafollicular cells/ Pseudounipolar cells, All ganglia / Adrenal Medulla, Schwann cells, Spiral Membrane.

45. Hemifacial Spasm

First described by Gowers in 1884, hemifacial spasm represents a segmental myoclonus of muscles innervated by the facial nerve. The disorder presents in the fifth or sixth decade of life, almost always unilaterally, although bilateral involvement may occur rarely in severe cases. Hemifacial spasm generally begins with brief clonic movements of the orbicularis oculi and spreads over years to other facial muscles (corrugator, frontalis, orbicularis oris, platysma, zygomaticus). Compressive lesions (e.g., tumor, arteriovenous malformation, Paget disease) and non-compressive lesions (e.g., stroke, multiple sclerosis plaque, basilar meningitis) may present as hemifacial spasm. Most instances of hemifacial spasm previously thought to be idiopathic were probably caused by aberrant blood vessels (e.g., distal branches of the anterior inferior cerebellar artery or vertebral artery) compressing the facial nerve within the cerebellopontine angle.

46. Intrasellar arachnoid cysts (IAC) are rare. The presenting clinical picture of IAC mimics that of a nonsecreting pituitary adenoma. With the use of sophisticated radiological studies, the differential diagnosis between the two conditions should be easy. However, the cysts can appear hyperintense compared with the cerebrospinal fluid (CSF) on T1-weighted magnetic resonance imaging (MRI) scans. In the literature, surgical morbidity for arachnoid cysts seems to be higher than that for pituitary adenomas after the transsphenoidal procedure.

In normal conditions, there is no arachnoid tissue below the diaphragma sellae. The pituitary gland is surrounded by a capsule that can be identified anatomically and during surgery as a membranous layer enveloping the two lobes of the gland and the pituitary stalk. At the histological level, this capsule is clearly not arachnoid but a derivative of the pia. There is no evidence of differentiation of a leptomeningeal layer surrounding the pituitary gland. During development, the sellar mesenchyma progressively transforms into dura mater and completely surrounds the gland and closes the aperture of the sella turcica (ST) to form the diaphragma. The diameter of the diaphragmatic aperture is highly variable. There are several types of diaphragmatic apertures: 1) the opening is very narrow, allowing passage of the stalk only (42%); 2) the aperture is larger than the stalk (37.5%); and 3) the diaphragm is reduced to a rim of dura or is nonexistent (20.5%). The presence of a large diaphragmatic aperture, or even the absence of diaphragm, and the discrepancy between the volume of the pituitary gland and that of the ST are factors that allow penetration of arachnoid into the ST. In the empty sella syndrome, arachnoid extends largely into the sella, freely communicating with the suprasellar SAS. No pressure gradient exists between the sellar and suprasellar compartments. They most commonly present ranging in age from 16 to 80 years and are not always non communicating.

47. Central nervous system (CNS) disease caused by Mycobacterium tuberculosis is an uncommon yet highly devastating manifestation of tuberculosis, which was universally fatal in the era before antituberculosis therapy. CNS tuberculosis accounts for approximately 1% of all cases of tuberculosis, carries a high mortality and a distressing level of neurological morbidity, and disproportionately afflicts children and human immunodeficiency virus (HIV)-infected individuals. CNS involvement was noted in 5 to 10% of extrapulmonary tuberculosis cases with more recent indicating that 6.3% of extrapulmonary cases (1.3% of total tuberculosis cases) involve the CNS. Adults with TBM often present with the classic meningitis symptoms of fever, headache and meningismus (stiff neck) along with focal neurological deficits, behavioral changes, and alterations in consciousness. Almost 10% patients of TBM present with optochiasmatic arachnoiditis. Often, a history of or current positive tuberculin skin test, history of exposure to tuberculosis, or the identification of particular risk factors for tuberculosis raises the concern of TBM, although a history of tuberculosis is elicited in only approximately 10% of patients. The presence of active pulmonary tuberculosis on chest X-ray ranges from 30 to 50%. Patients coinfected with HIV do not appear to have an altered presentation of TBM. The mortality rate associated with treated TBM is 20 to 50%.

49. On magnetic resonance imaging, some patients with clinical neuroendocrine disorders have thickened pituitary stalks, the anatomical structure which connects the hypothalamus to the pituitary. Causes of thickened stalk include Lymphocytic Hypophysitis / Infundibulitis, Sarcoidosis (inflammatory), Craniopharyngioma, Germ cell tumor, Metastases, Pituitary adenomas, Other primary CNS tumors (Neoplastic), Langerhans cell histiocytosis (uncertain classification), Syphilis, Tuberculosis (Infection).

50. An infundibulum is a funnel-shaped region of dilatation at the origin of an artery most commonly seen in the posterior communicating artery from the internal carotid artery. It may be round or conical, has a diameter of less than 2 mm, and is symmetric. The internal carotid artery is at its base, and the posterior communicating artery arises from its apex. An infundibulum must be distinguished from aneurysms of the posterior communicating artery and internal carotid artery.

51. Horner's syndrome (also known as Bernard-Horner syndrome and oculosympathetic palsy) is a combination of symptoms and signs that arises on the same side as the lesion of the sympathetic trunk.

Signs that are found in patients on the affected side of the face include

- Partial ptosis
- Upside-down ptosis (slight elevation of the lower lid)
- Anhidrosis
- Miosis
- Pseudoenophthalmos (the impression that the eye is sunk caused by a narrow palpebral aperture)
- Pupillary dilation lag
- Loss of ciliospinal reflex
- Bloodshot conjunctiva, depending on the site of lesion.
- Unilateral straight hair (in congenital Horner's syndrome)
- Heterochromia iridum (in congenital Horner's syndrome)

Interruption of sympathetic pathways leads to several implications. It inactivates the dilator muscle and thereby produces miosis. It inactivates the superior tarsal muscle which produces ptosis. It inactivates the orbitalis muscle which produces the effect of enophthalmos. It also reduces sweat secretion in the face. Sometimes there is flushing on the affected side of the face due to dilation of blood vessels under the skin. The pupil's light reflex is maintained as this is controlled via the parasympathetic nervous system. In children, Horner's syndrome sometimes leads to heterochromia, a difference in eye color between the two eyes. This happens because a lack of sympathetic stimulation in childhood interferes with melanin pigmentation of the melanocytes in the superficial stroma of the iris. Causes can be divided according to the presence and location of anhidrosis:

- Central (anhidrosis = face, arm and trunk)
- Syringomyelia
- Multiple sclerosis
- Encephalitis
- Brain tumors
- Lateral medullary syndrome
- Preganglionic (anhidrosis = face)
- Cervical rib traction on stellate ganglion
- Thyroid carcinoma
- Thyroidectomy
- Goiter
- Bronchogenic carcinoma of the superior fissure (Pancoast tumor) on apex of lung
- Klumpke paralysis
- Trauma - base of neck, usually blunt trauma, sometimes surgery.
- As a complication of tube thoracostomy
- Thoracic aortic aneurysm
- Postganglionic (no anhidrosis)
- Cluster headache - combination termed Horton's headache
- A Horner's syndrome may occur during a migraine attack
- Carotid artery dissection/carotid artery aneurysm
- Cavernous sinus thrombosis
- Middle ear infection
- Sympathectomy
- Nerve blocks, such as cervical plexus block, stellate ganglion or interscalene block

52. Downbeating nystagmus means that the eyes drift upward, and "beat" or jump downward. Explanations that have been offered for DBN include asymmetrical smooth pursuit and aberrant tone in the central pathways serving the anterior semicircular canals. Experimentally, ablation of the cerebellar flocculus in monkeys produces downbeating nystagmus. Generally patients with Fllocular disease, such as Chiari, have nystagmus that increases on lateral gaze. This is probably just one of the many mechanisms. Chiari may contribute to as many as 1/3 of cases, cerebellar degenerations, demyelinating disease, drug toxicity (e.g. amiodarone), neoplasia, and "idiopathic" are other common causes.

53. The geniculate ganglion is located within the temporal bone. The first branch from the ganglion is the greater superficial petrosal nerve which passes to the pterygopalatine ganglion innervates the nasal and palatine mucosa and the lacrimal gland of the eye; lesions proximal to the point produce hyperacusis.

54. Optic nerve injuries

The optic nerve is vulnerable to indirect and direct trauma causing functional impairment of vision. Optic nerve injuries occur in the setting of head injury which is often a consequence of road traffic accidents or falls. The diagnosis of optic nerve injury may be delayed by the presence of other life-threatening injuries. Direct injury to the optic nerve should be distinguished from indirect injury. Direct injury arises from penetrating trauma, especially orbital fractures associated with mid-facial fractures. Several varieties of direct optic nerve injury may be recognized ophthalmoscopically or with imaging techniques: optic nerve avulsion, transection, optic nerve sheath hemorrhage, orbital hemorrhage, and orbital emphysema. Indirect optic nerve injury is more common. The force of impact in a head injury may be transmitted to the optic nerve. The frequency of optic nerve injury occurring in closed head injury varies from 0.5 to 5%. Ocular examination is initially normal apart from a relative or absolute afferent pupillary defect. A wide variety of visual field defects may occur. Optic atrophy develops after 4–6 weeks. Optic nerve avulsion usually follows severe orbital trauma, but cases have been reported following relatively trivial injury. Vision loss is usually severe and immediate. Ophthalmoscopy shows absence of the optic disc and a ring of hemorrhage. Imaging may confirm the diagnosis but may show an intact sheath. Ultrasound may be helpful. The nerve tears at the lamina cribrosa, perhaps as a result of rotation of the globe, raised intraocular pressure or sudden retropulsion followed by anterior displacement.

Optic nerve transection occurs as a complication of midfacial trauma and orbital fracture. There is no light perception, corroborated by visual evoked potentials. CT scanning may show the bone fragment transecting the optic nerve. Optic nerve sheath hemorrhage may be difficult to recognize clinically and yet cause potentially reversible visual failure. An expanded nerve sheath associated with proptosis should raise the possibility of a hematoma in the optic nerve sheath, which can be drained via a sheath fenestration. Orbital hemorrhage may be diffuse or localized to the orbit. There is an associated proptosis and ophthalmoplegia. The injury to optic nerve function results from raised pressure in the orbit and may be relieved by elevating the head and administering acetazolamide to lower the intraocular pressure. If conservative measures fail, then a lateral canthotomy and drainage of orbital hemorrhage may restore function.

Orbital emphysema is a well-recognized clinical entity in the setting of injury to the paranasal sinuses. Hairline fractures of the thin bone lining the orbital walls may produce a ball-valve effect so that air accumulates in the orbit and causes proptosis and compression of the eye and nerve. Drainage of the air by a retrobulbar needle has been effective. The mechanism of damage to the optic nerve by closed head injury has been extensively studied. After blunt trauma to the superior orbital rim or frontotemporal region of the cranium, compression forces are transmitted to the orbital apex and optic canal. Within the canal, the optic nerve dura fuses with the periosteum of the bone. Since the vasculature of the optic nerve in the canal is pial, compression and contusion of the nerve produce a compartment syndrome whereby swelling exacerbates the ischemia. The optic nerve is also vulnerable to a shearing injury under the fixed edge of the falciform dural fold just before it enters the optic canal.

55. The bony margins of the orbital canal in humans do not derive from a single bone, but are rather a mosaic of seven embryologically distinct structures: the zygomatic bone laterally, the sphenoid bone, with its lesser wing forming the optic canal and its greater wing forming the lateral posterior portion of the bony orbital process, the maxillary bone inferiorly and medially which, along with the lacrimal and ethmoid bones, form the medial wall of the orbital canal. The ethmoid air cells are extremely thin, and form a structure known as the lamina papyracea, the most delicate bony structure in the skull, and one of the most commonly fractured bones in orbital trauma. The lacrimal bone also contains the nasolacrimal duct. The superior margin and orbital rim, otherwise known as the orbital process, is formed by the frontal bone.

The roof (superior wall) is formed primarily by the orbital plate frontal bone, and also the lesser wing of sphenoid near the apex of the orbit. The orbital surface presents medially by trochlear fovea and laterally by lacrimal fossa.

The floor (inferior wall) is formed by the orbital surface of maxilla, the orbital surface of zygomatic bone and the minute orbital process of palatine bone. Medially, near the orbital margin, is located the groove for nasolacrimal duct. Near the middle of the floor, located infraorbital groove, which leads to the infraorbital foramen. The floor is separated from the lateral wall by inferior orbital fissure, which connects the orbit to pterygopalatine and infratemporal fossa. The medial wall is formed primarily by the orbital plate of ethmoid, as well as contributions from the frontal process of maxilla, the lacrimal bone, and a small part of the body of the sphenoid. It is the thinnest wall of the orbit, evidenced by pneumatized ethmoidal cells. The lateral wall is formed by the frontal process of zygomatic and more posteriorly by the orbital plate of the greater wing of sphenoid. The bones meet at the zygomaticosphenoid suture. The lateral wall is the thickest wall of the orbit, important because it is the most exposed surface, highly vulnerable to blunt force trauma.

Borders

The base, which opens in the face, has four borders. The following bones take part in their formation:

1. **Superior margin:** frontal bone and sphenoid
2. **Inferior margin:** maxilla, palatine and zygomatic
3. **Medial margin:** ethmoid, lacrimal bone, and frontal
4. **Lateral margin:** zygomatic and sphenoid

56. The posteromedial middle fossa triangle, also known as Kawase's triangle, is defined between the lateral margin of the greater petrosal nerve (medial border), the lateral edge of the trigeminal nerve behind the point where the greater petrosal nerve passes below its lateral surface to the crest of the petrous apex (lateral border), and a line along the connection of the posterior border of the mandibular division of the trigeminal nerve and ganglion gasserian (the crest of petrous apex) to the center of the geniculate ganglion.

57. Apolipoprotein E (Apo-E)

Apolipoprotein E (Apo-E) is a major cholesterol carrier that supports lipid transport and injury repair in the brain. APOE polymorphic alleles are the main genetic determinants of Alzheimer disease (AD) risk: individuals carrying the ε4 allele are at increased risk of AD compared with those carrying the more common ε3 allele, whereas the ε2 allele decreases risk. Presence of the APOE ε4 allele is also associated with increased risk of cerebral amyloid angiopathy and age-related cognitive decline during normal ageing. Apo-E–lipoproteins bind to several cell-surface receptors to deliver lipids, and also to hydrophobic amyloid-β (Aβ) peptide, which is thought to initiate toxic events that lead to synaptic dysfunction and neurodegeneration in AD. Apo-E isoforms differentially regulate Aβ aggregation and clearance in the brain, and have distinct functions in regulating brain lipid transport, glucose metabolism, neuronal signaling, neuroinflammation, and mitochondrial function.

58. Hyperosmotic mannitol therapy is widely used in the clinical setting for acute and subacute reduction in brain edema, to decrease muscle damage in compartment syndrome, and to improve renal perfusion. Though beneficial rheological effects commonly are attributed to mannitol, its direct effects on endothelial cells are poorly understood. Mannitol is a cell-impermeant, non-metabolized, 6-carbon sugar administered intravenously as a hypertonic solution in the treatment of a number of clinical conditions. The beneficial clinical effects of mannitol have been attributed to the consequent increase in intravascular volume and coincident decrease in extracellular fluid volume. In brain edema resulting from closed-head trauma and ischemic brain swelling, mannitol is used to reduce intracranial pressure and to improve cerebral blood flow. Mannitol therapy of the compartment syndrome of crush injury has been found to decrease the need for fasciotomy and to increase limb survival. Mannitol has also been shown to decrease myocardial reperfusion injury and remains a therapy for acute renal failure, especially of the myoglobinuric type.

In addition to its osmotic diuretic action, poorly defined rheological benefits have been ascribed to mannitol. Mannitol has been advocated as a neuroprotective adjunct along with hypothermia during temporary occlusion of parent vessels in aneurysm surgery. It also has been reported to possess antioxidant properties, and has been used intra-arterially to disrupt the blood-brain barrier and improve delivery of pharmacological agents. Mannitol is customarily administered every 3 to 4 hours in bolus doses of up to 1 to 1.5 g/kg body weight, resulting in step increments in serum osmolarity of up to 320 mOsm.

59. Cytotoxic brain edema swelling of nerve and glial cells is among the very early pathophysiologic sequelae of focal cerebral ischemia. Once cell swelling has exhausted the cerebral compliance, intracranial pressure increases and, thereby, causes secondary ischemia. Hypertonic solutions, mannitol in particular, have long been used to reduce intracranial pressure. More recently, hypertonic saline has been used for treatment of increased intracranial pressure in particular because sodium chloride with a reflection coefficient of 1.0 is better excluded from brain with an intact blood brain barrier than mannitol (reflection coefficient 0.9).

60. Corticosteroids are usually indicated in any patient with a malignant brain tumor and symptomatic peritumoral edema. Dexamethasone is most commonly used by neuro-oncologists owing to its comparably minimal mineralocorticoid activity. The vasogenic edema surrounding brain tumors contributes significantly to the morbidity experienced by patients. Edema results from the flow of fluid into the extracellular space of the brain parenchyma through an incompetent blood–brain barrier (BBB). In high-grade gliomas and brain metastases, the BBB is typically disrupted, allowing passage of fluid into the extracellular space. The increased permeability of the BBB is primarily owing to opening of the interendothelial tight junctions, but also due to increased endothelial pinocytosis and endothelial fenestrations. Defective endothelial tight junctions result from deficiency of normal astrocytes (which produce factors required for the formation of a normal BBB) and the tumor cell-associated production of additional factors, such as VEGF and scatter factor/hepatocyte growth factor, which increase the permeability of tumor vessels.

It has been suggested that corticosteroids produce their anti-edema effect by reducing the permeability of tumor capillaries. As indicated previously, corticosteroids diffuse through the plasma membrane and bind to the cytoplasmic receptor, allowing the steroid–receptor complex to move to the nucleus where it directly affects transcription of genes and also interacts with other transcription factors, mediating non-transcriptional regulation of other signaling cascades. Corticosteroids decrease endothelial permeability by upregulation of the tight junction (TJ) component occludin in endothelial cells and partly by causing dephosphorylation of occludin.

61. Albumin is usually well tolerated. However, immediate allergic-type reactions are possible with fever, shivering, nausea, vomiting, urticaria, hypotension, increased salivation and effects on respiration and heart rate. Very fast infusions (20–50 mL/minute) can cause fall in systemic blood pressure and, in elderly subjects and those at risk of congestive heart failure, it can cause congestive heart failure especially when the more concentrated solutions of albumin are used. Albumin is considered a safe blood derivative from the point of view of transmission of infections, although there are some questions about the potential transmission of prions.

62. It has been suggested that phenytoin causes a reduction in folic acid levels, predisposing patients to megaloblastic anemia. Folate is presented in foods as polyglutamate, which is then converted into monoglutamates by intestinal conjugase. Phenytoin acts by inhibiting this enzyme, thereby causing folate deficiency. Other side effects may include: agranulocytosis, aplastic anemia, decreased white blood cell count and a low platelet count.

63. Diagnostic differences between SIADH and CEREBRAL SALT WASTING

SIADH

In general, 3 diagnostic criteria are: hyponatremia, inappropriately concentrated urine, and no evidence of renal or adrenal dysfunction.

1. Lowserum sodium hyponatremia usually<134 meq/l.
2. Lowserum osmolality < 210 mOsm/L
3. High urinary sodium (salt wasting) at least >18 mEq/Loften 50-150
4. High ratio of urine; serum osmolality often 1.5–2.5:1, but may be 1:1
5. Normal renal function (check BUN and creatinine): BUN commonly <10
6. Normal adrenal function (no hypotension, no hyperkalemia)
7. No hypothyroidism
8. No signs of over hydration or dehydration

CEREBRAL SALT WASTING

Cerebral salt wasting, renal loss of sodium due to intracranial disease producing hyponatremia and decrease in extracellular fluid volume. **CAUTION:** patients with aneurysmal SAH may have CSW with hyponatremia which mimics SIADH, however there is usually hypovolemia in CSW. In this setting, fluid restriction may exacerbate vasospasm induced ischemia. The mechanisms whereby the kidneys fail to conserve CSW is not known.

Laboratory Tests (serum and urinary electrolytes and osmolalities) may be identical with SIADH and CSW. Furthermore, hypovolemiain CSW may stimulate ADH release. To differentiate, CVP, Pulmonary capillary wedge pressure, and plasma volume (a nuclear medicine study) are low in hypovolemia (i.e., CSW). Comparing the features of CSW and SIADH. The two most important differences being extracellular volume and salt balance. An elevated Serum $K^+$with hyponatremia is incompatible with the diagnosis of SIADH.

65. Cerebral vasospasm produces a reduction of regional CBF to levels that result in cerebral ischemia, and the metabolic consequences of this ischemia produce neurological deficits that may be reversible or irreversible. Hypervolemic hemodilution therapy has been reported to be effective for preventing neurological deficits due to delayed cerebral vasospasm. Manipulation of blood viscosity offers an effective and rapid means of increasing the perfusion of ischemic regions in the brain, and hemodilution therapy improves the microcirculation of the ischemic penumbra by decreasing blood viscosity. It is generally thought that blood flow and blood viscosity in the microcirculation vary with hematocrit level, RBC aggregability and flexibility, platelet aggregability, and plasma viscosity. Hematocrit has a major influence on blood viscosity. Although the oxygen content of blood is reduced as the hematocrit decreases, the relative oxygen transport capacity increases as the hematocrit is lowered to 30 to 33%. At reduced driving pressures, blood flow is limited by the increase of viscosity that occurs at low shear rates. Since RBC aggregation is also shear-rate dependent, aggregation may be enhanced in the cerebral microcirculation, especially in ischemic areas where the shear rate is low. It has also been shown that at lower shear rates, erythrocyte aggregation plays the major role in determining blood viscosity. Hypercoagulability, platelet hyperactivity, and reduced RBC deformability occurs with vasospasm. Such systemic changes of intravascular components could promote cerebral ischemia through an increase of blood viscosity. Measurement of the hematocrit level alone does not give a precise estimate of blood viscosity, and monitoring of RBC aggregability is also desirable. The RBC aggregation rate is decreased by hypervolemic hemodilution therapy both because of a decrease in hematocrit and by the direct effect of the low-molecular-weight dextran, which reduces RBC aggregation, reduces blood viscosity, and improves microcirculatory flow at low shear rates. The cause of the increase in RBC aggregability after SAH is not clear, but it may be related to changes of plasma albumin, fibrinogen, α_2-macroglobulin, or RBC surface charge. SAH itself may alter the RBC surface charge and other RBC membrane properties. Evidence has accumulated that patients with cerebral vasospasm show good recovery from ischemic symptoms after intravascular volume expansion therapy.

66. MS affects one in every 500 persons, women twice as frequently as men. It is more common in young adults and causes a variety of neurological deficits (visual loss, paralysis, sensory loss, ataxia, brainstem signs, psychiatric disorders, dementia. Many MS cases evolve over a long period (20–30 years) with remissions and exacerbations. Some cases have an acute, fulminant, even fatal course, and others go into a relentlessly progressive phase after a period of remissions and exacerbations. The pathology is characterized by multifocal lesions, the MS plaques. With time, gliosis develops, and plaques reach a burned-out stage consisting of demyelinated axons. In H&E stains, plaques appear pale compared to normal white matter. Myelin stains show complete loss of myelin or pallor of myelin staining. The inflammatory cells in multiple sclerosis include primarily CD-8 lymphocytes, microglia, and macrophages.

67. The importance of early treatment of LMMC patients is paramount because the likelihood of avoiding or reversing a neurological deficit by surgical treatment is greatest early on and decreases with age, presumably indicating that with delayed treatment, chronic traction on the spinal cord ultimately leads to irreversible deficits. Surgery is relatively simple and its results rather beneficial in types I (dorsal) and II (caudal) LMMC, while it involves considerable risk in type III (transitional or mixed) LMMC, especially when its aim is extensive separation of the lipoma from the attached spinal cord.

68. Chiari malformations are usually caused by structural defects in the brain and spinal cord. These defects develop during fetal development. Much less commonly, Chiari malformations can occur later in life. Tethered cord is a frequent accompaniment, infact it also has been postulated that it in many cases it is because of the tethered cord that the tonsillar descent is seen.

69. Non-hindbrain related syrinx as a complication of meningitis is well documented. The imaging diagnosis is best made by MRI. In postmeningitic syringomyelia, syringo peritoneal/ pleural shunt insertion may give satisfactory results despite the duration of the neurological deficits. The mechanism of syrinx formation due to inflammatory arachnoiditis includes ischemic myelomalacia secondary to inflammatory occlusion of spinal cord vessels with subsequent syrinx formation. Focal scarring causes a block in the circulation of CSF, thus forcing CSF into the central canal of the spinal cord via Virchow-Robin spaces. Obstruction of Virchow-Robin spaces also emerges, focal cystic dilatations in the cord eventually coalesce to form a syrinx. Spontaneous opening of the syrinx into the subarachnoid space is a rare event but could occur in severe cases. In trauma patients, it is proposed that the presence of arachnoiditis at the level of trauma causes spinal cord tethering and plays an important role in the pathophysiology of progressive posttraumatic myelomalacic myelopathy. Spinal cord tethering alone may lead to progressive neurological deficits despite a decompressed subarachnoid space and a collapsed syrinx. However following a meningitic event arachnoid scarring is generally much more extensive.

70. Results of a landmark, seven-year National Institutes of Health-funded trial, Management of Myelomeningocele Study (MOMS), demonstrate clear benefit for babies who undergo fetal surgery to treat spina bifida, the most common birth defect in the central nervous system. It showed that babies who had corrective surgery for spina bifida (myelomeningocele) while still in the uterus, experience a reduction in potentially life-threatening hydrocephalus and have an increased ability to walk. www.cincinnatichildrens.org/

71. Topical hyaluronic acid application at the end of surgery is found to offer some reduction in secondary tethering in repair of spina bifida.

72. Children with neurofibromatosis type 1 (NF1) are at increased risk of developing plexiform neurofibroma throughout the body, including the cervical soft tissues.

73. Cerebellar abscess induced by a contiguous dermal sinus is a rare event. Otogenic suppuration is the cause in 93% of the cases, while hematogenous infection is infrequent.. Intracranial dermoid cysts are rare, but can cause recurrent bacterial or aseptic meningitis, abscesses or mass effect. The posterior fossa is the most common location for intracranial dermoids. Embryologically, these malformations occur between weeks 3–5 of gestation. They are thought to arise from a failure of cleavage between the ectoderm of the neuraxis and the cutaneous ectoderm, with a resultant incorporation of the cutaneous ectoderm into the neural tube. A dermal sinus develops when a cutaneous tract containing sebaceous material persists. Description of children who manifest as an occipital "lump" or discharging sinus of varied duration has been reported in literature. They have to underwent prompt surgical excision of the cyst and the sinus, and receive a prolonged course of antibiotics. A high index of suspicion for the detection of dermoid cysts is required when a congenital midline skin lesion such as a dimple or a scalp swelling is reported. Prophylactic excision is indicated to prevent serious sequelae.

74. Redundant nerve root syndrome of cauda equine is not a rare entity. Recognition of this entity is important as the nerves may cause unpleasant surprise for the surgeon if not well prepared. During surgery the nerves may herniate through a dural rent anf reposition may not be possible, a duraplasty may be needed. Materials for this kind of unexpected situation should be prepared beforehand. Therefore understanding the redundant nerve root syndrome and preparing the team for a potential situation are essential. Myelographic appearance is not specific and might be confusing since these filling defects might suggest the possibility of tumor, an AVM. Vascular filling defects are a normal feature of the thoracic myelogram. Filling defects greater than 1.4 mm diameter, which are excessively tortuous, long and multiple, serpiginous should be regarded as highly suspicious of an AVM. A lateral film is important when vascular filling defects are seen, for if these filling defects are anterior to the cord, an AVM is more likely. Filling defects in RNS change their position when the patient shifts his position but filling defects of AVM remain constant in position.

75. Symptomatic ventricular coaptation, or the slit ventricle syndrome, is frequently described and recognized as a clinical entity in the pediatric population. It is characterized by symptoms of shunt failure (i.e., ataxia, obtundation, nausea, vomiting, lethargy, irritability, and complaints of headache) and the CT findings of ventricular coaptation (slit-like ventricles). Mild forms are seen in adults and more severe forms are seen in children. Patients must be symptomatic to be diagnosed with slit ventricle syndrome.

Pathology

The exact etiology behind slit ventricle syndrome is debatable and include

- Intermittent proximal catheter obstruction with collapsed ventricles
- Shunt obstruction resulting with increased intracranial pressure from non-compliant ventricles
- Craniocerebral disproportion
- Venous hypertension

Radiographic appearance

CT and MRI: Small ventricles with a characteristic slit-like appearance.

76. The management of slit ventricle syndrome is difficult and challenging. In general, a neurosurgeon with expertise in the management of hydrocephalus is optimal. Various treatment options have been proposed and include:

Shunt revision.

- ❖ Change the ventricular catheter
- ❖ Change the shunt valve
- ❖ Add siphon controlling device (SCD)
- ❖ Programmable valve with or without SCD
- ❖ Converting to a lumboperitoneal shunt.

Temporarily blocking the flow of the shunt (via "externalization" of the shunt) in order to expand the ventricles.

- ❖ This should be done with ICP monitoring due to the risk of coma.
- ❖ Many patients have aqueductal stenosis, and therefore are candidates for endoscopic third ventriculostomy (ETV).
- ❖ In some cases, a special shunt configuration draining both the ventricles and the cisterns (space around the brain) can equalize the inner and outer brain pressures, thus reducing the chance of producing slit ventricles again. This type of shunt is called a ventriculocisternoperitoneal shunt.
  - ➢ Subtemporal decompression
- ❖ This procedure is rarely performed because improvements, if any, are typically short-lived.

77. Furosemide, like other loop diuretics, acts by inhibiting NKCC2, the luminal Na-K-2Cl symporter in the thick ascending limb of the loop of Henle. The action on the distal tubules is independent of any inhibitory effect on carbonic anhydrase or aldosterone; it also abolishes the corticomedullary osmotic gradient and blocks negative, as well as positive, free water clearance. Because of the large NaCl absorptive capacity of the loop of Henle, diuresis is not limited by development of acidosis, as it is with the carbonic anhydrase inhibitors.

Additionally, furosemide is a noncompetitive subtype-specific blocker of GABA-A receptors. Furosemide has been reported to reversibly antagonize GABA-evoked currents of $\alpha_6\beta_2\gamma_2$ receptors at μM concentrations, but not $\alpha_1\beta_2\gamma_2$ receptors. During development, the $\alpha_6\beta_2\gamma_2$ receptor increases in expression in cerebellar granule neurons, corresponding to increased sensitivity to furosemide. With respect to its use in lowering ICP it decreases the CSF production, increases free water excretion and in combined use with mannitol causes more sustained decrease in ICP.

78. The Wechsler Memory Scale (WMS) is a neuropsychological test designed to measure different memory functions in a person. Anyone with age 16-90 years is eligible to take this test. The current version is the fourth edition (WMS-IV) which was published in 2009 and which was designed to be used with the WAIS-IV. WMS-IV is made up of seven subtests: Spatial Addition, Symbol Span, Design Memory, General Cognitive Screener, Logical Memory (I and II), Verbal Paired Associates (I and II), and Visual Reproduction (I and II). A person's performance is reported as five Index Scores: Auditory Memory, Visual Memory, Visual Working Memory, Immediate Memory, and Delayed Memory.

The WMS-IV also incorporates an optional cognitive exam (Brief Cognitive Status Exam) that helps to assess global cognitive functioning in people with suspected memory deficits or those who have been diagnosed with a various neural, psychiatric and/or developmental disorders. This may include conditions such as dementias or mild learning difficulties. There is clear evidence that the WMS differentiates clinical groups (such as those with dementias or neurological disorders) from those with normal memory functioning and that the primary index scores can distinguish among the memory-impaired clinical groups.

79. Paget's disease of bone (also termed osteitis deformans or Paget's disease of bone, is a chronic disorder that can result in enlarged and misshapen bones. Paget's disease is rare in people less than 55 years of age. Men are more commonly affected than women (3:2). Paget's disease is caused by the excessive breakdown and formation of bone, followed by disorganized bone remodeling. This causes affected bone to weaken, resulting in pain, misshapen bones, fractures and arthritis in the joints near the affected bones. Rarely, it can develop into a primary bone cancer known as Paget's sarcoma. Often Paget's disease is localized to only a few bones in the body. The pelvis, femur, and lower lumbar vertebrae are the most commonly affected bones. Paget's disease typically is localized, affecting just one or a few bones, as opposed to osteoporosis, for example, which usually affects all the bones in the body. The first manifestation of Paget's disease is usually an elevated alkaline phosphatase in the blood. Overall, the most common symptom is bone pain. Although there is no cure for Paget's disease, medications (bisphosphonates and calcitonin) can help control the disorder and lessen pain and other symptoms. Loss of hearing in one or both ears may occur when Paget's disease affects the skull and the bone that surrounds the inner ear. Treating the disease may slow or stop hearing loss. In rare cases, involvement of the skull may lead to compression of the nerves that supply the eye, leading to vision loss. In skull, both the tables are involved and there is widening of diploe, patient may complain that his cap worn last year does not fit his head now.

Pathogenesis

The pathogenesis of Paget's disease is described in 4 stages:

1. Osteoclastic activity
2. Mixed osteoclastic - osteoblastic activity
3. Osteoblastic activity
4. Malignant degeneration

80. The site of injection is the crucial factor in determining the degree of nerve fiber injury. The degree of injury varies significantly, depending upon the specific agent injected. The most severe injuries have been associated with widespread axonal and myelin degeneration. Pathological alterations in the nerve are evident as early as 30-minutes following injection injury. Although post-injection injury can occur in both adults and children, children appear to be at higher risk. The postulated mechanisms of injury include direct needle trauma, secondary constriction by scar, and direct nerve fiber damage, due to both axon and Schwann cell, with a breakdown in the blood-nerve barrier by neurotoxic chemicals in the injected agent. Neurological sequelae can range from minor transient sensory disturbance to severe sensory disturbance and paralysis, with poor recovery. Medical treatments including administration of vitamins and alpha-chymotrypsine have been tried with varying results, depending on the extent of the lesion. Early (within 2 months) physiotherapy may provide a better chance of recovery. The recommended treatment ranges from a conservative approach to immediate operative exposure and irrigation and has included early neurolysis or delayed exploration with neurolysis or resection and anastamosis. Current recommendations go in favor conservative treatment of 3-4 months before repair is planned.

81. Guillain–Barré syndrome also known as Guillain–Barré–Strohl syndrome or Landry's paralysis, is a rapid-onset muscle weakness as a result of damage to the peripheral nervous system. It is a demyelinating polyneuropathy. The first symptoms of Guillain–Barré syndrome are numbness, tingling, and pain, alone or in combination. This is followed by weakness of the legs and arms that affects both sides equally and worsening over time. The weakness can take half a day to over two weeks to reach maximum severity, and then becomes steady. The muscles of the neck may also be affected, and about half experience involvement of the cranial nerves, which supply the head and face; this may lead to weakness of the muscles of the face, swallowing difficulties and sometimes weakness of the eye muscles. Involvement of the muscles that control the bladder and anus is unusual. Many people with Guillain–Barré syndrome have experienced the signs and symptoms of an infection in the 3–6 weeks prior to the onset of the neurological symptoms. This may consist of upper respiratory tract infection (rhinitis, sore throat) or diarrhea. In children, particularly those younger than six years old, the diagnosis can be difficult and the condition is often initially mistaken (sometimes for up to two weeks) for other causes of pains and difficulty walking, such as viral infections, or bone and joint problems. On neurological examination, characteristic features are the reduced power and reduced or absent tendon reflexes (hypo- or areflexia, respectively). In the "Miller Fisher variant" subtype of Guillain–Barré syndrome weakness of the eye muscles (ophthalmoplegia) is more pronounced and may occur together with abnormalities in coordination (ataxia).

A characteristic finding in Guillain–Barré syndrome is an elevated protein level with low numbers of white blood cells ("albumin-cytological dissociation"); this distinguishes it from a number of other conditions (such as lymphoma and poliomyelitis) where both the protein and the cell count are elevated.

82. Stereotactic radiosurgery (SRS) treats brain disorders with a precise delivery of a single, high dose of radiation in a one-day session. Focused radiation beams are delivered to a specific area of the brain to treat tumors or AVMs.

Stereotactic radiosurgery is limited to the head and neck, because these areas can be immobilized with skeletal fixation devices that completely restrict the head's movement, permitting the most precise and accurate treatment. Radiosurgery (one-session treatment) has such a dramatic effect in the target zone that the changes are considered "surgical." Through the use of three-dimensional computer-aided planning and the high degree of immobilization, the treatment can minimize the amount of radiation that passes through healthy brain tissue.

Stereotactic radiosurgery is routinely used to treat brain tumors and lesions. It may be the primary treatment, used when a tumor is inaccessible by surgical means; or as a boost or adjunct to other treatments for a recurring or malignant tumor. Stereotactic radiosurgery works the same as all other forms of radiation treatment. It does not remove the tumor or lesion, but it distorts the DNA of the tumor cells. The cells then lose their ability to reproduce and retain fluids. The tumor reduction occurs at the rate of normal growth for the specific tumor cell. In lesions such as AVM radiosurgery causes the blood vessels to thicken and close off. The shrinking of a tumor or closing off of a vessel occurs over a period of time. For benign tumors and vessels, this will usually be 18-months to 2-years. For malignant or metastatic tumors, results may be seen in a few months, because these cells are very fast-growing.

Types: There are three basic forms of stereotactic radiosurgery represented by three different technological instruments. Each instrument operates differently, has a different source of radiation and may be more effective under different circumstances. The three are:

- Particle beam (proton)
- Cobalt-60 based (photon)
- Linear accelerator based (linac)

83. Intracavitary balloon catheter brain brachytherapy is localized temporary high-dose radiotherapy in the brain that requires placement of an inflatable balloon catheter in the surgical cavity after resection of a malignant brain mass. A radiation source is then placed in the balloon to expose surrounding brain tissue to radiation, either continuously or in a series of brief treatments. After the patient completes therapy, the radiation source is permanently removed, and the balloon catheter is surgically explanted.

At present, the Gliasite is the only device marketed in the United States for intracavitary balloon catheter brachytherapy in the brain. It includes a catheter tray with a double balloon catheter and accessories used for implantation of an aqueous saline solution of molecularly bound radioactive iodine [sodium 3-(I-125) iodo-4-hydroxybenzenesulfonate; Iotrex™ as the radiation source; and an access tray with items used for after loading and retrieving the radioactive material. One to three weeks after resection and balloon implantation, the Iotrex™ solution is loaded through a subcutaneous port and left in for 3 to 6 days. Prescribed radiation doses are usually 40–60 Gy measured at 0.5–1.0 cm from the balloon surface.

85. Stroop Color–Word Test

One measure of executive function is the Stroop Interference Test, originally developed in 1935 by Stroop to measure selective attention and cognitive flexibility. It is most often described as measuring the individual's ability to shift cognitive set); it is believed to provide a measure of cognitive inhibition) or the ability to inhibit an overlearned (i.e., dominant response) in favor of an unusual one. The Stroop is a quick measure that is used frequently in screening for brain damage. There are three components to this task. First, the individual is asked to name a series of color words (Word task). This component is believed to reflect basic reading rate and may be affected by speech motor problems or learning. Second, the individual is asked to name the color of a bar (Color task) of X's (e.g., XXX in red, blue, or green ink). As with the Word task, performance may be affected by speech motor function; it also may be impacted by the individual's inability to name colors. The final task is the Color–Word task on which the individual is shown the names of colors printed in conflicting ink colors (e.g., the word "blue" in red ink) and is asked to name the color of the ink rather than the word. Theoretically, when other factors are accounted for, the Color–Word task is the component that is believed to be measuring both mental flexibility and the ability to inhibit a dominant response. It also is believed to provide a measure of the individual's ability to inhibit stimulus-bound responses and deal with interference.

86. In statistics, a receiver operating characteristic (ROC), or ROC curve, is a graphical plot that illustrates the performance of a binary classifier system as its discrimination threshold is varied. The curve is created by plotting the true positive rate (TPR) against the false positive rate (FPR) at various threshold settings. The true-positive rate is also known as sensitivity. The false-positive rate is also known as the fall-out and can be calculated as (1 - specificity).

87. A persistent vegetative state is a disorder of consciousness in which patients with severe brain damage are in a state of partial arousal rather than true awareness. It is a diagnosis of some uncertainty in that it deals with a syndrome. After four weeks in a vegetative state (VS), the patient is classified as in a persistent (or 'continuing') vegetative state. This diagnosis is classified as a permanent vegetative state (PVS) some months after a non-traumatic brain injury (3 months in the US, 6 months in the UK, or one year after traumatic injury). Nowadays we prefer to call the state of consciousness an unresponsive wakefulness syndrome, primarily because of ethical questions about whether a patient can be called 'vegetative' or not.

88. Intracranial germinomas, also known as dysgerminomas or extra-gonadal seminomas, are a type of germ cell tumor, and are predominantly seen in pediatric populations. They tend to occur in the midline, either at the pineal region (majority) or along the floor of the third ventricle/suprasellar region. Usually the mass enhances brightly.

91. Mucopolysaccharidosis IV A also known as Morquio-Brailsford or Morquio syndrome, is a lysosomal storage disorder caused by a deficiency of the enzyme N-acetyl-galactosamine-6-sulphate sulphatase (GALNS). MPS IVA is multisystemic but manifests primarily as a progressive skeletal dysplasia. Spinal stenosis is a prominent feature.

Hurler syndrome, also known as mucopolysaccharidosis type I (MPS I), Hurler's disease, also gargoylism, is a genetic disorder that results in the buildup of glycosaminoglycans (formerly known as mucopolysaccharides) due to a deficiency of alpha-L iduronidase, an enzyme responsible for the degradation of mucopolysaccharides in lysosomes. Mental retardation, spinal stenosis and entrapment neuropathy are some of the features.

Achondroplasia is a common cause of dwarfism. It occurs as a sporadic mutation in approximately 80% of cases (associated with advanced paternal age) or it may be inherited as an autosomal dominant genetic disorder. Skeletal manifestations include a narrow foramen magnum, lumbar canal stenosis and metaphyseal cupping.

92. Cervical canal stenosis can be acquired (e.g. trauma, discs, and ossification of the posterior longitudinal ligament) or congenital. It refers to narrowing of the spinal canal, nerve root canals, or intervertebral foramina of the cervical spine.

Radiographic assessment

- Normal AP diameter is approximately 17 mm
- Relative stenosis 10–13 mm
- Absolute stenosis <10 mm

The width of the canal is not however constant, and progressively decreases as one moves down the cervical spine.

- C1: 23 mm
- C2: 20 mm
- C3-C6: 17 mm
- C7: 15 mm

The canal-to-body ratio of Torg and Pavlov:

This method uses the ratio of the diameter of cervical canal to the width of cervical body, with a ratio of < 0.8 on lateral view taken as an indication of cervical stenosis.

This ratio is variously referred to as the Torg ratio, the Pavlov ratio, the Torg-Pavlov ratio, or the canal-to-body ratio

93. Spinal stenosis is a well-defined clinical entity that is occasionally encountered in patients with acromegaly. Persistent elevation of growth hormone promotes hypertrophy of the bones and ligaments, resulting in widening of the thoracolumbar vertebral bodies, and developmental narrowing of the spinal canal.

94. Hypertension is the most powerful risk factor for aneurysm formation, regardless of age and sex, followed by hypercholesterolemia, heart disease, and cigarette smoking, whereas diabetes mellitus and daily drinking are insignificant for aneurysm formation. Hypertension and daily drinking are not related to the risk of aneurysm rupture, regardless of age and sex, whereas cigarette smoking is associated with an increased risk of aneurysm rupture in patients 60 years or older and in men. Radiation exposure can induce moya-moya syndrome however aneurysm formation per se has no relation to it.

96. A spinal epidural abscess threatens the spinal cord or cauda equina by compression and also by vascular compromise. If untreated, an expanding suppurative infection in the spinal epidural space impinges on the spinal cord, producing sensory symptoms and signs, motor dysfunction, and, ultimately, paralysis and death. Intervention early in the course of the disease undoubtedly improves the outcome. Frequently, diagnosis is understandably delayed because the initial presentation may be only nonspecific back pain. One half of cases are estimated to be misdiagnosed or have a delayed diagnosis. Most spinal epidural abscesses occur in the dorsal spine area, which is anatomically the longest of the spinal regions. Hematogenous spread with seeding of the epidural space is the suspected source of infection direct extension of infection from vertebral osteomyelitis occurs in adults and rarely in children. Staphylococcus aureus is the most commonly reported pathogen. Treatment is medical and surgical.

97. Glucocorticoid-induced osteoporosis (GIO) is the most prevalent form of secondary osteoporosis. Of the multiple side effects that can occur with glucocorticoid therapy, osteoporotic fractures are one of the most devastating, affecting 30–50% of patient. Glucocorticoids have a detrimental effect on bone formation, turnover and integrity. The primary action is on osteoblasts, decreasing replication and impairing differentiation and maturation, leading to decreased bone formation. Osteocytes are also affected, with decreased cell function and increased apoptosis resulting in impairment of their ability to detect and repair bone microdamage. GIO also involves an element of increased bone resorption. Other actions of glucocorticoids that negatively affect bone include decreased calcium absorption by the gastrointestinal tract and renal calcium loss. Steroid myopathy results in muscle weakness and therefore increased risk of falls and fractures. Prolonged glucocorticoid therapy may lead to hypogonadism by altering hypothalamic gonadotropin-releasing-hormone release, inhibiting pituitary release of gonadotropins, suppressing adrenal androgen production, and directly affecting ovarian and testicular hormone production.

98. Paget's is caused by the excessive breakdown and formation of bone, followed by disorganized bone remodeling. This causes affected bone to weaken, resulting in pain, misshapen bones, fractures and arthritis in the joints near the affected bones. Rarely, it can develop into a primary bone cancer known as Paget's sarcoma. The pathogenesis of Paget's disease is described in 4 stages: Osteoclastic activity, Mixed osteoclastic - osteoblastic activity, Osteoblastic activity and Malignant degeneration. There is release of hydroxyprolene in urine. Mithramycin is one of the drugs for treatment.

99. Myofascial pain syndrome (MPS), also known as chronic myofascial pain (CMP), is a syndrome characterized by chronic pain in multiple myofascial trigger points ("knots"). Characteristic features of a myofascial trigger points include: focal point tenderness, reproduction of pain upon trigger point palpation, hardening of the muscle upon trigger point palpation, pseudo-weakness of the involved muscle, referred pain, and limited range of motion following approximately 5 seconds of sustained trigger point pressure.

100. Hemangiopericytomas were described in 1942 by Stout and Murray. Begg and Garret first described meningeal hemangiopericytoma and proposed the term hemangiopericytoma.

The most common sites of involvement are bones of the lower extremity, pelvis, and retroperitoneum. Meninges are uncommon sites of presentation. Intracranial hemangiopericytomas were earlier classified as angioblastic meningioma, but now they are considered a separate entity with different biologic characteristics and immunohistochemistry profile as compared to meningioma.

101. Adie syndrome, sometimes known as Holmes–Adie syndrome or Adie's tonic pupil, is a neurological disorder characterized by a tonically dilated pupil that reacts slowly to light but shows a more definite response to accommodation (i.e., light-near dissociation). It is frequently seen in females with absent knee or ankle jerks and impaired sweating. It is named after the British neurologist William John Adie. It is caused by damage to the postganglionic fibers of the parasympathetic innervation of the eye, usually by a viral or bacterial infection which causes inflammation.

102. Ménière's disease also called endolymphatic hydrops, is a disorder of the inner ear that can affect hearing and balance. It is characterized by episodes of vertigo, tinnitus, and hearing loss. The hearing loss comes and goes for some time, alternating between ears, then becomes permanent.

104. Diagnosis of TB meningitis is made by analyzing cerebrospinal fluid collected by lumbar puncture. When collecting CSF for suspected TB meningitis, a minimum of 1 ml of fluid should be taken (preferably 5 to 10 ml).[9] The CSF usually has a high protein, low glucose and a raised number of lymphocytes. Acid-fast bacilli are sometimes seen on a CSF smear, but more commonly, M. tuberculosis is grown in culture. A spider web clot in the collected CSF is characteristic of TB meningitis, but is a rare finding.

105. Endoscopic third ventriculostomy (ETV) is a surgical procedure for treatment of hydrocephalus in which an opening is created in the floor of the third ventricle in the pre-mammillary area using an endoscope placed within the ventricular system. This allows the cerebrospinal fluid to flow directly to the pre-pontine cistern by bypassing any obstruction. The ETV procedure is used as an alternative to a cerebral shunt mainly to treat certain forms of noncommunicating obstructive hydrocephalus (such as aqueductal stenosis), but since the ETV was introduced as an accepted treatment modality the range of etiologies for which it is used has grown significantly.

106. Engel Epilepsy Surgery Outcome Scale

- *Class I*: Free of disabling seizures
- *Class II*: Rare disabling seizures ("almost seizure-free")
- *Class III*: Worthwhile improvement
- *Class IV*: No worthwhile improvement

108. Vagus nerve stimulation (VNS) is an adjunctive treatment for certain types of intractable. The proposed mechanisms include alteration of norepinephrine release by projections of solitary tract to the locus ceruleus, elevated levels of inhibitory GABA related to vagal stimulation and inhibition of aberrant cortical activity by reticular activation system The cyberonics VNS devices consist of a titanium-encased generator about the size of a pocket watch with a lithium battery to fuel the generator, a lead wire system with electrodes, and an anchor tether to secure leads to the vagus nerve. The battery life for the pulse generator varies and depends how frequently the device stimulates the nerve.

109. Deep brain stimulation (DBS) is a surgical procedure used to treat a variety of disabling neurological symptoms—most commonly the debilitating symptoms of Parkinson's disease (PD), such as tremor, rigidity, stiffness, slowed movement, and walking problems. DBS surgery offers important symptomatic relief in patients with moderate disability from Parkinson's disease who still retain some benefit from antiparkinsonian medications and who are cognitively intact. Patients who fluctuate between "ON" and "OFF" medication states are usually good surgical candidates, as are those who have troublesome dyskinesias. DBS is not used for control of seizures, among stimulation procedures it is vagal nerve stimulation which is used to control seizures.

110. Complex partial seizures (CPS) are seizures which impair consciousness to some extent: they alter the person's ability to interact normally with their environment. Temporal lobe epilepsy (TLE) is the most common symptomatic partial epilepsy in adolescents and adults but, extratemporal or neocortical epilepsy is more common in young children. Mesial temporal sclerosis (MTS), hippocampal sclerosis (HS), is the most common cause of TLE, representing greater than 80%. Other causes include perinatal injury, malformations of cortical development (MCD), arteriovenous malformations (cavernous hemangiomas, meningioangiomatosis), infections of the central nervous system (CNS), glial tumors (e.g., ganglioglioma, dysembryoplastic neuroepithelial tumors, astrocytomas, oligodendrogliomas, meningiomas, or CNS metastasis), hamartomas, head trauma, and limbic encephalitis. MTS involves neuronal loss in the hilar region of the hippocampus (CA1, CA3, CA4, and the dentate gyrus, with relatively sparing of the CA2 region. It is typically bilateral but greater on one side. Temporal lobe epilepsy with mesial temporal sclerosis usually presents between 6–10 years of age but can present from infancy to the 30s. MTS is usually a progressive disorder and seizures initially controlled with antiepileptic drugs can later become intractable in 60–90%.

112. Absence seizures are sometimes referred to as petit mal seizures. Absence seizures are characterized by a brief loss and return of consciousness, generally not followed by a period of lethargy. Absence seizures are easily induced by hyperventilation in more than 90% of people with typical absences. This is a reliable test for the diagnosis of absence seizures: a patient suspected of typical absences should be asked to hyperventilate for 3 minutes. Intermittent photic stimulation may also precipitate absence seizures.

115. Pseudoseizures (also called non-epileptic, hysterical, or psychogenic seizures) are paroxysmal changes in behavior that resemble epileptic seizures, but are without organic cause and are without simultaneous electroencephalogram (EEG) changes suggestive of epilepsy. An elevated prolactin level (usually 2 times baseline or 3 standard deviations above normal) is fairly predictive of a seizure or other major neurologic events, such as syncope. Patients with pseudoseizures usually do not have elevations in prolactin levels.

116. Frontal lobe epilepsy is characterized by recurrent seizures arising from the frontal lobes. Frequently, seizure types are simple partial or complex partial, often with secondary generalization. Status epilepticus may be associated more commonly with frontal lobe seizures than with seizures arising from other areas. The following features help to distinguish frontal lobe seizures from non-epileptic events: Stereotyped semiology, occurrence during sleep, brief duration (often < 30 seconds), rapid secondary generalization, prominent motor manifestations, complex automatisms.

117. Mesial temporal sclerosis (MTS), also commonly referred to as hippocampal sclerosis, is the most common association with intractable temporal lobe epilepsy (TLE). It is seen in up to 65% of autopsy studies in patients of intractable seizures. Findings include:

- Reduced hippocampal volume: hippocampal atrophy
- Increased T2 signal of medial temporal lobe
- When severe and long standing, additional associated findings include;
- Atrophy of the ipsilateral fornix and mammillary body
- Increased signal and or atrophy of the anterior thalamic nucleus
- Atrophy of the cingulate gyrus
- Increased signal and/or reduction in volume of the amygdala
- Reduction in volume of the subiculum
- Dilatation of temporal horn and temporal lobe atrophy
- Collateral white matter and entorhinal cortex atrophy
- Thalamic and caudate atrophy
- Ipsilateral cerebral hypertrophy
- Contralateral cerebellar hemiatrophy
- Loss of grey-white matter interface in the anterior temporal lobe
- Reduced white matter volume in the parahippocampal gyrus

118. Gorlin syndrome, also known as nevoid basal cell carcinoma syndrome, is a condition that affects many areas of the body and increases the risk of developing various cancerous and noncancerous tumors. Most people with Gorlin syndrome also develop noncancerous (benign) tumors of the jaw, called keratocystic odontogenic tumors. These tumors usually first appear during adolescence, and new tumors form until about age 30. Keratocystic odontogenic tumors rarely develop later in adulthood. If untreated, these tumors may cause painful facial swelling and tooth displacement. Seizure is not a feature.

119. Temporal lobe epilepsy is a chronic neurological condition characterized by recurrent, unprovoked epileptic seizures (epilepsy) which originate in the temporal lobe of the brain. The seizures involve sensory changes; for example, smelling an unusual odor that is not there (an olfactory illusion), or a memory disturbance. The most common cause is mesial temporal sclerosis. Treatment is through medication or surgery and prognosis is variable. Simple partial seizures (SPS) involve small areas of the temporal lobe such as the amygdala and hippocampus. The term "simple" means that the level of consciousness of the patient is not altered during the seizure. In temporal lobe epilepsy, a simple partial seizure usually causes abnormal sensations only. Complex partial seizures (CPS) are seizures which impair consciousness to some extent: they alter the person's ability to interact normally with their environment. They usually begin with a single partial seizure, then spread to a larger portion of the temporal lobe, resulting in impaired consciousness. Signs may include motionless staring, automatic movements of the hands or mouth, altered ability to respond to others, unusual speech, or other unusual behaviors.

120. In acute disconnection of a right-handed, left-hemisphere dominant patient, there often is mild akinesia and mutism as well as competitive movements between the two hands. There is left hand apraxia to verbal command, left-arm hypotonia, well-coordinated but repetitive reaching, groping or grasping with the left hand, and bilateral Babinski responses and urge incontinence. It is suggested by some that complete callosotomy cases where speech and manual dominance are in opposite hemispheres may result in prolonged loss of spontaneous speech. Patients sometimes complain that their left hand behaves in a "foreign" or "alien" manner, and they often express surprise at apparently purposeful left-hand actions.

121. Childhood and adult herpes encephalitis is usually due to HSV-1 (90%) with the rest due to HSV-2. There is no particular age, sex or seasonal predilection. HSV is an obligatory intracellular virus which enters via infecting nasopharyngeal cells into sensory branch of lingual nerve then ascends to trigeminal ganglion and remains latent for lifetime. Reactivation in case of immunosuppression, trauma, or other stresses can result in fulminant hemorrhagic necrotizing encephalitis. HSV has strong affinity for limbic system with bilateral but asymmetrical involvement. DWI/ADC is more sensitive than T2 weighted images, restricted diffusion is common due to cytotoxic edema.

122. Nasal gliomas, also known as nasal glial heterotopia, are a rare congenital lesion composed of dysplastic glial cells which have lost their intracranial connections and present as an extranasal or intranasal mass. Nasal gliomas are rare congenital lesions. These masses occur sporadically with no familial tendency. Nasal gliomas are composed of dysplastic glial tissue, and are congenital non-neoplastic lesions best categorized as heterotopia. They are rarely associated with other congenital malformations. A nasal glioma may be connected to the brain by a stalk of tissue in up to 15% of cases, but the stalk does not contain a direct fluid-filled tract that communicates with the subarachnoid spaces; therefore, a nasal glioma is distinct from an nasoethmoidal encephalocoele.

124. A Snellen chart is an eye chart that can be used to measure visual acuity. Snell's chart is used for testing distant visions only. Snellen chart is named after the Dutch ophthalmologist Herman Snellen who developed the chart in 1862. Many vision scientists and clinicians now use an improved chart known as the LogMAR chart.

The Jaeger chart is an eye chart used in testing for near-sightedness. It is a card on which a text is printed, with the various paragraphs of the text having sizes of type increasing from 0.37 mm to 2.5 mm. This card is to be held by a patient at a fixed distance from the eye. The smallest print that the patient can read determines their visual acuity.

125. The visual fields of both eyes overlap; therefore each eye is tested independently. The patient should cover their right eye with their right hand (vice versa when testing the opposite eye). With the examiner seated directly across from the patient, the patient should direct their gaze to the corresponding eye of the examiner. The testing itself can be performed using stationary or moving targets (disk mounted on a stick or examiner's fingers). A moving target should start outside the usual 180° visual field, then move slowly to a more central position until the patient confirms visualization of the target. Since it is easier to detect appearances of objects than disappearances hence the object is moved from periphery to the center of vision. To perform stationary testing, the examiner holds up a certain number of fingers peripherally, equidistant between himself and the patient. The patient is asked to correctly identify the number of fingers. All 4 quadrants (upper and lower, temporal and nasal) should be tested. Stationary targets are more precise because they present a finer stimulus to the retina and are less easily identifiable relative to a moving target.

126. Tuberculous meningitis is a feared manifestation of tuberculous infection, because it is often difficult to diagnosis, requires a long course of therapy, and is associated with significant morbidity and mortality. Its most common signs and symptoms include fever, headache, changes in mentation, and meningismus in most patients. Other signs include focal neurologic deficits, such as, cranial nerve palsies, paresis, seizures, and diminished cognition. Cranial nerve palsies occur in 20–30% of patients and may be the presenting manifestation of TBM. The 3rd cranial nerve is most commonly affected after optic nerve. Vision loss due to optic nerve involvement may occasionally be a dominant presenting symptom. Involvement of the oculomotor nerve can occur due to basal meningitis due to the long course of this nerve in the base of brain, due to vasculitis in the arteries supplying the midbrain region, or due to a tuberculoma situated in the midbrain region.

128. The applause sign has been previously reported to be indicative of neurodegenerative disorders, such as progressive supranuclear palsy (PSP). It is seen in patients with PSP, Parkinson's disease, multiple system atrophy (MSA), corticobasal degeneration (CBD), and Huntington's disease. The applause sign is done using the three clap test. Applause sign is a feature of frontal lobe dysfunction.

129. Parkinsonian gait (or festinating gait, from Latin festinare [to hurry]) is the type of gait exhibited by patients suffering from Parkinson's disease (PD). This disorder is caused by a deficiency of dopamine in the basal ganglia circuit leading to motor deficits. Gait is one of the most affected motor characteristics of this disorder although symptoms of Parkinson's disease are varied. Falls and freezing of gait are two episodic phenomena that are common in Parkinsonian gait. Falls and freezing of gait in PD are generally thought to be closely intertwined for several reasons, most importantly: both symptoms are common in the advanced stages of the disease and are less common in the earlier stages, with freezing of gait leading to falls in many instances. Marche a petit pas gait (gait with little steps) is seen in: bilateral diffuse cortical dysfunction, diffuse cerebrovascular disease, multiple sclerosis, muscle weakness.

130. Most patients with multiple system atrophy (MSA) develop the disease when they are older than 40 years (average 52–55 years), and they experience fast progression. Usually autonomic and/or urinary dysfunction develops first. Patients with MSA may have parkinsonian symptoms with poor or non-sustained response to levodopa therapy. Autonomic symptoms are the initial feature in 41–74% of patients with MSA; these symptoms ultimately develop in 97% of patients. Orthostatic hypotension is common in MSA, being present in at least 68% of patients. Patients are also susceptible to postprandial hypotension. Altered venous capacitance and baroreflex dysfunction have been reported as a cause.

131. Molecular misreading of the ubiquitin-B (UBB) gene results in a dinucleotide deletion in UBB mRNA. The resulting mutant protein UBB accumulates in diseases viz. Pick disease, frontotemporal dementia, progressive supranuclear palsy, and argyrophilic grain disease. Creutzfeldt–Jakob disease is a degenerative neurological disorder that is incurable and invariably fatal. CJD is at times called a human form of mad cow disease (bovine spongiform encephalopathy or BSE. CJD is caused by an agent called a prion. Prions are misfolded proteins that replicate by converting their properly folded counterparts, in their host, to the same misfolded structure they possess. CJD causes the brain tissue to degenerate rapidly, and as the disease destroys the brain.

132. Vertigo caused by problems with the inner ear or vestibular system, which is composed of the semicircular canals, the vestibule (utricle and saccule), and the vestibular nerve is called "peripheral", "otologic" or "vestibular" vertigo. The most common cause is benign paroxysmal positional vertigo (BPPV). Any cause of inflammation such as common cold, influenza, and bacterial infections may cause transient vertigo. Skull fractures also are a cause. Patients with peripheral vertigo typically present with mild to moderate imbalance and nausea. Vomiting is unusual.

133. Mycotic aneurysms are aneurysms arising from the infection of the arterial wall, usually bacterial. It is a complication of the hematogenous spread of bacterial infection, classically from the heart. The vessel wall becomes infected with bacteria, is digested and a false aneurysm forms, which is unstable and highly prone to rupture. The commonest organisms is Streptococcus. In drug addicts who make use of intravenous route staphylococcus may be the cause.

136. Neurocutaneous melanosis is a rare non-familial disorder generally characterized by congenital intradermal benign pigmented nevi and leptomeningeal melanosis. It is thought to represent an embryonal neuroectodermal dysplasia with excessive proliferation of melanin producing cells, either focal or diffuse, in both skin and leptomeninges. The diagnostic criteria described by Fox are: (a) abnormal skin pigmentation with giant or multiple pigmented nevi, (b) absence of malignant change in any skin lesion, and (c) absence of malignant melanoma in any organ other than the leptomeninges. However, Leaney et al stated that 2 to 13% of cases have malignant degeneration of skin nevi and Kaplan et al reported a case with distant organ metastases from leptomeningeal melanoma.

Melanocytes that originate from neural crest are normally found within the basal layer of the epidermis, piamater, reticular formation of the medulla, and substantia nigra. The pial melanocytes are more prominent on the inferior surfaces of the cerebellum, frontal, temporal, and occipital lobes, ventral aspect of the medulla, pons, cerebral peduncles, and upper cervical cord. Sometimes they may be seen macroscopically, even in healthy patients.

The melanocytes within the pia mater are responsible for the development of leptomeningeal melanosis. The dura is generally spared. Pigmented thickening of the leptomeninges is most frequent in the areas of physiologic melanocytic distribution. Diffuse intracranial leptomeningeal, intraspinal leptomeningeal, ventricular ependymal, and choroid plexus involvement also may occur. Melanin, which has a paramagnetic effect, shortens T1 and T2 relaxation times. Areas of melanin deposition appeared hyperintense on T1-weighted and spin-density images and hyperintense T2-weighted images. [AJNR 1995;16:603-6].

137. An epidural blood patch is a surgical procedure that uses autologous blood in order to close one or many holes in the dura mater of the spinal cord, usually as a result of a previous lumbar puncture. The procedure can be used to relieve post dural puncture headaches caused by lumbar puncture. A small amount of the patient's blood is injected into the epidural space near the site of the original puncture; the resulting blood clot then "patches" the meningeal leak. The procedure carries the typical risks of any epidural puncture. However, even though it is often effective, further intervention is sometimes necessary.

138. The Panda appearance in neuroimaging refers to the appearance of the midbrain, when the red nucleus and substantia nigra are surrounded by high T2 signal. It is classically seen in Wilson disease, although whenever the white matter is diffusely abnormal in the region a similar appearance will be perceived such as in Japanese encephalitis. Wilson's disease is an inborn error of copper metabolism that is characterized by deficiency of ceruloplasmin, the serum transport protein for copper. Copper is deposited in the liver, and after hepatic binding sites are saturated, it is released. Systemic disease then develops and there is abnormal accumulation of copper in the brain, particularly in the putamen and globus pallidus. A Kayser-Fleischer ring (the brown ring on the edge of the iris) is common in Wilson's disease, especially when neurological symptoms are present.

139. Episodic movement disorders are characterized by circumscribed attacks of disturbed movement without loss of consciousness. Neurological examination between attacks is usually, although not necessarily, normal. In many cases the beginning and end of the movement disturbance is abrupt. Usually attacks are repetitive. The primary indication for AEDs remains certainly epilepsy, even if other neurological conditions may be treated with these drugs when the typical treatments are ineffective. Several pathophysiological mechanisms inducing a neuronal excitability seems to be involved in an imbalance of both GABAergic and glutamatergic neurotransmissions and therefore could be similar in epilepsy and episodic movement disorders.

140. Numerous studies have been performed to determine the degree of cerebellar tonsillar ectopia necessary for diagnosis of Chiari I malformation. MRI is the definitive imaging study for diagnosis of Chiari I malformation. The position of the cerebellar tonsils is measured on sagittal T_1 or T_2-weighted images of the cervical spine or brain by drawing a line at the foramen magnum from the inner margin of the opisthion to the basion, and then measuring the distance from that line to the inferior most margin of the cerebellar tonsils. Normal descent of tonsils below foramen magnum is up to 5 mm.

141. Chiari malformation is associated with a wide range of symptoms which vary by type.

Type I Chiari malformation usually causes no symptoms. Most people with the condition don't even know that they have it unless it is incidentally discovered during a diagnostic imaging test. But if the malformation is severe, type I may cause symptoms such as pain in the lower back of the head and neck; it usually develops quickly and intensifies with any activity that increases pressure in the brain, such as coughing and sneezing, Dizziness and problems with balance and coordination, Swallowing difficulties, Sleep apnea.

Most children born with type II Chiari malformation have hydrocephalus. Older children with type II Chiari malformation may develop headache associated with coughing or sneezing, bending over, strenuous physical activities. Some of the most common symptoms are linked to problems with the function of nerves in the brain stem. These include weakness of vocal cords, swallowing difficulties, breathing irregularities.

142. There are four types of Chiari malformations:

***Type I*:** This is by far the most commonly observed type in children. In this type, the lower part of the cerebellum —but not the brain stem—extends down to some extent through the foramen magnum.

Type II: This is usually only seen in children born with spina bifida. Spina bifida is the incomplete development of the spinal cord and/or its protective covering. Type II is also known as "classic" Chiari malformation. In type II Chiari malformation, both the cerebellum and the brain stem extend into the foramen magnum.

***Type III*:** This is the most serious form of Chiari malformation. It involves the protrusion or herniation of the cerebellum and brain stem through the foramen magnum and into the spinal cord. This usually causes severe neurological defects. Type III is incompatible with life.

***Type IV*:** This involves an incomplete or undeveloped cerebellum. It sometimes is associated with exposed parts of the skull and spinal cord. Type IV is a rare type.

143. **Probst bundles** denote white matter fibers normally destined to cross the corpus callosum parallel the interhemispheric fissure in patients with agenesis of the corpus callosum, leading to widely spaced lateral ventricles, in a "racing car" configuration.

144. Ultrasound may be a useful screening exam and may be of use in the pediatric population. The lack of ossification of the posterior arch of the spine in normal infants and the presence of a bony defect in patients with spina bifida permit sonographic examination. MRI is useful in visualizing the conus medullaris, assessing the thickness of the filum terminale, identifying traction lesions, and evaluating associated bony dysraphisms.

146. Neural tube defects (NTD), with a birth incidence of approximately 1/1000 in Americans are the second most common type of birth defect after congenital heart defects. In humans, the most common NTD is myelomeningocele.

These common birth defects vary in frequency depending on the geographical localization. They occur at frequencies ranging from 0.9 in Canada to 7.7 in the United Arab Emirates and 0.7 in central France to 11.7 in South America per 10,000 births. The maximum incidence is seen in Hispanics.

147. Red cell folate is assayed by radioisotope dilution or immunological methods. This is to be preferred to serum folate which fluctuates with dietary intake. An erythrocyte folate level less than 317 nmol/L (140 ng/mL) indicates reduced body stores.

148. Multifactorial disturbances in embryonic neurulation have been identified as causes of NTDs. Incidence of different NTDs varies according to geographic conditions, race/ethnicity, sex of the newborn, as well as high caffeine intake, low calorie diet, alcohol consumption, lack of folate supplementation at any time of pregnancy, oral contraceptive usage, obesity and passive smoking. In addition, other factors associated with one or both NTDs include maternal birthplace, parity, timing of prenatal care initiation, socio-economic status, as well as maternal age, education, nutritional status, drug usage, presence of maternal chronic diseases, and acute infections during pregnancy

149. **Lemon sign**, noted on antenatal imaging, is one of the many notable fruit inspired signs. It is a feature when there appears to be an indentation of the frontal bone (depicting that of a lemon). It is classically seen as a sign of a Chiari II malformation and also seen in the majority (90–98%) of fetuses with spina bifida. **Banana sign** is seen on axial imaging through the posterior fossa of fetus and is associated with the Chiari II malformation. It describes the way the cerebellum is wrapped tightly around the brain stem as a result of spinal cord tethering and downward migration of posterior fossa contents. The cisterna magna gets obliterated and the shape of the cerebellum has the appearance of a banana. The sign persists into the second and third trimesters.

150. Closure of a myelomeningocele is a deceptively simple operation; however, attention to several subtle details can significantly reduce operative complications. Operative intervention should be directed toward preserving neurological function and optimizing the subsequent repair of a tethered spine should this become necessary. Careful attention to the vascular supply to the placode, precise separation of neural from cutaneous tissues, a diligent search for associated tethering anomalies such as diastematomyelia and a thickened filum terminale, careful pia to pia reconstruction of the placode, and simple but meticulous wound closure all help in achieving these aims. The timely management of associated hydrocephalus will help to avoid cerebrospinal fluid leakage and wound breakdown. Close attention to these details will ameliorate many of the immediate and delayed complications of myelomeningocele closure.

151. Because the vertebral column grows longer than the spinal cord, spinal cord segments do not correspond to vertebral segments, especially in the lower spinal cord. In the fetus, vertebral segments do correspond with spinal cord segments upto 6-month. At tern spinal cord lies at the level of L3 vertebrae. In the adult, however, the spinal cord ends around the L1/L2 vertebral level, forming a structure known as the conus medullaris.

152. In a patient with tuft of hair at back look for a spinal problem such as a lipoma (fatty tumor), spinal cord abnormality called diastematomyelia (split spinal cord), tethered cord, other types of spinal tumor, and spina bifida.

153. Pang divided SCM into two types. Type I SCM consists of two hemicords, each contained within its own dural sheath and being separated by a rigid osseocartilaginous median septum. A type II SCM consists of two hemicords housed in a single dural sheath being separated by a non-rigid, fibrous median septum. Split cord is 3-times commoner in girls than boys.

154. Dandy-Walker Syndrome is a congenital brain malformation involving the cerebellum and the fluid-filled spaces around it. The key features of this syndrome are an enlargement of the fourth ventricle, a partial or complete absence of the cerebellar vermis, and cyst formation near the lowest part of the skull. An increase in the size of the fluid spaces surrounding the brain as well as an increase in pressure may also be present.

The syndrome can appear dramatically or develop unnoticed. Symptoms, which often occur in early infancy, include slow motor development and progressive enlargement of the skull. In older children, symptoms of increased intracranial pressure such as irritability and vomiting, and signs of cerebellar dysfunction such as unsteadiness, lack of muscle coordination, or jerky movements of the eyes may occur. Other symptoms include increased head circumference, problems with the nerves that control the eyes, face and neck, and abnormal breathing patterns. Dandy-Walker Syndrome is frequently associated with absent corpus callosum and malformations of the heart, face, limbs, fingers and toes.

156. VGM can be classified into the mural or choroidal type, depending on the characteristic of the fistula. The mural type consists of high-flow shunts, supplied by the collicular and posterior choroidal arteries, ending directly within the aneurysmal wall of the median prosencephalic vein. The choroidal type involves the interposition of an extensive arterial network between the arterial feeder, supplied by the choroidal, subfornical, or pericallosal arteries or thalamoperforator arteries, and the venous aneurysm. The choroidal form usually leads to more severe symptoms whereas the mural form is better tolerated clinically. Mixed forms combining direct shunts and arterial networks may also occur.

Vein of Galen malformations should be differentiated from the vein of Galen aneurysmal dilatation (VGAD), which represents a normally formed vein of Galen that dilates as a result of outflow obstruction. The dilated venous structure drains an arteriovenous malformation located in the subarachnoid space, either supra- or infratentorially, in addition to the adjacent normal cerebral parenchyma. The degree of dilatation is variable and depends on the extent of stenosis or thrombosis. The frequency of VGADs in neonates and infants is low and patients with VGAD often present in later age during childhood, with intracranial hemorrhage, focal neurological deficits, and in the very young, with delayed psychomotor development. The pathophysiological consequences of VGM most often manifests as high-output cardiac failure and neurological symptoms secondary to cerebral venous congestion and abnormal CSF flow. The severity of the symptoms is variable and dependent on the underlying angioarchitecture of the VGM as well as the age of the child. Typically neonates present with congestive heart failure, infants present with hydrocephalus, and the older children or adults present with headache and, frequently, with signs and symptoms of subarachnoid hemorrhage.

157. An arachnoid cyst is identified in 1.4% of adult patients undergoing an MRI scan and in 2.6% of children undergoing MRI scan. It has been estimated that arachnoid cysts account for 1% of intracranial masse. In children, arachnoid cysts occur more commonly in boys but apparently are equally distributed in the elderly. Temporal lobe cysts are more commonly found on the left side (2.5:1), and there seems to be a significant male preponderance of temporal arachnoid cysts. For all other sites, there does not appear to be any gender predilection apart from the cerebellar pontine angle, which may be more common in women.

The **Galassi classification system** is one used for classifying arachnoid cysts.

***Type I*:** small, spindle-shaped, limited to the anterior portion of the middle cranial fossa, usually with free communication on CT cisternography.

***Type II*:** superior extent along sylvian fissure with displacement of the temporal lobe.

***Type III*:** large, fills the whole middle cranial fossa, with displacement of not only the temporal lobe but also the frontal and parietal lobes. Little communication with subarachnoid space on CT cisternography.

158. The following features are observed with VACTERL association

- V - Vertebral anomalies
- A - Anal atresia
- C - Cardiovascular anomalies
- T - Tracheoesophageal fistula
- E - Esophageal atresia
- R - Renal (Kidney) and/or radial anomalies
- L - Limb defects

Although it was not conclusive whether VACTERL should be defined by at least two or three component defects, it is typically defined by the presence of at least three of the above congenital malformations.

Vertebral defects

Vertebral anomalies, or defects of the spinal column, usually consist of small (hypoplastic) vertebrae or hemivertebra where only one half of the bone is formed. About 80 percent of patients with VACTERL association will have vertebral anomalies. In early life these rarely cause any difficulties, although the presence of these defects on a chest x-ray may alert the physician to other defects associated with VACTERL. Later in life these spinal column abnormalities may put the child at risk for developing scoliosis, or curvature of the spine.

Anal defects

Anal atresia or imperforate anus is seen in about 55% of patients with VACTERL association. These anomalies are usually noted at birth and often require surgery in the first days of life. Sometimes babies will require several surgeries to fully reconstruct the intestine and anal canal.

Cardiac defects

Up to 75 percent of patients with VACTERL association have been reported to have congenital heart disease. The most common heart defects seen with VACTERL association are ventricular septal defect (VSD), atrial septal defects and tetralogy of Fallot. Less common defects are truncus arteriosus and transposition of the great arteries.

Tracheoesophageal fistula defects

Esophageal atresia with tracheoesophageal fistula (TE fistula) is seen in about 70% of patients with VACTERL association, although it can frequently occur as an isolated defect. Fifteen to 33% of patients with TE fistulas will also have congenital heart disease. However these babies usually have uncomplicated heart defects, like a ventricular septal defect, which may not require any surgery.

Renal / Kidney defects

Renal (kidney) defects are seen in approximately 50% of patients with VACTERL association. In addition, up to 35% of patients with VACTERL association have a single umbilical artery (there are usually two arteries and one vein) which is often associated with additional kidney or urologic problems. Renal abnormalities in VACTERL association can be severe, with incomplete formation of one or both kidneys or urologic abnormalities such as obstruction of outflow of urine from the kidneys or severe reflux (backflow) of urine into the kidneys from the bladder. These problems can cause kidney failure early in life and may require kidney transplant.

Limb defects

Limb defects occur in up to 70% of babies with VACTERL association and include a displaced or hypoplastic thumb, extra digits (polydactyly), fusion of digits (syndactyly) and forearm defects such as radial aplasia. Babies with limb defects on both sides tend to have kidney or urologic defects on both sides, while babies with limb defects on only one side of the body tend to have kidney problems on that same side.

Other features

Features secondary to VACTERL components including single umbilical artery, ambiguous genitalia, abdominal wall defects, diaphragmatic hernia, and anomalies like intestinal and respiratory anomalies, and oligohydramnios sequence defects are frequent enough to be considered an extension of VACTERL. Cardiac defects are thought to fit in this category.

Growth

Many babies with VACTERL are born small and have difficulty with gaining weight. Babies with VACTERL association, however, do tend to have normal development and normal intelligence. Although, children with VACTERL may have a more active brain. Some children are said to have a higher IQ and are able to work through word/number/shape problems more easily.

159. **Fåhræus–Lindqvist effect** is an effect where the viscosity of a fluid, in this case blood, changes with the diameter of the tube it travels through; in particular there's a decrease of viscosity as the tube's diameter decreases (only if the vessel diameter is between 10 and 300 micrometers). This is because erythrocytes move over the center of the vessel, leaving plasma at the wall of the vessel.

160. The cerebrospinal fluid **(CSF)** is produced from arterial blood by the choroid plexuses of the lateral and fourth ventricles by a combined process of diffusion, pinocytosis and active transfer. A small amount is also produced by ependymal cells. The **choroid plexus** consists of tufts of capillaries with thin fenestrated endothelial cells. These are covered by modified ependymal cells with bulbous microvilli. The total volume of CSF in the adult ranges from 140 to 270 ml. The volume of the ventricles is about 25 ml. CSF is produced at a rate of 0.3–0.5 ml per minute or 400–500 ml per day. The circulation of CSF is aided by the pulsations of the choroid plexus and by the motion of the cilia of ependymal cells. CSF is absorbed across the arachnoid villi into the venous circulation and a significant amount probably also drains into lymphatic vessels around the cranial cavity and spinal canal. The arachnoid villi act as one-way valves between the subarachnoid space and the dural sinuses. The rate of absorption correlates with the CSF pressure. CSF acts as a cushion that protects the brain from shocks and supports the venous sinuses (primarily the superior sagittal sinus, opening when CSF pressure exceeds venous pressure). It also plays an important role in the homeostasis and metabolism of the central nervous system. CSF from the lumbar region contains 15 to 45 mg/dl protein (lower in children) and 50–80 mg/dl glucose (two-thirds of blood glucose). Protein concentration in cisternal and ventricular CSF is lower. Normal CSF contains 0–5 mononuclear cells. The CSF pressure, measured at lumbar puncture (LP), is 100–180 mm of H_2O (8-15 mm Hg) with the patient lying on the side and 200-300 mm with the patient sitting up.

161. Normal pressure hydrocephalus (NPH), AKA Hakim-Adams syndrome, is clinically important because it may cause treatable symptoms, including one of the few forms of remediable dementia. As originally described, the hydrocephalus of NPH was considered to be idiopathic. However, in some cases a predisposing condition ("secondary NPH") may be identified: 1. post-SAH 2. post-traumatic 3. post-meningitis 4. following posterior fossa surgery 5. tumors, including carcinomatous meningitis.

The triad is not pathognomonic, and similar features may also be seen e.g. in vascular dementia, Alzheimer's dementia and Parkinson's disease.

1. **Gait disturbance:** usually precedes other symptoms. Wide based with short, shuffling steps and unsteadiness on turning. Patients often feel like they are "glued to the floor" (so-called "magnetic gait") and may have difficulty initiating steps or turns.
2. **Dementia:** Primarily memory impairment with bradyphrenia (slowness of thought) and bradykinesia.
3. Urinary incontinence.

162. The most likely symptom to improve with shunting is incontinence, then gait disturbance, and lastly dementia. The following are Indicators of good prognosis: presence of the classic triad, also 77% of patients with gait disturbance as the primary symptom improved with shunting. Patients with dementia and no gait disturbance rarely respond to shunting.

LP: OP > 100 mm H_2O. Isotope cisternogram: typical NPH pattern. Continuous CSF pressure recording: pressure > 180 mm H_2O or frequent Lundberg B waves.

CT or MRI: Large ventricles with flattened sulci. Response is better when symptoms have been present for a shorter time.

163. Neurofibrillary Tangles (NFTs) are aggregates of hyperphosphorylatedtau protein that are most commonly known as a primary marker of Alzheimer's Disease. Their presence is also found in numerous other diseases viz.

- Progressive supranuclear palsy
- Dementia pugilistica (chronic traumatic encephalopathy)
- Frontotemporal dementia and parkinsonism linked to chromosome 17 however without detectable β-amyloid plaques.
- Lytico-Bodig disease (Parkinson-dementia complex of Guam)
- Ganglioglioma and gangliocytoma
- Meningioangiomatosis
- Subacute sclerosing panencephalitis
- Lead encephalopathy, Tuberous Sclerosis, Hallervorden-Spatz disease, and Lipofuscinosis

164. Schwannoma arise from all cranial nerve except first two because they are myelinated by oligodendrocyte not schwann cell.

Acoustic schwannomas account for 80 to 90% of tumors found in the CPA and are common tumors of the posterior fossa, second only to the gliomas. Overall, they account for 6 to 8% of all intracranial tumors. Typically benign, slowly growing tumors, the inferior vestibular nerve is involved in 50%, superior vestibular in 50%. Cystic changes are rare. The site of origin of the tumor is believed to be the point of transition between the central and peripheral myelin, where Schwann cells meet oligodendrocytes (Obesteiner-Redlich zone) inside the internal auditory canal (IAC).

165. Meningiomas are slow growing, extra-axial tumor, usually benign, arise from arachnoid (not dura) imaging (MRI or CT): classically broad based attachment on dura often with dural tail, typically enhance densely, may cause hyperostosis of adjacent bone.

Meningiomas account for 14.3-19% of primary intracranial neoplasms. Incidence peaks at 45 years age. Female: male ratio is 1.8:1. most common location Is convexity (20%), followed by parasagittal (15%), tuberculum sellae 12%), sphenoid wing (11%).

WHO graded each of these meningioma subtypes into one of three categories based primarily upon the likelihood of recurrence and the rate of growth exhibited by each. The overall classifications are benign (Grade I), atypical (Grade II) and malignant (Grade III).

166. Idiopathic intracranial hypertension (IIH), sometimes called by the older names benign intracranial hypertension (BIH) or pseudotumor cerebri (PTC), is a neurological disorder that is characterized by increased intracranial pressure in the absence of a tumor.

The main symptoms are headache, nausea, and vomiting, as well as pulsatile tinnitus, double vision and other visual symptoms. If untreated, it may lead to vision loss.

CAUSE

Idiopathic" means "of unknown etiology". Therefore, IIH can only be diagnosed if there is no alternative explanation for the symptoms.

Intracranial pressure may be increased due to medications such as high-dose vitamin A derivatives (e.g. isotretinoin for acne), long-term tetracycline antibiotics (for a variety of skin conditions) and hormonal contraceptives.

If there is an underlying cause, the condition is termed "secondary intracranial hypertension". [1]Common causes of secondary intracranial hypertension include obstructive sleep apnea (a sleep-related breathing disorder), systemic lupus erythematosus (SLE), chronic kidney disease, and Behçet's disease. Pregnancy is also associated with peudotumor cerebri.

167. The average cerebral blood flow in humans is approximately 55 mL per 100 g of brain tissue per minute. Thus while the human brain comprises only about 2.5% of the body's weight, it receives almost 15 percent of the cardiac output, attesting to the high vascular demands of this organ. A reliable and frequently used method of determining cerebral blood flow is the method of Kety and Schmidt. It is based on the Fick principle. The cerebral blood flow is higher in children than in adults, typically exceeding 100 mL per 100 g per minute. The brain utilizes fully 25 percent of the body's total oxygen consumption. The arteriovenous O_2 difference is relatively high since the brain receives only 15 percent of the cardiac output. The arteriovenous difference is 6.6 mL per 100 ml., falling from 19.6 to 13 mL per 100 mL as blood passes through the brain. Thus we can calculate a cerebral oxygen consumption of approximately 3.5 mL per 100 g per minute. The utilization of oxygen by the brain is not uniform throughout its mass. The gray matter consumes as much as 94% of cerebral oxygen and white matter which makes up fully 60 percent of the brain's mass consumes only 6%. Oxygen consumption, and hence oxygen need, increases as we move up the neuraxis. It is lowest in the spinal cord and increases through the medulla, midbrain, thalamus, cerebellum, and cerebral cortex. Thus it is not surprising to find that the sensorimotor functions of the cerebral cortex are more sensitive to hypoxic damage than are the vegetative functions of the pontomedullary areas. Progressive decreases in cerebral oxygen consumption are always accompanied by progressive decreases in the level of mental alertness. Compared to the mentally alert young man with an O_2 consumption of 3.5 mL per 100 g per minute, the mentally confused states associated with diabetic acidosis, insulin hypoglycemia, and some forms of cerebral arteriosclerosis might typically show O_2 consumptions rates down to 2.8 mL per 100 g per minute. Finally, the comatose states of diabetic coma, insulin coma, and anesthesia can show consumption rates as low as 2.0 mL per 100 g per minute. On the other hand. O_2 consumption by the brain increases during convulsions.

169. The mechanism(s) by which mannitol provides its beneficial effects is still controversial, but probably includes some combination of the following:

1. Lowering ICP
   A. *Immediate plasma expansion:* reduces the hematocrit and blood viscosity (improved rheology) which increases CBF and O_2 delivery. This reduces ICP within a few minutes, and is most marked in patients with CPP < 70 mmHg.
   B. *Osmotic effect:* increased serum tonicity draws edema fluid from cerebral parenchyma. Takes 15–30 minutes until gradients are established. Effect lasts 1.5–6 hours, depending on the clinical condition.

2. Supports the microcirculation by improving blood rheology.
3. Possible free radical scavenging.

The overall effect of mannitol is that cerebral blood volume (CBV) decreases and cerebral blood flow (CBF) increases. With bolus administration, onset of ICP lowering effect occurs in 1–5 minutes; peaks at 20–60 minutes. When urgent reduction of ICP is needed, an initial dose of 1 gm/ kg should be given over 30 minutes. When long-term reduction of ICP is intended, the infusion time should be lengthened to 60 minutes and the dose reduced (e.g. 0.25–0.5 gm/kg q 6 hours).

170. CBF is equal to the cerebral perfusion pressure (CPP) divided by the cerebrovascular resistance (CVR):

CBF = CPP / CVR

Cerebral blood flow (CBF) is the blood supply to the brain in a given period of time. In an adult, CBF is typically 750 milliliters per minute or 15% of the cardiac output. This equates to an average perfusion of 50 to 54 milliliters of blood per 100 grams of brain tissue per minute. CBF is tightly regulated to meet the brain's metabolic demands. Too much blood (a condition known as hyperemia) can raise intracranial pressure (ICP), which can compress and damage delicate brain tissue. Too little blood flow (ischemia) results if blood flow to the brain is below 18 to 20 mL per 100 g per minute, and tissue death occurs if flow dips below 8 to 10 mL per 100 g per minute. Cerebral blood flow is determined by a number of factors, such as viscosity of blood, how dilated blood vessels are, and the net pressure of the flow of blood into the brain, known as cerebral perfusion pressure, which is determined by the body's blood pressure. Cerebral blood vessels are able to change the flow of blood through them by altering their diameters in a process called autoregulation; they constrict when systemic blood pressure is raised and dilate when it is lowered. Arterioles also constrict and dilate in response to different chemical concentrations. For example, they dilate in response to higher levels of carbon dioxide in the blood and constrict to lower levels of carbon dioxide. For example, assuming a person with an arterial partial pressure of carbon dioxide ($PaCO_2$) of 40 mm Hg (normal range of 38 - 42 mm Hg) and a CBF of 50 mL per 100 g per min. If the $PaCO_2$ dips to 30 mm Hg, this represents a 10 mm Hg decrease from the initial value of $PaCO_2$. Consequently, the CBF decreases by 1 mL per 100 g per min for each 1 mm Hg decrease in $PaCO_2$, resulting in a new CBF of 40 mL per 100 g of brain tissue per minute. In fact, for each 1 mm Hg increase or decrease in $PaCO_2$, between the range of 20–60 mm Hg, there is a corresponding CBF change in the same direction of approximately 1–2 mL/100g/min, or 2–5% of the CBF value. This is why small alterations in respiration pattern can cause significant changes in global CBF, specially through $PaCO_2$ variations.

171. Poor prognostic factor after head injury are: low GCS score, extremes of age, hypotension, hyperthermia, hyperglycemia, hypoxia, hypercarbia, coagulopathy, mydriasis, increase in ICP.

172. The most affected CN involved in head injury is the olfactory nerve (CN I), when more than 1 CN is involved, the most frequent association is between CNs VII and VIII.

173. A perilymph fistula is an abnormal opening in fluid filled inner ear. There are several possible places that there can be an opening–between the air-filled middle ear/mastoid sinus, into the intracranial cavity, or into other spaces in the temporal bone. In most instances it is a tear or defect in one or both of the small, thin membranes between the middle and inner ears. These membranes are called the oval window and the round window.

Head trauma is a common cause of fistulas, usually involving a direct blow to the ear. Fistulas may also develop following rapid or profound changes in intracranial or atmospheric pressure, such as may occur with scuba diving, or even just dives into a swimming pool. Forceful coughing, sneezing or straining as in lifting a heavy object may rarely cause a fistula. In pregnancy, collagen changes throughout the body and fistulae may arise spontaneously or in association with delivery. Children are likely more prone to develop fistulae.

174. Fornix is part of the limbic system. While its exact function and importance in the physiology of the brain is still not entirely clear, it has been demonstrated in humans that surgical transection – the cutting of the fornix along its body – can cause memory loss. There is some debate over what type of memory is affected by this damage, but it has been found to most closely correlate with recall memory rather than recognition memory. This means that damage to the fornix can cause difficulty in recalling long-term information such as details of past events, but it has little effect on the ability to recognize objects or familiar situations.

175. Auditory brainstem response (ABR) audiometry typically uses a click stimulus that generates a response from the basilar region of the cochlea. The signal travels along the auditory pathway from the cochlear nuclear complex proximally to the inferior colliculus. ABR waves I and II correspond to true action potentials. Later waves may reflect postsynaptic activity in major brainstem auditory centers that concomitantly contribute to waveform peaks and troughs. The positive peaks of the waveforms reflect combined afferent (and likely efferent) activity from axonal pathways in the auditory brain stem.

Wave I: The ABR wave I response is the far-field representation of the compound auditory nerve action potential in the distal portion of cranial nerve (CN) VIII. The response is believed to originate from afferent activity of the CN VIII fibers (first-order neurons) as they leave the cochlea and enter the internal auditory canal.

Wave II: The ABR wave II is generated by the proximal VIII nerve as it enters the brain stem.

Wave III: The ABR wave III arises from second-order neuron activity (beyond CN VIII) in or near the cochlear nucleus. Literature suggests wave III is generated in the caudal portion of the auditory pons. The cochlear nucleus contains approximately 100,000 neurons, most of which are innervated by eighth nerve fibers.

Wave IV: The ABR wave IV, which often shares the same peak with wave V, is thought to arise from pontine third-order neurons mostly located in the superior olivary complex, but additional contributions may come from the cochlear nucleus and nucleus of lateral lemniscus.

Wave V: Generation of wave V likely reflects activity of multiple anatomic auditory structures. The ABR wave V is the component analyzed most often in clinical applications, it is believed to originate from the vicinity of the inferior colliculus. The second-order neuron activity may additionally contribute in some way to wave V. The inferior colliculus is a complex structure, with more than 99% of the axons from lower auditory brainstem regions going through the lateral lemniscus to the inferior colliculus.

Waves VI and VII: Thalamic (medial geniculate body) origin is suggested for generation of waves VI and VII, but the actual site of generation is uncertain.

176. A striatal toe has been defined as an apparent extensor plantar response, without fanning of the toes, in the absence of any other signs suggesting dysfunction of the corticospinal tract.

Striatal deformities of the hand and foot are abnormal postures that are common in patients with advanced Parkinson's disease (PD); they can present in the early stages of PD and in other parkinsonian disorders. The term striatal is used because pathology in the neostriatum (putamen and caudate) has been suggested to cause the deformities, but the pathogenesis is unknown. Misdiagnosis of the deformities is common-particularly when they occur early and in the absence of cardinal parkinsonian signs, such as tremor, bradykinesia, and rigidity-because the hand deformities are similar to those in rheumatoid arthritis, equinovarus foot deformity typically suggests an orthopedic problem, and toe extension may be thought to be the Babinski sign of upper-motor-neuron syndromes.

177. **Jaeger chart** is an eye chart used in testing for near-sightedness. It is a card on which a text is printed, with the various paragraphs of the text having sizes of type increasing from 0.37 mm to 2.5 mm. This card is to be held by a patient at a fixed distance from the eye. The smallest print that the patient can read determines their visual acuity.

Snellen chart is an eye chart that can be used to measure distant visual acuity.

Hess charts are used in diagnosis of strabismus.

178. The ptosis caused by the oculomotor palsy can be unilateral or bilateral, as the subnucleus to the levator muscle is a shared, midline structure in the brainstem. In cases in which the palsy is caused by the compression of the nerve by a tumor or aneurysm, it is highly likely to result into an abnormal ipsilateral papillary response and a larger pupil. Surgical third nerve palsy is characterized by a sudden onset of unilateral ptosis and an enlarged or sluggish pupil to the light. In this case, imaging tests such as CTs or MRIs should be considered. Medical third nerve palsy, contrary to surgical third nerve palsy, usually does not affect the pupil and it tends to slowly improve in several weeks. Surgery to correct ptosis due to medical third nerve palsy is normally considered only if the improvement of ptosis and ocular motility are unsatisfactory after half a year. Patients with third nerve palsy tend to have diminished or absent function of the levator. When caused by Horner's syndrome, ptosis is usually accompanied by miosis and anhidrosis. In this case, the ptosis is due to the result of interruption innervations to the sympathetic, autonomic Muller's muscle rather than the somatic levator palpebrae superioris muscle. The lid position and pupil size are typically affected by this condition and the ptosis is generally mild, no more than 2 mm. The pupil might be smaller on the affected side. While 4% cocaine instilled to the eyes can confirm the diagnosis of Horner's syndrome, hydroxyamphetamine eye drops can differentiate the location of the lesion. Patients show wrinkled forehead if ptosis is because of oculomotor nerve palsy and wrinkling is lost in sympathetic paralysis.

179. Horner's syndrome (HS) is caused by interruption of sympathetics to the eye and face anywhere along their path, Possible Sites of Disruption of Sympathetics.

1st order neuron (central neuron): Interruption is often accompanied by other brainstem abnormalities. Etiologies of dysfunction: infarction from vascular occlusion (usually PICA), syringobulbia, intra parenchymal neoplasm.

2nd order neuron (preganglionic): Etiologies of dysfunction: lateral sympathectomies, significant chest trauma, apical pulmonary neoplasms (Pancoast tumor), high thoracic or cervical neuroblastoma.

3rd order neuron (postganglionic): The most common type. Etiologies of dysfunction: neck trauma, carotid vascular disease/studies (e.g. carotid dissections, cervical bony abnormalities, migraine, skull base neoplasms, cavernous sinus lesions (e.g. meningioma). With involvement only of fibers on ICA, anhidrosis does not occur (i.e. sweating is preserved) on ipsilateral face since fibers to facial sweat glands travel with ECA.

Unilateral findings on the involved side in a fully developed Horner's syndrome are

1. Miosis in Horner's syndrome is only 2–3 mm. This will be accentuated by darkening the room, which causes the normal pupil to dilate.
2. Ptosis is due primarily to paralysis of the superior and inferior tarsal muscles (weakness of the inferior tarsal muscle is technically called ~inverse ptosis"). Ptosis in HS is partial, as compared to complete ptosis which is due to weakness of levator palpebra superioris which is not involved in Homer's syndrome.
3. Enophthalmos is due to Muller's muscle paralysis, which also contributes a maximum of 2 mm to the ptosis.
4. Hyperemia of eye
5. Anhydrosis of half of face

180. Optokinetic nystagmus (OKN) is nystagmus that occurs in response to a rotation movement. It is present normally. The nystagmus consists of initial slow phases in the direction of the stimulus (smooth pursuits), followed by fast, corrective phases (saccade). Presence of nystagmus indicates an intact visual pathway. OKN can be used as a crude assessment of the visual system particularly in infants. When factitious blindness or malingering is suspected, check for optokinetic nystagmus to determine whether there is an intact visual pathway. The response is absent in parietal lobe lesions.

181. Decorticate posturing: Classically attributed to disinhibition by removal of corticospinal pathways above the midbrain. Abnormal flexion in upper limbs and extension in lower limbs: slow flexion of arm, wrist and fingers with adduction in the upper limb. Extension, internal rotation, plantarflexion in lower limb.

Decerebrate posturing: Classically attributed to disinhibition of vestibulospinal tract (more caudal) and pontine reticular formation (RF) by removing inhibition of medullary RF (transection at intercollicular level, between vestibular and red nuclei). Abnormal extension in upper limb and lower limb. Detail: opisthotonus (head and trunk extended), teeth clenched, arms extended, adducted and hyperpronated (internally rotated), wrists flexed, fingers flexed. Legs extended and internally rotated, feet plantar flexed and inverted, toes plantar flexed. **Pyramidal tracts** include both the corticospinal and corticobulbar tracts. These are aggregations of upper motor neuron nerve fibres that travel from the cerebral cortex and terminate either in the brainstem (corticobulbar) or spinal cord (corticospinal) and are involved in control of motor functions of the body. If fibers of the corticospinal tracts are damaged anywhere along their course from the cerebral cortex to the lower end of the spinal cord, this will give rise to an upper motor neuron syndrome. A few days after the injury to the upper motor neurons, a pattern of motor signs and symptoms appears, including spasticity, hyperactive reflexes, a loss of the ability to perform fine movements, and an extensor plantar response known as the Babinski sign. Abductors and extensors of the upper limbs and flexors of the lower limb are the muscle groups mostly involved in pyramidal lesions.

185. Dravet syndrome is a genetic disorder, most often due to a mutation in the SCN1A sodium channel gene. Many children with treatment-resistant epilepsies have been reported to benefit from marijuana.

Among the more than 400 chemical compounds in C. sativa, there are at least 85 terpenophenolic compounds referred to as cannabinoids. Isolation and characterization of these lipophilic compounds led to studies that found that psychotropic effects are due to Δ^9-tetrahydrocannabinol (THC). By contrast, cannabidiol (CBD) is the most abundant non-psychoactive cannabinoid in cannabis. Both THC and CBD have been demonstrated to have anticonvulsant efficacy in multiple species and animal models. However, while THC has been found to be provconvulsant in some models of epilepsy, CBD has not.

Neurosurgery 2015;76(4)357-61

187. Anterior plagiocephaly is produced by unilaterial coronal suture involvement. Unilateral lambdoid suture involvement causes posterior plagiocephaly and bilambdoid suture involvement causes posterior brachycephaly; while as anterior brachycephaly is caused by bicoronal suture involvement. *(Youman's p. 3305)*

189-191. Hypertrophic olivary degeneration is a rare phenomenon that occurs after an insult to the dentato-rubro-olivary tract (Guillain-Mollaret triangle), constituted by the dentate, rubro and inferior olivary nuclei, which are interconnected via the central tegmental tract and superior and inferior cerebellar peduncles. This is a degenerative disorder that initially develops with hypertrophy. Injury to any of such components may result in axonal interruption to the inferior olivary nucleus, leading to its degeneration. In cases where the alterations are restricted to the central tegmental tract, the HOD is ipsilateral and in cases where there is involvement of the dentate nucleus or of the dentate nucleus or superior cerebellar peduncle, the condition is contralateral.

193. Krabbe disease, also known as globoid cell leukodystrophy (GLD), is a rare, autosomal recessive disorder caused by mutations in the gene coding for the lysosomal enzyme galactocerebrosidase (GALC). GALC is responsible for the catabolism of galactocerebroside; enzymatic deficiency results in accumulation of the metabolite psychosine, which is cytotoxic to oligodendrocytes, the myelin-producing cells of the central nervous system.

194. Adrenomyeloneuropathy (AMN) is the adult form of the progressive neurodegenerative condition, X-linked adrenoleukodystrophy. Mutation in the ABCD1 gene results in a disrupted peroxisomal beta oxidation causing accumulation of the saturated very long chain fatty acids.

195. Meckels cave meningoceles are localized in the lateral sphenoid wing lateral to V2 and the foramen rotundum underneath the semilunar ganglion, reaching to the superior orbital fissure, pterygopalatine fossa, and medial orbital space, mostly emerging from an enlarged Meckel cave and giving rise to osseous erosion of the sphenoid wing. Most commonly seen as asymptomatic incidental finding.

196. Paraneoplastic syndrome is defined as a collection of symptoms and clinical signs occurring in cancer patients involving systemic effects taking place remotely from the tumor. They are not attributable to direct compression or invasion by the tumor or to adverse effects from infection, nutritional deficits, or treatment. PNS are classified according to their clinical manifestations (i.e, endocrine, hematologic, neurologic, dermatologic, inflammatory). Neurologic PNS occur in 6% of all patients with cancer.

197. Malignant hyperthermia is a rare, but life-threatening, autosomal-dominant inherited disorder that may lead to metabolic crisis of skeletal muscle in susceptible individuals following exposure to triggering agents, such as volatile anesthetics or depolarizing muscle relaxants. Functionally altered calcium release channels cause dysfunction of intracellular calcium homeostasis and uncontrolled calcium release from the sarcoplasmic reticulum, which may lead rapidly to a fatal hypermetabolic state known as malignant hyperthermia crisis.

198. Vincristine-induced peripheral neuropathy occurs in nearly all children receiving vincristine for acute lymphoblastic leukemia. It is characterized by progressive motor, sensory, and autonomic nerve damage. Microtubule structure disruption and subsequent neuronal axon dysfunction, as well as inflammatory processes, have been suggested as possible pathophysiologic mechanisms. Common VIPN signs and symptoms include numbness and tingling in the hands and feet with associated neuropathic pain, asymptomatic hyporeflexia and muscle weakness.

199. Lead encephalopathy can present in acute or chronic forms. In acute lead encephalopathy the patient presents with headache, vomiting, ataxia, convulsions, paralysis, stupor and coma. In chronic lead encephalopathy, the patient presents with loss of memory, behavioral abnormalities, depression, ataxia, seizures, drowsiness, restlessness and loss of sensory perception. Chronic neurocognitive signs can be observed at lower lead levels than those associated with frank encephalopathy.

201. Cocaine is a powerfully addictive stimulant drug made from the leaves of the coca plant. It produces short-term euphoria, energy, and talkativeness in addition to potentially dangerous physical effects like raising heart rate and blood pressure. Cocaine is a strong central nervous system stimulant that increases levels of the dopamine. Cocaine prevents the dopamine reuptake causing excessive amounts to build up in the synapse. This amplifies the dopamine signal and ultimately disrupts normal brain communication. The effects of cocaine depend on the method of taking it. Regular snorting of cocaine, for example, can lead to loss of the sense of smell, nosebleeds, problems with swallowing, hoarseness, and a chronically runny nose. Ingesting cocaine by the mouth can cause severe bowel gangrene as a result of reduced blood flow. Cocaine is more dangerous when combined with other drugs or alcohol, the combination of cocaine and heroin (known as a "speedball") carries a particularly high risk of fatal overdose.

202. Frontotemporal dementia is a common early-onset dementia, usually presenting with behavioral or language impairment and associated with atrophy of the frontal and/or temporal lobes. There is prominent neuronal loss in the frontal and temporal cortex, subiculum, and amygdala. Both gray and white matter show abundant GGIs (globular glial inclusions) composed of abnormal filaments present mostly in oligodendrocytes. The severity of white matter tau abnormalities correlated with a reduction in myelin and axons and with microglial activation.

203. Progressive supranuclear palsy (PSP) is a neurodegenerative syndrome that is clinically characterized by progressive postural instability, supranuclear gaze palsy, parkinsonism and cognitive decline. Pathologically, diagnosis of PSP is based on characteristic features, such as neurofibrillary tangles, neutrophil threads, tau-positive astrocytes and their processes in basal ganglia and brainstem, and the accumulation of 4 repeat tau protein.

204. Friedreich's ataxia is the most common autosomal recessive inherited ataxia, with onset before 25 year of age. It is characterized by progressive limb and truncal ataxia, lower limb areflexia, extensor plantars, dysarthria and loss of joint position and vibration sensations. Other important features are skeletal deformity, hypertrophic cardiomyopathy and diabetes mellitus. Friedreich's ataxia is due to the mutation of frataxin gene on the long arm of chromosome 9.

205. Wallenberg syndrome was first mentioned in a report by Adolf Wallenberg in 1895 on the clinical symptoms of a patient. He later performed a pathological analysis on this same autopsy case in 1901, reporting a detailed pathological lesion. In this autopsy report, Adolf Wallenberg verified that the disease is caused by the obstruction of the posterior inferior cerebellar artery (PICA The criteria are pathological obstruction of the PICA or VA, infarct in the lateral medulla, correspondence between the clinical symptoms and the neuropatholoical lesions.

206. In more advanced disease, there is reduced brain weight, frontal and temporal atrophy with prominent medial temporal atrophy with compensatory dilation of the lateral and third ventricles. There is also atrophy of the thalamus, hypothalamus, and mammillary body, thinning of the corpus callosum, and reduction in subcortical white matter. On the microscopic level, neurofibrillary tangle (NFT)—intracellular aggregates of phosphorylated tau protein—are the hallmark of dementia pugilistica.

207. Tuberous sclerosis complex has a wide range of mucocutaneous manifestations that includes adenoma sebaceum (angiofibroma), connective tissue nevi, hypomelanotic macules, periungual fibromatous lesions, fibromatous plaque on forehead, and oral mucosal fibromas. Adenoma sebaceum is the best-known cutaneous manifestation of tuberous sclerosis. It is clinically characterized by multiple, discrete, translucent, reddish waxy papules that are distributed symmetrically around the nose and over the cheeks and forehead. Shagreen patches are connective tissue nevi on lower back. Patients with tuberous sclerosis and Indian origin have higher prevalence than patients in the west.

209. Wilson's disease also known as hepatolenticular degeneration, is an autosomal recessive disorder resulting from abnormal copper metabolism, subsequently leading to the accumulative deposition of copper in the target organs and impairing the normal functions of the affected organs. The exact molecular mechanisms leading to the abnormal copper metabolism is unknown. Liver is the major organ for copper deposition in patients with Wilson's disease. Excessive copper deposition in the liver causes hepatic dysfunction, resulting in a large spectrum of manifestations ranging from mild abnormalities in liver function tests, to acute or chronic hepatitis, cirrhosis, or even fulminant hepatitis. Excessive deposition of the copper in brain may cause neurological disorders such as Parkinson-like symptoms, including bradykinesia, tremor and dystonia, or neuropsychiatric symptoms.

210. It is a life-threatening disorder caused by thiamine (vitamin B1) depletion, has historically been associated with a classic triad of acute neurological symptoms: confusion, ataxia, and ophthalmoplegia. Thiamine deficiency disease can affect primarily the central and peripheral nervous systems (dry beriberi) or the cardiovascular system (wet beriberi).

211. ALS can be defined as a neurodegenerative disorder characterized by progressive muscular paralysis with degeneration of motor neurons in the primary motor cortex, brainstem and spinal cord. Amyotrophy refers to the atrophy of muscle fibers, which are denervated as their corresponding anterior horn cells degenerate, leading to weakness of affected muscles and visible fasciculation. "Lateral sclerosis" refers to hardening of the anterior and lateral corticospinal tracts as motor neurons in these areas degenerate and are replaced by gliosis.

212. Retinitis pigmentosa is characterized by a progressive neuro-degenerative damage mostly affecting rods, which are the retinal photoreceptors able to ensure both the nocturnal and the peripheral visions. Patients have a decreasing visual ability in the dark (nyctalopia), a slight to moderate shrinking of the visual field. Moreover, because the cones are prevalently involved, these individuals usually complain about diminution of both quantity and quality of central vision.

216. Loss of consciousness following cough was first described in 1876 as "laryngeal vertigo" Since then, several hundred cases of what is now most commonly termed cough syncope have been reported, often in association with various medical conditions. Some early authors assumed this entity to be a form of epilepsy, but by the mid-20th century, general consensus reflected that post-tussive syncope was a consequence of markedly elevated intrathoracic pressures induced by coughing. A typical profile of the cough syncope patient emerging from the literature is that of a middle-aged, large-framed or overweight male with obstructive airways disease. Presumably, such an individual would be more likely to generate the extremely high intrathoracic pressures associated with cough-induced fainting. The precise mechanism of cough syncope remains a matter of debate. Theories proposed include various consequences of the marked elevation of intrathoracic pressures induced by coughing: diminished cardiac output causing decreased systemic blood pressure and, consequently, cerebral hypoperfusion; increased cerebrospinal fluid (CSF) pressure causing increased extravascular pressure around cranial vessels, resulting in diminished brain perfusion; or, a cerebral concussion-like effect from a rapid rise in CSF pressure. More recent mechanistic studies suggest a neurally mediated reflex vasodepressor-bradycardia response to cough. Since loss of consciousness is a direct and immediate result of cough, elimination of cough will eliminate the resultant syncopal episodes. *(Resp Med 2014;108(2):244-51)*

217. Nocturnal frontal lobe epilepsy is characterized by frequent, sometimes violent, and often brief seizures at night, that usually commence during childhood. It can arise sporadically or be inherited in an autosomal dominant fashion. Clinical features associated with nocturnal seizures include vocalizations, complex and often violent automatisms, and ambulation, making the condition sometimes difficult to distinguish from parasomnias.

221. Migraine is a predominantly female disorder. Menarche, menstruation, pregnancy, and menopause, and also the use of hormonal contraceptives and hormone replacement treatment may influence migraine occurrence. Migraine usually starts after menarche, occurs more frequently in the days just before or during menstruation, and ameliorates during pregnancy and menopause. There is increased risk of ischemic and hemorrhagic stroke, cardiac disease, retinal vasculopathy, and mortality in patients with migraine. Headache is usually unilateral but can be holocranial also.

224. The conventional definition of myofascial pain syndrome is characterized by regional pain originating from hyperirritable spots located within taut bands of skeletal muscle, known as myofascial trigger points. Common etiologies of myofascial pain and dysfunction may be from direct or indirect trauma, spine pathology, exposure to cumulative and repetitive strain, postural dysfunction, and physical deconditioning. Injections into the trigger points are a common and effective treatment, presumably due to mechanical disruption by the needle and termination of the dysfunctional activity of involved motor endplates. Ultrasound is a technique that has been proposed to treat myofascial pain by converting electrical energy to sound waves in order to provide heat energy to muscles. Transcutaneous electric nerve stimulation (TENS) is a treatment modality that utilizes an electrical current to stimulate nerve fibers in order to provide pain relief. Magnetic stimulation and laser therapy has also been used in the treatment.

225. Nystagmus is an involuntary, rapid and repetitive movement of the eyes. Usually the movement is side-to-side (horizontal nystagmus), but it can also be up and down (vertical nystagmus) or circular (rotary nystagmus). The movement can vary between slow and fast, and it usually involves both eyes. There are two types of nystagmus: congenital and acquired. Congenital nystagmus develops in infancy, usually between 6-weeks and 3-months of age. Acquired nystagmus occurs later in life and has a variety of causes, including an association with serious medical conditions. Unlike children with nystagmus, adults who acquire nystagmus may see images as shaky. Pendular nystagmus is a sinusoidal oscillation. The waveform of pendular nystagmus may occur in any direction; it can be torsional, horizontal, vertical, or a combination of these, resulting in circular, oblique, or elliptical trajectories. It may be different in the two eyes, sometimes even monocular. Pendular nystagmus is less common than jerk nystagmus.

CHAPTER

Neuroanatomy

Rumana Makhdoomi, Arif Sarmast, Irfan Bhat

IMPORTANT THEORY

TEMPORAL LOBE ANATOMY

Dr J Todd, an English psychiatrist, wrote in The Syndrome of Alice in Wonderland (1955) that, "There is wide appreciation of the fact that epileptic subjects, and their blood relatives, are prone to experience bizarre disturbances of the body image". Lewis Carroll, who wrote Alice in Wonderland, is thought to have had epilepsy. He may very likely have been describing his own symptoms as he penned the transformations of his characters.

EMBRYOLOGY

The forebrain (prosencephalon) divides into telencephalon and diencephalon. The telencephalon develops a diverticulum on each side and its cavity is called the lateral ventricle. The telencephalon forms the anterior end of the 3rd ventricle and the diverticulum on either side forms the cerebral hemisphere. Each hemisphere arises at the beginning of the 5th embryonic week. They grow in all directions rapidly. The inferior expansion forms the temporal lobes. The medial wall of the hemisphere remains thin. This area is invaginated by vascular mesoderm, forming the choroid plexus.

GROSS ANATOMY

The temporal lobe lies inferior to the lateral sulcus (sylvian fissure). Limited posteriorly by an imaginary line joining the pre-occipital incisura to the parieto-occipital sulcus. The parieto-occipital sulcus runs along the medial aspect of the hemisphere and meets the superomedial margin of the hemisphere approx. 5 cm from the occipital pole.

LATERAL ASPECT

Lateral surface is divided into three parallel gyri by two sulci.

- Superior temporal gyrus
- Middle temporal gyrus
- Inferior temporal gyrus
- Superior temporal sulcus
- Inferior temporal sulcus

The lateral temporal surface has three gyri:

Superior temporal gyrus [STG] → Area 22.

Middle temporal gyrus [MTG] → Area 21.

Inferior temporal gyrus [ITG] → Area 20.

These gyri terminate anteriorly at the temporal pole → Area 38.

The superior temporal gyrus lies between the sylvian fissure and the superior temporal sulcus. The angular gyrus, a parietal lobe structure, caps the upturned posterior end of the superior temporal sulcus. Along its superior margin, the STG is continuous with the gyri on the floor of the posterior ramus of the sylvian fissure. These gyri vary in number and they extend anterolaterally around the insula as transverse temporal gyri of Heschl. Gyri of Heschl and adjoining area of STG form the primary auditory cortex (Area 42). The MTG lies between the superior and inferior temporal sulci. The temporal horn and the ambient and the crural cisterns are located deep to the MTG. The ITG lies below the inferior temporal sulcus and continues around the inferior border of the hemisphere to form the lateral part of the basal surface.

Planum temporale is a part of posterior aspect of STG which takes part in language related auditory processing. Gyrus of Heschl and planum temporale are more prominent on the left side. The temporal lobe is enormously expanded in humans. Commonly studied old world monkeys lack MTG and hence poses problems in relating physiological and anatomical studies in non-human primates to human brain topography.

MEDIAL ASPECT

Most complex of the medial cortical areas. Formed predominantly by the rounded medial surfaces of the parahippocampal gyrus and uncus. Three longitudinal strips of neural tissue, one located above the other, which are interlocked with the hippocampal formation. The most inferior strip is formed by the rounded medial edge of the parahippocampal gyrus. The middle strip is formed by the dentate gyrus, a narrow serrated strip of gray matter located on the medial surface of the hippocampal formation. The superior strip is formed by the fimbria of the fornix, a white band formed by the fibers emanating from the hippocampal formation and directed posteriorly into the crus of the fornix. The parahippocampal and dentate gyri are separated by the hippocampal sulcus. The dentate gyrus and the fimbria are separated by the fimbriodentate sulcus. The amygdala and the hippocampal formation lie intimate to each other. The parahippocampal gyrus also extends around the lower border to form the medial part of the basal surface of the temporal lobe, where it is separated from the medially projecting uncus by the rhinal sulcus.

Uncus, is the medially projecting anterior part of the parahippocampal gyrus. When viewed from above or below, it has an angular shape with anterior and posterior segments that meet at a medially directed apex. The anterior segment of the uncus faces anteromedially and the posterior segment faces posteromedially. The anterior segment has an undivided medial surface, but the posterior segment is divided into upper and lower parts by the uncal notch, a short sulcus. Medial face of the anterior segment faces the proximal part of the sylvian, the carotid cistern, and the ICA and the proximal MCA.

Posterior segment faces the cerebral peduncle and, with the peduncle, forms the lateral and medial walls of the crural cistern through which the posterior cerebral, anterior choroidal and medial posterior choroidal arteries pass. The apex between the anterior and posterior segment is located lateral to the oculomotor nerve. The amygdaloid nucleus forms almost all of the interior and comes to the medial surface of the upper part of the anterior segment.

The upper part of the posterior segment is formed largely by the medial aspect of the head of the hippocampus. The inferior choroidal point is the lower end of the choroidal fissure along which the choroid plexus is attached. Located just behind the upper edge of the posterior uncal segment, immediately behind the head of the hippocampus. It is the site where the anterior choroidal artery passes through the choroidal fissure to enter the temporal horn.

Dentate gyrus, is named for its characteristic tooth-like elevations. Extends posteriorly from the upper part of the posterior segment of uncus. Continues posteriorly below and behind the splenium of the corpus callosum with the fascicular gyrus, a smooth grayish band that blends above into the indusium griseum. Amygdaloid nucleus is named so because it resembles an almond. Situated entirely within uncus. Forms anterior wall of the temporal horn. It fuses with the tip of the tail of the caudate nucleus. The amygdala gives rise to the stria terminalis, which courses between the thalamus and caudate nucleus deep to the thalamostriate vein.

Hippocampus is a curved elevation of gray matter; approximately 5 cm long. It runs along entire length of the medial part of floor of the temporal horn. Dentate gyrus runs along its medial edge. A curved collection of gray matter lies inferiorly (Ammon's horn). Sits above and is continuous below with the rounded medial surface of the parahippocampal gyrus. The hippocampus blends into and forms the upper part of the posterior uncal segment. The hippocampus, the parahippocampal gyrus and the dentate gyrus together form the hippocampal formation. The hippocampus is divided into three parts: head, body and tail. The head, directed anteriorly, has 3–4 digitations, resembling paw of sea-horse; hence called *pes hippocampus*. The body of the hippocampus extends along the medial part of the floor of the temporal horn, narrowing into the tail that disappears as a ventricular structure. The convex ventricular surface is covered with ependyma. Beneath this lies a thin layer of white matter; alveus. The alveus consists of nerve fibers which originated in the hippocampus. These fibers converge medially to form a bundle, viz. fimbria. The fimbria becomes continuous with the crus of fornix. The temporal horn extends into the medial part of the temporal lobe to just anterior to the hippocampal head and to just behind the amygdala. The temporal horn ends approximately 2.5 cm from the temporal pole. The inferior choroidal point, at the lower end of the choroidal fissure, is located just behind the head of the hippocampus and immediately lateral to the lateral geniculate body.

BASAL ASPECT

The basal surfaces of the temporal and occipital lobes are formed by the same gyri that continue from anterior to posterior across their uninterrupted border. From medial to lateral are the parahippocampal and occipitotemporal gyri and the lower surface of the inferior temporal gyrus. The parahippocampal gyrus extends backward from the temporal pole to the posterior margin of the corpus callosum. Continues posteriorly to blend into the isthmus of the cingulate gyrus and lingual. The collateral sulcus, one of the most constant cerebral sulci, begins near the occipital pole and extends anteriorly, parallel and lateral to the calcarine sulcus. Posteriorly, it separates the lingual and occipitotemporal gyrus, and anteriorly, it courses between the parahippocampal and the occipitotemporal gyri. The collateral sulcus is located below the temporal horn and indents deeply into the basal surface producing a prominence, the collateral eminence, in the floor of the temporal horn, viz. collateral eminence. The occipitotemporal sulcus courses parallel and lateral to the collateral sulcus and separates the occipitotemporal gyrus and basal surface of the inferior temporal gyrus. A short rhinal sulcus is often found anteriorly lateral to the uncus.

BLOOD SUPPLY AND VENOUS DRAINAGE

The lateral aspect is perfused mainly by the branches of the MCA:

- Anterior temporal A
- Middle temporal A
- Temporo-occipital A

The ITG is supplied by branches of the PCA. The choroid plexus of the temporal horn is supplied by the branches of the anterior choroidal artery. The superficial middle cerebral vein drains most of the lateral aspect. It follows the sylvian fissure to end at the cavernous sinus. A superior anastomotic vein of Trolard connects the sup middle cerebral vein to the superior sagittal sinus. An inferior anastomotic vein of Labbe runs over the temporal lobe and connects the sup. middle cerebral vein to the transverse sinus. A few inferior cerebral veins drain the inferior aspect. They anastomose with basal veins and middle cerebral veins and drain into cavernous, transverse and superior petrosal sinuses.

Vein of Labbe (Inferior Anastomotic Vein)

Largest anastomotic channel that crosses the temporal lobe between the sylvian fissure and the transverse sinus. Usually arises from the middle portion of the sylvian fissure and is directed posteriorly and inferiorly toward the anterior part of the transverse sinus. May cross the temporal lobe as far back as the posterior limit of the lobe or as far forward as the anterior third of the lateral surface. There may be double veins of Labbé, in which case the posterior vein is usually larger. Although the veins of Trolard and Labbé and the superficial sylvian vein may be of nearly equal size, it is more common for one or two of them to predominate and the other to be small or absent. Usually, there is asymmetry between the right and left hemispheres in the size of these channels.

PAPEZ CIRCUIT

Takes part in memory and also controls emotion, behavior and drive. Connects structures of the limbic system. Cingulate gyrus > parahippocampal gyrus and amygdala > hippocampus > fornix > manmillary body > anterior nucleus of thalamus > cingulate gyrus.

CORTICAL STRUCTURE

Predominantly 6-layered Cortex

Gyrus of Heschl forms the primary auditory cortex (AI). Surrounding areas form auditory association areas (AII). Geniculocortical fibers from medial geniculate body terminate in layer IV of the cortex. Auditory cortex connects with the prefrontal cortex, anterior cingulate gyrus and to corresponding areas in the opp. hemisphere. Auditory association areas connect with other sensory association areas around the sup. temporal sulcus. Injury to auditory cortex produces cortical deafness, auditory agnosia, with contralateral predominance. Patient is unaware of the deficit. Difficulty in localizing source of sound. Noticeable deficit occurs only when there is b/l damage. Damage to temporoparietal junction causes auditory inattention. Damage to posterior superior temporal area on dominant side causes Wernicke's aphasia.

Middle temporal cortex (area 21) is polysensory, connects with auditory (sup temporal gyrus), visual and somatosensory association pathways. Also has connections with pulvinar areas of the thalamus. Lesion to middle temp. gyrus (esp. dominant side) causes visuospatial difficulties, prosopagnosia and severe sensory dysphasia. Inferior temporal cortex (area 20) is a higher visual association area. Receives fibers from ipsilateral occipitotemporal visual areas (V4). Sends efferent fibers to paralimbic areas on medial aspect of temporal lobe. Also connected to prefrontal cortex and frontal eye field. Cortex of the temporal pole receives fibers from widespread areas of temporal association cortex. Dorsal part receives auditory input and inferior part receives visual input. Sends efferent fibers to limbic and paralimbic areas and also to prefrontal cortex. Related to behavioral performance and recognition of high-level aspects of social stimuli.

Superior, middle and inferior temporal gyri and parahippocampal gyrus are phylogenetically 6-layered neocortex. Hippocampus and dentate gyri are part of the older 3-layered allocortex. Damage to the limbic system results in disturbance of emotional behavior, pattern of rage, anger and sexual behavior.

Klüver-Bucy syndrome: Experimental damage to b/l amygdala in monkeys. Visual agnosia or psychic blindness, loss of fear or rage reaction, hypersexuality, bulimia.

Hippocampus is related to converting recent memory to long-term memory. Lesion in hippocampus causes affected person unable to convert newly acquired memory into long-term memory [Anterograde amnesia]. Memory of remote past events before the lesion developed is unaffected.

Visual memory → Picture/scene recall [Rt parahippocampal cortex]. Verbal memory → Word recall [Lt parahippocampal cortex]. Periamygdaloid area: Primary olfactory cortex. Entorhinal area (area 28): it is a part of anterior portion of parahippocampal gyrus and is olfactory association area. Lesion in it causes olfactory hallucination.

Neoplasms or space occupy lesions of the temporal lobe present with:

Vague personality change to frank behavioral disturbances, anxiety, depression, fear and anger, paranoia, memory deficit, learning and cognitive disabilities, apathy.

Meyer's Loop

Contains optic radiation fibers from LGB to calcarine cortex. Inferior retinal fibers, representing contralateral superior visual field arch anteriorly in the temporal lobe, sweeping forward and laterally above the temporal horn, runs 5–7 cm from the temporal tip. Damage causes contralateral superior quadrantanopia. Light reflex preserved.

TEMPORAL LOBE EPILEPSY

Very common in humans. Commonest type of seizure originates from temporal lobe, approx. 25% of all epilepsies. Often resistant to pharmcotherapy. Most commonly associated with amygdaloid and hippocampal sclerosis [medial temporal sclerosis]. Both are deep structures → 3–4 cm below the surface. Electrophysiological studies sometimes miss it. Ipsilateral temporal horn may show dilatation.

Complex Partial/Psychomotor Seizure

Described by Hughlings-Jackson (uncal fits). Lesion mostly in antero-medial parts of temp. lobe i.e., hippocampus, uncus, amygdala, parahippocampal gyrus.

Formed visual hallucination – macropsia/micropsia, olfactory hallucination, auditory hallucination, autonomic disturbances viz. *déjà vu, déjà entendu or jamais vu.* Anxiety, fear, rage, obsessive thoughts, speech or action.

TEMPORAL LOBECTOMY

Landmarks

- Dominant side → Anterior 4 cm from temporal tip.
- Non-dominant side → Anterior 5 cm from temporal tip.

A layer of cortex bordering the sylvian fissure is preserved to prevent disruption of the vasculature. In the dominant side, superior temporal gyrus is preserved to minimize disruption of speech function.

Surgery in Temporal Lobe Epilepsy

Extent of dissection depends on exact site of origin of seizure and probable neurologic and neuropsychological deficits that can result from such resection. Usual sites of origin → Superior, middle, inferior temporal gyri, parahippocampal gyrus, hippocampus, amygdala and uncus. Ammon's horn sclerosis is found in 85% of resected specimens.

When Seizure Focus Lies in the Lateral Temporal Lobe

More extensive resection of lateral temporal lobe is done. For dominant side awake craniotomy is preferred to permit language mapping. Recording from amygdalo-hippocampal complex is also done simultaneously and resection done in presence of epileptiform activity. Solely resecting lesion in lateral temporal neocortex while sparing mesial structures is often ineffective.

When Preoperative MRI Reveals Hippocampal Sclerosis

Resection of lateral temporal neocortex → up to 3 cm of anterior most part of middle and inferior temporal gyri. Relatively aggressive resection of the mesial temporal structures, tailored to intra-operative electrophysiological recordings. Neocortical resection provides generous exposure for hippocampal resection.

Anterolateral Temporal Lobectomy

Structures to be preserved -Superior temporal gyrus on the dominant side. Vein of Labbe (4–6 cm from temporal tip). Branches of MCA (which leave the sylvian fissure and run over superior and middle temporal gyri within anterior 4 cm of temporal lobe, to supply posteriorly located language areas. Veins draining from sylvian fissure to sphenoparietal sinus. Resection should be kept anterior to petrous ridge. Resection carried on till temporal horn is entered. Resection of amygdala, hippocampus and parahippocampal gyrus are next completed. Structures to be aware of: Internal capsule, lying medial to temporal horn, PCA, 3rd and 4th cranial nerves, lying in the incisura.

Complications: Transient dysphasia. Transient paresis of cranial nerves III and IV with subtle diplopia. Contralateral superior quadrantanopia – in 50% patients – incidence can be lowered if lateral temporal lobe resection is restricted to less than 4 cm. Acute psychosis – rare but well recognized complication. Anxiety (5% patients) – responds to psychotropic medications. Memory and attention deficits.

Seizure control: Patients with Ammon's horn sclerosis have the best outcome. About 68% turned seizure-free and another 24% had significant improvement in seizure frequency. Patients with atypical sclerosis have the poorest outcome.

ANATOMY AND SURGICAL APPROACHES TO LATERAL VENTRICLES

Anatomy

Two paired cavities, C-shaped, each cavity contains about 10-ml CSF.

Divided into: Frontal horn (Length 6 cm), Body between IVF and atrium, temporal horn (length 4 cm), occipital horn, atrium

Frontal Horn

Boundaries

Medial wall by septum pellucidum, roof, anterior wall and floor by anterior wrapping of the corpus callosum, genu, rostrum and trunk, lateral wall by internal aspect of the head of the caudate nucleus.

Body

Boundaries

Medial wall: Septum pellucidum and body of fornix

Roof: Body of corpus callosum

Lateral wall: Medial part of the body of caudate nucleus

Floor: Dorsal surface of thalamus between thalamo-caudate sulcus and tenia thalami (attachment line of choroid plexus on thalamus).

Atrium

Confluence of Horns

Communicates cranially, ventrally and medially with frontal horn, dorsally with occipital horn, and caudally, ventrally and laterally with inferior horn. Overlies the pulvinar, posterior pole of thalamus which constitutes the anterior wall.

Roof: Fibers coming from the splenium.

Medial wall: choroidal fissure with choroidal plexus (glomus).

Occipital Horn

2 prominences formed cranially and inferiorly by fibers of splenium of corpus callosum and deep part of calcarine sulcus

Floor is bulged by collateral sulcus forming collateral eminence,

Lateral Wall

White matter of tapetum formed by external fibers of the splenium of corpus callosum, overlaid laterally by optic radiations and then inferior longitudinal fasciculus.

Temporal Horn

Floor-hippocampus and caudally collateral eminence

Roof: Inferior aspect of thalamus, tail of the caudate nucleus and deep white matter of temporal lobe

Medial wall: Choroidal fissure and choroid plexus clinging to the fimbria and to the inferior aspect of the hemisphere. The anterior extremity is situated just behind the amygdaloid nucleus.

Interventricular foramen-bounded on each side by anterior pole of thalamus and ventrally by anterior crus fornicis. Diameter 3–4 mm and presents a posterior concavity. Marked by reflexion of choroidal plexus of the roof of the third ventricle which continues with choroidal plexus of lateral ventricle and venous angle between thalamostriate vein and internal cerebral vein.

Arterial Vasculature of the Lateral Ventricle

Anterior Choroidal Artery

Arises from terminal segment of ICA closer to the origin of the PCom. Two segments: cisternal and plexal. Frequently anastomoses with branches of other choroidal arteries. Sends branches to adjacent nervous structures viz., optic tract, cerebral peduncle, globus pallidus, origin of optic radiations.

Posterior Choroidal Artery

The medial posterior choroid artery; gives few feeding vessels to the choroidal plexus of the lateral ventricle. Arises from the posterior cerebral artery (P1 segment), anastomoses are often found between the medial posterior choroidal artery and the lateral posterior choroidal artery.

The lateral posterior choroidal artery, number per hemisphere ranges from 1 to 9 (average 4). Arises from either P2 or P3 segment of the PCA, runs laterally to the PCA and enters the choroidal fissure. Area of distribution is cerebral peduncle, fornix, pulvinar and caudate nucleus.

Veins of the Lateral Ventricles

Provide valuable landmarks in directing the surgeon to the foramen of Monro and choroidal fissure during operations on the ventricles. The choroidal veins are bulky and tortuous, easily seen, run over the plexus. Superior choroid vein, very bulky, runs ventrally towards the ventricle body to join either the thalamostriate vein or internal cerebral vein. Inferior choroid vein ends in the inferior ventricular veins and also in the basal vein at the same place. Medial choroid veins course from the plexus of the ventricular body to the ICV.

Veins of the Ventricular Walls

Medial wall of the LV-anterior septal vein- the most constant vein, drains into the venous confluence near the foramen. Vein of the amygdaloid body drain into the basal vein or into the transverse vein of the hippocampus which drains into the basal vein.

Lateral wall is drained by anterior caudate veins which drain into the thalamostriate vein. Posterior caudate veins also drain into the thalamostriate vein.

Thalamostriate vein, the most constant, runs in the thalamo-caudate sulcus and forms the venous angle with the ICV through the IVF.

SURGICAL APPROACHES TO LATERAL AND THIRD VENTRICLES

Transcallosal Approach

Indications are frontal horn tumors located mainly in the ventricle, tumor extending to both frontal horns and to third ventricle. Intraventricular orientation is gained by choroid plexus and thalamostriate veins, foramen of Monro, tumor identification, resection of tumor as internal debulking followed by dissection. Advantages are less chances of neural injury, access to both ventricles, less chances of epilepsy (?), entry to third ventricle easy if required. Disadvantages are more chances of vascular injury, theoretical risks of callosotomy, superiorly located tumors are generally cannot be tackled. Complications include vascular injury, corpus callosal syndrome, reduced spontaneity of speech to frank mutism, interhemispheric transfer syndromes.

Transcortical Approach

Indication are tumor growing outside the ventricle, tumor located mainly antero-superiorly in frontal horn, non-dominant hemisphere. Disadvantages are more chances of epilepsy and porencephalic cysts, limited entry to opposite ventricles. Complications include epilepsy, direct cortical incision and damage, memory loss, retraction of caudate nucleus, hemiplegia, retraction of centrum semiovalis. Combined transcallosal and transcortical approach is needed for large tumors involving both ventricles.

Atrial Tumors

Transcortical approach is favored. Lateral decubitus position with face turned towards the floor. Superior parietal lobule is identified, 1–2 cm cortisectomy.

Transcortical approach preferred as ventricles diverge posteriorly. Splenium sacrifice has physiological risks which is avoided in this approach. Complications include speech problems, acalculia, apraxia, visual field deficits, homonymous hemianopia, splenium syndrome, interhemisphere disconnection syndrome.

Occipital Approach

Suitable for tumors situated in part of the pulvinar, medial occipital lobe, and medial atrial wall facing the quadrigeminal cistern, three-quarter prone position with occipital area to be operated lowermost and face turned toward the floor. An atrial tumor that extends into the medial occipital cortex, near the junction of the vein of Galen and straight sinus, can be exposed by opening through the isthmus of the cingulate gyrus in front of the calcarine sulcus.

Transtemporal/Subtemporal Approaches

Used for a lesion in the middle or posterior third of the temporal horn. Supine with head turned almost laterally. Small temporal craniotomy. Dura opened based on base. Cortical incision in the middle or inferior temporal gyrus anterior to the optic radiations. An alternative route is the subtemporal route, in which an incision is made in the inferior temporal or occipitotemporal gyrus or the collateral sulcus on the lower surface of the temporal lobe. Minimizes the possibility of damage to the optic radiations and speech centers of the dominant hemisphere. Complications include visual field deficits, superior quadrantanopia, language deficits dyslexia, agraphia, acalculia.

THE CEREBRAL VENOUS ANATOMY AND MANAGEMENT OF POSTOPERATIVE VENOUS INFARCT

Gross Anatomy

Cerebral venous drainage comprises of 3 segments:

1. *Outer/superficial segment:* Drains scalp/muscles/tendons by scalp veins.
2. *Intermediate segment:* Draining skull/diploe/duramater by diploe veins, emissary veins, meningeal veins and dural venous sinuses.
3. *Cerebral segment:* Draining the brain proper by means of superficial cortical veins and deep venous system.

Cerebral Venous System

Scalp veins.

Diploic veins. The diploic veins and scalp veins can function as collateral pathways for venous outflow from I/C structures.

- Emissary veins.
- The meningeal veins.
- The bridging veins.

Cortical veins. The superficial cortical veins are divided into three groups based on whether they drain the lateral, medial, or inferior surface of the hemisphere.

- The cortical veins on the three surfaces are further subdivided on the basis of the lobe and cortical area that they drain.
- The largest group of cortical veins terminate by exiting the subarachnoid space to become bridging veins that cross the subdural space and empty into the venous sinuses in the dura mater.
- A smaller group of cortical veins terminate by directly joining the deep venous system of the brain.

Dural Sinuses and Bridging Veins

The bridging veins are divided into four groups based on their site of termination:

Superior sagittal group, which drains into the superior sagittal sinus;

Tentorial group, which drains into the transverse or lateral tentorial sinus;

Sphenoidal group, which drains into the sphenoparietal or cavernous sinus;

Falcine group, which drains into the straight or inferior sagittal sinus either directly or through the basal, great, or internal cerebral veins.

The dural sinuses into which the cortical veins empty are:

Superior and inferior sagittal, straight, transverse, tentorial, cavernous, sphenoparietal, sphenobasal, and sphenopetrosal sinuses.

These sinuses form the terminal part of the superficial cortical venous system.

Major Anastomotic Veins

The **vein of Trolard** is the largest vein connecting he superficial sylvian vein with the superior sagittal sinus.

The **vein of Labbé** is the largest vein connecting the superficial sylvian vein with the transverse sinus.

The superficial sylvian vein drains the areas along the sylvian fissure and empties into the sinuses along the sphenoid ridge.

Different patterns:

a. All three anastamatic veins are present, but the veins of Labbé and Trolard are dominant.
b. Dominant superficial sylvian and vein of Trolard.
c. Dominant superficial sylvian vein.
d. Dominant vein of Labbé.

The vein of Labbé predominates in the dominant hemisphere nearly twice as often as it predominates in the non-dominant hemisphere, and the vein of Trolard predominates in the non-dominant hemisphere with approximately the same frequency.

Deep Cerebral Veins

Gross Anatomy

The deep venous system of the brain consists of the internal cerebral, basal, and great vein and their tributaries.

These veins drain the deep white and gray matter surrounding the lateral and third ventricles and the basal cisterns.

The deep veins are divided into a ventricular group, composed of the veins draining the walls of the lateral ventricles, and a cisternal group, which includes the veins draining the walls of the basal cisterns.

The deep cerebral veins may pose a major obstacle to operative approaches to deep-seated lesions, especially in the pineal region, where multiple veins converge on the great vein. The fact that sacrifice of the major trunks of the deep venous system only infrequently leads to venous infarction with mass effect and neurological deficit is attributed to the diffuse anastamoses between the veins. Dandy noted that, not infrequently, one internal cerebral vein has been sacrificed without effect and, on a few occasions, both veins and even the great vein have been ligated with recovery without any apparent disturbance of function. On the other hand, injury to this complicated venous network has caused diencephalic edema, mental symptoms, coma, hyperpyrexia, tachycardia, tachypnea, miosis, rigidity of limbs, and exaggeration of deep tendon reflexes. Occlusion of the thalamostriate and other veins at the foramen of Monro may cause drowsiness, hemiplegia, mutism, and hemorrhagic infarction of the basal ganglia.

Functional Anatomy

The dural sinuses are designed to maintain the patency in the face of negative pressure. Their triangular shape make them relatively non compressible. Bridging vein entering the sinuses opposite the direction of sinus blood flow. There are no valves. Their wall contain noradrenergic and peptinergic fibers.

Physiology

Role in maintainance of ICP:

Of the 3 major intracranial components, cerebral blood volume can change most rapidly.

70–80% of cerebral blood volume is located in venous system.

Regulators of cerebral venous flow are: Pco2, sympathetic system

At high ICP: Sympathetic tone increase— veins constricts—cerebral blood. Vol. decrease—tends to lower ICP into venous sinuses.

Role in CSF absorption:

CSF absorbed through arachnoid villi.

The flow across villus is unidirectional and a pressure differential is required for flow.

Applied Aspects

- The distribution of the superficial cortical veins is not as irregular and variable as is generally supposed, and their examination during the venous phase of the cerebral angiogram may prove helpful in localizing expanding lesions by revealing poor filling and displacement and alteration in the direction of flow.
- The fact that sacrifice of the individual cortical veins only infrequently leads to venous infarction, hemorrhage, swelling, and neurological deficit is attributed to the diffuse anastomoses between the individual cortical veins and b/n the sup. Cortical and the deep ventricular and cisternal veins.
- In subtemporal approaches the various bridging veins encountered include the temporal, occipital, temporobasal, and occipitobasal veins and the vein of Labbé.
- Sacrifice of these veins, which pass from the lower part of the hemisphere to the transverse and tentorial sinuses, frequently causes some degree of venous infarction and edema of the temporal lobe.
- A contralateral hemiparesis, more marked in the face and arm than the leg, with an aphasia if the dominant hemisphere is affected, may follow occlusion of these veins.
- The ventricular veins provide valuable landmarks in directing the surgeon to the foramen of Monro and the choroidal fissure during operations on the ventricles.
- This is especially true if hydrocephalus, a common result of ventricular tumors, is present, because the borders between the neural structures in the ventricular walls become less distinct as the ventricles dilate.
- The thalamostriate vein is helpful in delimiting the junction of the caudate nucleus and the thalamus because it usually courses along the sulcus separating these structures.

Surgical Management of Sinus Wall Injuries

- **Small laceration:** Can often be closed with small interrupted sutures.
  - Up to 50% stenosis is well tolerated.
- **Large tears/laceration:**
  - Ligation in non-critical sinuses like anterior 1/3rd of SSS, non-dominant transverse/sigmoid sinus, inferior sagittal sinus and straight sinus.
  - Autogenous venous graft in critical sinuses like posterior 2/3rd of SSS, torcula, dominant transverse/sigmoid sinus.

Control of Bleeding from Venous Sinuses

- Digital pressure in case of small hemorrhage.
- Intraluminal balloon occlusion using fogarty catheter.
- Rarely a shunt fashioned from pediatric endotracheal tube preoperatively, can be used to provide control of bleeding as well as diversion of blood.

VENOUS LACUNAE

- The lacunae may extend along the medial extent of the hemisphere adjacent to the falx and as far as 3 cm laterally over the convexity.
- Entering or occluding a lacuna at operation does not necessarily result in occlusion of the cortical veins or the superior sagittal sinus because most of the veins course deep to the lacunae and usually empty directly into the sinus.

- ❖ In opening the dura mater adjoining the superior sagittal sinus, one should attempt to preserve the meningeal sinuses, which may arise as far as 2.5 cm lateral to the superior sagittal sinus.
- ❖ These sinuses may receive the terminal end of numerous cortical veins.
- ❖ In removing a parasagittal tumor deep to these sinuses, the dura is opened along the edges of the sinus while preserving the sinus' proximal junction with the cortical veins and its distal junction with the superior sagittal sinus.
- ❖ The tumor is then separated from the lower margin of the meningeal sinus without sacrificing the sinus.
- ❖ The operative approach directed along the falx toward the anterior part of the corpus callosum may require the sacrifice of a bridging vein to the superior sagittal sinus.
- ❖ Occasionally, the corpus callosum may be reached in the area between the anterior and posterior frontal veins without sacrificing any bridging veins.
- ❖ Obliteration of the bridging veins to the superior sagittal sinus in the region of the precentral, central, or postcentral gyri frequently causes a contralateral hemiparesis that is more prominent in the lower than the upper extremity and is usually transient.
- ❖ Spontaneous occlusion of the veins in this region causes a hemiparesis that is commonly accompanied by headache and seizures
- ❖ In occipital transtentorial operative approach, the occipital pole can usually be retracted from the straight sinus and the junction of the falx and the tentorium without sacrificing any veins to the superior sagittal or transverse sinuses.
- ❖ The superior sagittal sinus is commonly devoid of bridging veins in the area just in front of the torcular herophili.

Postoperative Venous Infarct

Etiologies

1. Inadvertent coagulation/tear of bridging veins/meningeal sinuses during cranial surgeries.
2. Resection of malignant tm/meningioma invading major venous sinus.
3. Repair of traumatic dural venous sinus injuries.
4. Even following cannulation of neck veins.
5. Intraoperative/postoperative dehydration.

Various surgeries implicated in literature are:

- ❖ Acoustic neuroma surgeries.
- ❖ Clipping of ACA aneurysm.
- ❖ Tumors firmly adherent to cortex.
- ❖ Open surgical excision of cortex cyst of 3rd ventricle.

Venous occlusion-elevated cerebral venous pressure, dilated venous/capillary beds, interstitial edema develops. Increased CSF production and decreased CSF absorption.

Pathophysiology

Extensive collateral in venous system leads to compensation in early stage of venous occlusions.

Ultimately rupture of venous structure with hematoma formation.

Presentation

Nakase et al in ActaNeurochir (Wien). 2005 has found that there are 2 types of infarcts:

- ❖ Severe onset (severe type)
- ❖ Gradual onset (mild type)

The former needs immediate treatment from the intra-operative period onward, and the prevention of the ongoing venous thrombosis is essential in the latter.

Varied Clinical Features: acc. to specific sites:

- **Cavernous sinus thrombosis:** chemosis, proptosis and painful ophthalmoplegia.
- **Deep venous system:** diencephalic dysfunction and death, abulia, disorientation, vertical gaze paresis, etc.
- **Midportion of SSS:** spastic hemiparesis/quadriparesis
  - Raised ICT features
- **Posterior portion of SSS:** Visual field defects
- **Diffuse sinus thrombosis:** Symptom/signs of acutely raised ICT with herniation.
  - Cortical blindness
  - Coma

Diagnostic Investigations

NCCT: positive delta sign in acute SSS thrombosis.

Hemorrhage in hemisphere.

Diagnosed by DWI.

DSA: Detects venous sinus thrombosis as filling defects.

CECT: Negative delta sign in acute SSS thrombosis -gyral/tentorial enhancement

Cord sign in cortical venous thrombosis.

MRI: Investigation of choice, special sequences used:

Gradient refocused echo–MRA (GRE)

DWI

THERAPY

General Measures

Regular clinical and radiological follow-up:

Avoid dehydration/hypotension/hyperglycemia -seizure prophylaxis.

Symptomatic treatment of raised ICT:

- Head elevation
- Hyperventilation
- Osmotic agent-mannitol/furosemide ventricular drainage for hydrocephalous.

Most of the venous infarcts will improve with these measures and can be followed-up. Thrombosed channels shows recanalization and collateral channels open-up.

Role of Anticoagulants

- Anticoagulants (heparin and acitrom) inhibits the progression of thrombosis, but has the inherent danger of increasing hemorrhagic complications.
- Sepulveda JM et al in Neurologia. 2004 has advocated the use of anticoagulant treatment in hemorrhagic brain infarcts due to large venous sinus thrombosis.

Role of Surgical Treatment

1. Ventricular drainage in cases presenting as acute hydrocephalous.
2. **Decompressive hemicraniectomy:** If severe mass effect is present and patient condition is deteriorating inspite of all medical measures.

MULTIPLE CHOICE QUESTIONS

1. **All the following statements about anterior choroidal artery are true, except:**
   a. It arises from internal carotid artery ICA posteromedially
   b. It runs medially below the optic tract
   c. It travels in quadrigeminal cistern
   d. It enters the choroidal fissure
   Ref. Rhoton, p89-90

2. **The bulkiest lobe of brain is:**
   a. Left occipital lobe b. Right frontal lobe
   c. Left frontal lobe d. Right temporal lobe
   Ref. Rhoton, p34-5

3. **Which of the cerebellar peduncle is the thickest?**
   a. Superior peduncle b. Middle peduncle
   d. Inferior peduncle d. All are equal
   Ref. Snells Neuroanatomy, 3rd/e, p218-9

4. **The correct order of naming of different segments of middle cerebral artery MCA is:**
   a. Sphenoidal-insular-opercular-cortical
   b. Insular-sphenoidal-opercular-cortical
   c. Opercular-sphenoidal-insular-cortical
   d. Sphenoidal -opercular-insular-cortical
   Ref. Rhoton, p127

5. **All the following statements about vein of Labbe are correct, except:**
   a. It is also known as inferior anastamotic vein
   b. It courses across the temporal lobe posteriorly and superiorly
   c. It joins the transverse sinus at the level of pre-occipital notch
   d. None of the above
   Ref. Rhoton, p200

6. **Which of the segments of the posterior cerebral artery extends from the lateral part of the quadrigeminal cistern up to the anterior part of calcarine sulcus?**
   a. P_1 segment b. P_2 segment
   c. P_3 segment d. P_4 segment
   Ref. Rhoton, p136-9

7. **The recurrent artery of Heubner usually arises from:**
   a. Proximal A_1 b. Distal A_1
   c. Proximal A_2 d. Distal A_2
   Ref. Rhoton, p119

8. **The largest cerebellar nucleus is:**
   a. Dentate nucleus b. Emboliform nucleus
   c. Fastigial nucleus d. Globose nucleus
   Ref. Snells Neuroanatomy, 3rd/e, p217

9. **The paired internal cerebral veins join the basal veins to form:**
   a. Straight sinus
   b. Thalamostriate vein
   c. Vein of Galen
   d. Superficial middle cerebral vein
   Ref. Rhoton, p221

10. **All the following statements about vertebral artery are true, except:**
    a. It supplies the structures in the posterior fossa predominantly
    b. The two vertebral arteries join to form the basilar artery
    c. The right vertebral artery is usually dominant
    d. One segment or the entire length of a vertebral artery may be hypoplastic
    Ref. Greenberg, 4th/e, p54-5

11. **Dolichoectasia of basilar artery is defined if on angiography the diameter of the artery is:**
    a. >2.5 mm b. >3.5 mm
    c. >4.5 mm d. >5.5 mm
    Ref. Journal of Neurology Neurosurgery and Psychiatry 2004;75:22-6

ANSWERS

1. c. **2.** c. **3.** b. **4.** a. **5.** b. **6.** c. **7.** c. **8.** a. **9.** c. **10.** c.
11. c.

12. All the following statements are true, except:

a. The biceps of brachi tendon reflex involves C5 root
b. D-10 dermatome includes the skin of the groin
c. Neurotendinous spindles are innervated by myelinated nerve fibers
d. The gamma motor efferent fibers innervate the intrafusal fibers of a muscle spindle

Ref. Bickerstaff, 6th/e, p181, 208

13. Which of the following statements is/are true?

a. The archicerebellum is the oldest part of the cerebellum
b. The archicerebellum receives input from vestibular nuclei
c. Both 'a' and 'b' are correct
d. None of the above

Ref. Snells Neuroanatomy, 3rd/e, p211-5

14. Which of the following statements is/are true?

a. The floor of the fourth ventricle is also known as rhomboid fossa
b. The floor of the fourth ventricle is divided into 2 assymetrical halves
c. On each sides of the median sulcus, there is an elevation known as medial eminence
d. 'a' and 'c' are correct

Ref. Rhoton, p439-40

15. All the following statements are true, except:

a. The midbrain is composed of 2 cerebral peduncles
b. Each cerebral peduncle is divided into anterior crus and posterior tegmentum
c. The 3rd cranial nerve exits from the lateral side of crus cerebri
d. The tectum is situated posterior to the aqueduct of sylvius

Ref. Snells Neuroanatomy, 3rd/e, p237-41

16. All the following statements are true, except:

a. The superior colliculus is a mass of white matter of midbrain
b. It is connected to the lateral geniculate body
c. It has a role in eye movements
d. It receives input from the optic nerve

Ref. Snells Neuroanatomy, 3rd/e, p241, and Patten, p94-6

17. All the following statements about pineal gland are true, except:

a. The pineal gland lies along the posterior 3rd ventricle
b. The gland is attached to telencephalon by pineal stalk
c. It lies posterior to the midbrain
d. The pineal stalk is in close relation with Habenular and posterior commissure

Ref. Snells Neuroanatomy, 3rd/e, p252

18. All the following statements are true, except:

a. The corpus callosum is the largest commissure of brain
b. The cingulate gyrus lies superior to the corpus callosum
c. The cingulate gyrus lies between cingulate sulcus inferiorly and calossal sulcus superiorly
d. Sectioning the corpus callosum in the midline leads to disconnection syndromes

Ref. Snells Neuroanatomy, 3rd/e, p274

19. The motor speech area lies in:

a. Left anterior temporal area
b. Right superior frontal gyrus
c. Left posterior inferior frontal gyrus
d. Left inferior temporal gyrus

Ref. Snells Neuroanatomy, 3rd/e, p299

20. All the following about hippocampus are true, except:

a. Its anterior end is expanded to form pes hippocampus
b. The nerve fibers arising from the white matter form the fimbria
c. Hippocampus forms part of the papez circuit
d. It is named hippocampus as it resembles hippopotamus

Ref. Snells Neuroanatomy, 3rd/e, p269-70

Answers

12. b. **13.** c. **14.** d. **15.** c. **16.** a. **17.** b. **18.** c. **19.** c. **20.** d.

21. Which of the following statements is true?
a. Light touch and pressure get transmitted through anterior spinothalamic tract
b. Pain and temperature sensation ascend through the lateral spinothalamic tract
c. Vibration and position sense ascend through the posterior column
d. All the above are true
Ref. Bickerstaff, 6th/e, p185-92

22. All the following statements are true, except:
a. Lesion in the caudate nucleus causes chorea
b. Lesion in the lentiform nucleus causes dystonia
c. Athetosis occurs in lesions of the corpus striatum
d. Hemiballismus occurs in lesions of globus pallidus
Ref. Patten, 2nd/e, p181-2

23. All the following statements about neurons of cerebellum are true, except:
a. There are two types of afferent fibers which enter the cerebellum
b. The climbing fibers are the terminal fibers of the rubrocerebellar tract
c. The climbing fibers enter the molecular layer
d. The mossy fibers have multiple branches
Ref. Snells Neuroanatomy, 3rd/e, p215-6

24. Which of the following structures is not involved in direct and consensual light reflexes?
a. Pretectal nucleus
b. Edinger-Westphal nucleus
c. Ciliary ganglion
d. Medial longitudinal fasciculus
Ref. Snells Neuroanatomy, 3rd/e, p425

25. Which nucleus of 5th cranial nerve lies in the lateral gray matter around the cerebral aqueduct?
a. Spinal nucleus
b. Mesencephalic nucleus
c. Motor nucleus
d. Sensory nucleus
Ref. Snells Neuroanatomy, 3rd/e, p430-3

26. The main nerve supply of dura mater is from:
a. Accessory nerve
b. Trigeminal nerve
c. Vagus nerve
d. None of the above
Ref. Snells Neuroanatomy, 3rd/e, p522-3

27. Which of the following cranial nerves lies within the cavernous sinus?
a. Oculomotor nerve
b. Trochlear nerve
c. Trigeminal nerve
d. Abducent nerve
Ref. Rhoton, p403-7

28. All the following statements about dentate ligament are true, except:
a. It basically is thickened arachnoid membrane
b. It consists of teeth like processes in pairs
c. It separates anterior spinal nerve roots from the posterior roots
d. It anchors the spinal cord
Ref. Snells Neuroanatomy, 3rd/e, p172

29. A 35-year-old female demonstrates facial weakness especially of perioral region during emotional changes. The most likely site of lesion is:
a. Frontal lobe
b. Temporal lobe
c. Parietal lobe
d. None of the above
Ref. Bickerstaff, 6th/e, p80

30. All the following statements about anterior longitudinal ligament of spine are correct, except:
a. It consists of 2 layers of collagen
b. It prevents hyperextension of spine
c. The ALL at upper dorsal spine is weaker than at lower dorsal spine
d. It prevents overdistraction of spine
Ref. Youmans, 5th/e, p4186

Answers

21. d. **22.** d. **23.** b. **24.** d. **25.** b. **26.** b. **27.** d. **28.** a. **29.** a. **30.** a.

31. All the following statements about ligamenta flava are correct, except:
a. These are paired ligaments connecting the spinal laminae
b. These are attached to the dorsal surface of the lower vertebra and anterior surface of the upper vertebra
c. These ligaments are yellow in color
d. These ligaments contain lot of elastin
Ref. Youmans, 5th/e, p4186

32. The area between the greater superficial petrosal nerve, the carotid artery and the semicircular canals is known as:
a. Trutman's triangle
b. Kawases triangle
c. Parkinson's triangle
d. None of the above
Ref. Schmidek and Sweet, 4th/e, p959

33. Pacchinonian bodies are:
a. Histopathological feature of meningiomas
b. Histopathological feature of pilocytic astrocytomas
c. Arachnoid villi
d. Calcified structures near the pineal recess
Ref. Youmans, 5th/e, p1100

34. Arachnoid villi are maximum in density near:
a. Lamina cribrosa
b. Superior sagittal sinus
c. Torcula
d. Cavernous sinus
Ref. Youmans, 5th/e, p1100

35. The medial posterior choroidal arteries arise from:
a. Posterior cerebral arteries in the interpeduncular cistern
b. Posterior cerebral arteries in the quadrigeminal cistern
c. Posterior communicating arteries
d. Basilar artery
Ref. Rhoton, p141

36. The hippocampus is separated medially from the brainstem by:
a. Crural cistern
b. Ambient cistern
c. Quadrigeminal cistern
d. Chiasmatic cistern
Ref. Rhoton, p719-28

37. All the following statements are true, except:
a. Fibers subserving pain and temperature pass through spinothalamic tract
b. The fibers carrying vibration and joint position sense tract through the posterior column
c. In the spinothalamic tract, the fibers from lower limb lie lateral and fibers from upper limb lie medially
d. In the posterior column, the fibers from lower limb lie lateral and fibers from upper limb lie medially
Ref. Bickerstaff, 6th/e, p196-202

38. A young female on neurological examination was found to have loss of pain and temperature on right side of face and left side of body. Most likely the lesion is involving the:
a. Descending root of the right trigeminal nerve and lateral spinothalamic tract in the medulla
b. Descending root of the right trigeminal nerve and the posterior column in the medulla
c. Sensory nucleus of the right trigeminal nerve and the lateral spinothalamic tract in the pons
d. None of the above
Ref. Bickerstaff, 6th/e, p73

39. All the following statements about trigeminal nerve sensations are correct, except:
a. Touch fibers ascend and enter the main sensory nucleus of midbrain
b. Pain and temperature fibers reach up to the descending nucleus up to the second cervical segment
c. Ophthalmic division fibers reach up to the lowest level of the descending nucleus and mandibular division fibers reach up to highest level
d. Sensory nucleus lies lateral to the motor nucleus in the brainstem
Ref. Patten, 2nd/e, p167-9

ANSWERS

31. b. **32.** b. **33.** c. **34.** b. **35.** a. **36.** b. **37.** d. **38.** a. **39.** a.

40. If right cornea is touched and only the right eye blinks without blinking on left side, the lesion lies with:

a. Ophthalmic division of right trigeminal nerve
b. Right facial nerve
c. Ophthalmic division of left trigeminal nerve
d. Left facial nerve

Ref. Bickerstaff, 6th/e, p74-5

41. The normal height of adenohypophysis in prepuberal and postpubertal individuals respectively is:

a. 2 mm and 5 mm
b. 2.5 mm and 6 mm
c. 3 mm and 7 mm
d. None of the above

Ref. American journal of Radiology 1984;143: 377-81

42. The three eminencies in the floor of the 4th ventricle from medial to lateral are:

a. Hypoglossal eminence – intermediate eminence– eminence over area vestibularis
b. Eminence over area vestibularis – intermediate eminence – hypoglossal eminence
c. Hypoglossal eminence – eminence over area vestibularis – eminence over dorsal motor nucleus of vagus
d. None of the above

Ref. Snells Neuroanatomy, 3rd/e, p230

43. All the following statements about area postrema are true, except:

a. It lies in the 4th ventricle floor below the obex
b. It is sensitive to apomorphine
c. It receives afferents from nucleus solitarius
d. It is a chemoreceptor

Ref. Snells Neuroanatomy, 3rd/e, p231, 356

44. All the following statements about primary visual cortex are true, except:

a. It is located in the lateral occipital lobe
b. The macular field is represented at the pole
c. The superior field is represented inferiorly
d. The left visual field is represented on the right hand side

Ref. Snells Neuroanatomy, p300

45. On a routine neurological examination, a young collegiate was found to have normal visual activity but both pupils failed to react to the light. MRI brain most likely shall show a:

a. Pontine lesion
b. Midbrain lesion
c. Chiasmal lesion
d. Bilateral occipital lesion

Ref. Bickerstaff, 6th/e, p58

46. A 40-year-old female had a generalized tonic convulsion followed by loss of consciousness. During the seizure, she was noticed to have deviation of eyes to right side. The most likely site and nature of the lesion is:

a. Left frontal astrocytoma
b. Right frontal tuberculoma
c. Brainstem lesion
d. None of the above

Ref. Patten, 2nd/e, p94-5

47. All the following statements about examination of fundus are correct, except:

a. The nasal side of the disk is normally paler than the temporal side
b. The disk in optic nerve sheath meningioma is chalky white in appearance
c. The myopic disk looks normally pale
d. The nasal edge of the disk is normally blurred

Ref. Bickerstaff, 6th/e, p43-9

48. A middle aged man reports to his family physican with atrophy of left side of tongue. On examination, the hemitongue shows fasciculations and the tongue is deviated to the left side. MRI brain shows a lesion involving the left hypoglossal canal. The pathological possibilities of the lesion is/are:

a. Schwannoma
b. Glomus jugulare
c. Meningioma
d. All the above

Ref. Bickerstaff, 6th/e, p108

ANSWERS

40. d.	**41.** a.	**42.** a.	**43.** a.	**44.** a.	**45.** b.	**46.** d.	**47.** a.	**48.** d.

49. All the following statements regarding the blood supply of spinal cord are true, except:

a. It is supplied by one anterior spinal artery and two posterior spinal arteries
b. The posterior spinal arteries arise from the anterior inferior cerebellar arteries
c. The anterior spinal artery supplies the anterior two-thirds of the spinal cord
d. The artery of Adamkiewicz arises from the aorta at the level of lower dorsal or upper lumbar vertebral level

Ref. Snells Neuroanatomy, 3rd/e, p173-4

50. All the following statements regarding subthalamus are true, except:

a. The cranial ends of red nucleus and substantia nigra are situated in subthalamus
b. The subthalamic nucleus is biconcave in shape
c. The subthalamic nucleus is involved in control of muscle activity
d. The subthalamic nucleus is an important target for deep brain stimulation for movement disorders

Ref. Snells Neuroanatomy, 3rd/e, p252

51. All the following statements about superior petrosal sinus are true, except:

a. SPS courses within the attachment of the tentorium to the petrous ridge
b. Its medial end connects with the cavernous sinus and its lateral and joins the junction of the transverse and sigmoid sinuses
c. The bridging views that join it arise from the cerebrum, cerebellum and brainstem
d. The sinus may cause overt, under or around the posterior root of the trigeminal nerve

Ref. Rhoton, p197

52. All the following statements about vein of Trolard are true, except:

a. The vein of Trolard is the largest anastamotic vein crossing the cortical surface of the frontal and parietal lobes between the superior sagittal sinus and the sylvian fissure
b. The vein of Trolard usually joins the supper sagittal sinus as a single channel
c. Its lower end is usually a single channel that anastamosis with the veins along the sylvian fissure
d. It is directed backwards towards the direct of flow as it joins the sinus

Ref. Rhoton, p199

53. All the following statements about caudate nucleus are true, except:

a. The caudate nucleus is a C-shaped cellular mass that wraps around the thalamus
b. The head bulges into the lateral wall of the frontal horn
c. The body of the nucleus forms part of the lateral wall of atrium
d. The tail extends from the atrium into the tip of the occipital horn

Ref. Rhoton, p235

54. All the following statements about velum interpositum are correct, except:

a. It is located in the floor of the 3rd ventricle
b. It is usually a closed space
c. It is widest posteriorly
d. The upper end and lower walls of it are formed by the 2-membranous layers of tela choroidea

Ref. Rhoton, p213

55. All the following statements about temporal horn of the lateral ventricle are true, except:

a. The temporal horn extends forwards from the atrium below the pulvinar into the medial part of the temporal lobe and ends in the anterior wall behind the amygdaloid nucleus
b. The floor is formed by the hippocampus and collateral eminence, roof by the thalamus and lateral wall by the tapetum
c. The medial wall is formed by caudate tail
d. The veins from the temporal horn join the basal vein or its tributaries

Ref. Rhoton, p219

ANSWERS

49. b. **50.** b. **51.** c. **52.** d. **53.** d. **54.** a. **55.** c.

56. All the following statements regarding superior orbital fissure are true, except:

a. The superior orbital fissure provides a communication between the orbit and the middle cranial fossa
b. The cavernous sinus is situated behind
c. The superior orbital fissure is located between the greater and lesser wings of sphenoid bone
d. The fissure slopes gently downwards from its medial to lateral border

Ref. Rhoton, p337

57. All the following statements regarding ciliary ganglion are true, except:

a. The ciliary ganglion is situated on the superomedial aspect of the optic nerve
b. It receives 3-branches: motor, sensory and sympathetic
c. The parasympathetic fibers synapse in the ciliary ganglion
d. The short ciliary nerve passes from the ganglion to the globe

Ref. Rhoton, p345

58. All the following statements about fornix are true, except:

a. Fornix is a C-shaped structure and wraps around the thalamus in the wall of the ventricle
b. The fornix consists mainly of hippocampo-manmillary tract
c. The fimbra arise in the floor of the 3rd-ventricle and passes posteriorly to become the crus of the fornix
d. At the junction of the atrium and the body of the lateral ventricle, the paired crura meet to form the body of the fornix

Ref. Rhoton, p235

59. All the following statements regarding optic canal are true, except:

a. The intracranial optic canal has an ovoid-shape with a slight greater diameter in the mediolateral than in the supero-inferior dimension
b. It is situated lateral to the anterior clinical process and optic strut
c. The medial margin is formed by the body of the sphenoid bone
d. The upper margin is formed by the anterior root of the lesser wing of the sphenoid bone

Ref. Rhoton, p335

60. Which of the following statements about posterior cranial fossa are correct?

a. It is the largest and deepest of the 3-cranial fossae
b. It is about one-eighth of the intracranial space
c. Only 2 of the 12 pairs of cranial nerves are located outside it; the 10 other pairs have a segment within the posterior fossa
d. All the above are correct

Ref. Rhoton, p439

61. All the following statements about 4th ventricle are true, except:

a. It is a broad tent-shaped midline cavity located between the cerebellum and the brainstem
b. It is connected rostrally through the aqueduct with the 3rd ventricle, caudally through the foramen of Magendie with the cisterna magna and laterally through the foraminae of Luschka with the cerebellopontine angles
c. It has a roof, a floor and 2-lateral recesses
d. Most of the cranial nerves arise from its roof

Ref. Rhoton, p443

62. All the following statements regarding cavernous sinus are true, except:

a. the cavernous sinus is narrowest anteriorly and widest posteriorly
b. It is connected to the orbit by the superior and inferior ophthalmic veins, to the cerebral hemispheres through the middle and inferior cerebral veins, to the retina by the central retinal vein
c. the basilar sinus is the largest and most constant intercavernous connection across the midline which passes anterior to the dorsum sella
d. The 3-main venous spaces within the sinus are medial, antero inferior and the postero superior compartments by their relation to the carotid artery

Ref. Rhoton, p426

ANSWERS

56. d. **57.** a. **58.** c. **59.** b. **60.** d. **61.** d. **62.** c.

63. All the following statements regarding sphenoid sinus are true, except:

a. The sphenoid sinus separates the cavernous sinuses, the cavernous segments of the carotid arteries
b. It is present as minute cavities at birth but its main development takes place after puberty
c. It may sometimes partially encircle the optic canals
d. As age advances, the sinus decreases in size

Ref. Rhoton, p369

64. All the following statements regarding diaphragm sellae are correct, except:

a. The diaphragm is more rectangular than circular
b. It is more convex or concave rather than flat
c. It is thicker around the infundibulum and thinner at the periphery
d. A deficiency of diaphragm sella is a precondition for empty sella syndrome

Ref. Rhoton, p383

65. All the following statements about pons are correct, except:

a. The belly of the pons is convex from side to side as well as from top to bottom
b. The pons is continuous on each side with the middle cerebellar peduncles
c. It has a shallow midline groove, the basilar sulcus which extends from its superior to its inferior border
d. The posterior root of the trigeminal nerve emerges from the lower position of the middle cerebellar peduncle

Ref. Rhoton, p454

66. Which of the following statements regarding veins of the brainstem are true?

a. The veins of the brainstem are divided into 2 groups based whether they course longitudinally or transversally
b. The longitudinal veins are the median anterior pontomesencephalic, median anterior medullary, lateral anterior pontomesencephalic, lateral anterior medullary
c. The transverse veins are the veins of the pontomesencephalic and the pontomedullary sulci and the transverse pontine, transverse medullary and posterior communicating vein
d. All are true

Ref. Rhoton p515

67. All the following statements about tentorial incisura are correct, except:

a. The tentorial incisura is roughly triangular
b. The incisura is filled with midbrain, uncus and parahippocampal gyrus
c. The width of the incisura usually varies from 26 to 36 mm
d. The posterior part of the 3rd ventricle projects into the anterior incisural space

Ref. Rhoton p567

68. All the following statements regarding petrous bone are true, except:

a. The petrous part of the temporal bone is wedged between the sphenoid and occipital bones
b. It contains the acoustic and vestibular labyrinth
c. It has a base, apex, 4 surfaces
d. The tympanic segment of the facial nerve begins at the geniculate ganglion and ends at the level of the stapes

Ref. Rhoton p653

69. Which of the following statements about temporal bone are correct?

a. The temporal bone is divided into squamous, petrous, mastoid, tympanic and styloid parts
b. The mastoid part is trabeculated and pneumatized and contains the mastoid antrum
c. The petrous part is compact and encloses the cochlea, the vestibule, facial and carotid canals
d. The styloid process projects downwards and serves as the site of attachment of various muscles
e. All are correct

Ref. Rhoton p643

ANSWERS

63. d. **64.** c. **65.** d. **66.** d. **67.** d. **68.** c. **69.** e.

70. Which of the following statements about floor of the 4th ventricle are true?

a. The floor has a rhomboid shape and its cranial apex is at the level of the aqueduct and caudal tip is located at the rostral end of the remnant of the spinal canal, anterior to the foramen of Magendie
b. The floor is divided into 3 parts vertically, the superior and inferior parts are triangular in shape
c. The floor is divided longitudinally into 2 symmetrical halves by the median sulcus
d. All are true

Ref. Rhoton p455

71. All the following statements about vascular relations of 4th ventricle are true, except:

a. Superior cerebellar artery is intimately related to the superior half of the roof
b. The PICA is related to the inferior half of the roof
c. The AICA is related to the lateral recess and the foramen of Luschka
d. The choroidal branches of AICA supply the choroid plexus in the roof of the 4th ventricle

Ref. Rhoton p456

72. Which of the following statements regarding SCA (superior cerebellar artery) are correct?

a. The SCA is divided into 4 segments; anterior pontomesencephalic, lateral pontomesencephalic, cerebellomesencephalic and cortical
b. Anterior pontomesencephalic is located between dorsum sellae and the upper brainstem
c. Lateral pontomesencephalic begins at the anterolateral margin of the brainstem and frequently dips caudally into the lateral side of upper pons
d. Cerebellomesencephalic segment courses within the cerebellomesencephalic fissure
e. All are true

Ref. Rhoton p462

73. All the following statements about tentorial arteries are true, except:

a. The artery of Bernasconi and Cassinari arise from the meningohypophyseal trunk
b. The marginal tentorial artery arises from the inferolateral trunk
c. The marginal tentorial artery passes laterally below the abducens nerves
d. Superior cerebellar artery and posterior cerebellar artery also are sources of tentorial arteries

Ref. Rhoton p575

74. All the following statements about foramen magnum are true, except:

a. The occipital bone surrounds the foramen magnum
b. The foraminal opening is oval shaped and is wider anteriorly than posteriorly
c. The structures located in it are lower cranial and upper spinal nerves, caudal brainstem, rostral spinal cord
d. The most common surgical approach to access the foramen is the posterior route

Ref. Rhoton p587

75. Which of the following statements regarding veins of the brainstem are true?

a. The veins of the brainstem are divided into 2 groups based whether they course longitudinally or transversally
b. The longitudinal veins are the median anterior pontomesencephalic, median anterior medullary, lateral anterior pontomesencephalic, lateral anterior medullary
c. The transverse veins are the veins of the pontomesencephalic and the pontomedullary sulci and the transverse pontine, transverse medullary and posterior communicating vein
d. All are true

Ref. Rhoton p515

ANSWERS

70. d. **71.** d. **72.** e. **73.** c. **74.** b. **75.** d.

76. All the following statements about tentorial incisura are correct, except:

a. The tentorial incisura is roughly triangular
b. The incisura is filled with midbrain, uncus and parahippocampal gyrus
c. The width of the incisura usually varies from 26 to 36 mm
d. The posterior part of the 3rd ventricle projects into the anterior incisural space

Ref. Rhoton p567

77. All the following statements regarding petrous bone are true, except:

a. The petrous part of the temporal bone is wedged between the sphenoid and occipital bones
b. It contains the acoustic and vestibular labyrinth
c. It has a base, apex, 4 surfaces
d. The tympanic segment of the facial nerve begins at the geniculate ganglion and ends at the level of the stapes.

Ref. Rhoton p653

78. Which of the following statements about temporal bone are correct?

a. The temporal bone is divided into squamous, petrous, mastoid, tympanic and styloid parts
b. The mastoid part is trabeculated and pneumatized and contains the mastoid antrum
c. The petrous part is compact and encloses the cochlea, the vestibule, fcial and carotid canals
d. The styloid process projects downwards and serves as the site of attachment of various muscles
e. All are correct

Ref. Rhoton p643

79. Which of the following statements about floor of the 4th ventricle are true?

a. The floor has a rhomboid shape and its cranial apex is at the level of the aqueduct and caudal tip is located at the rostral end of the remnant of the spinal canal, anterior to the foramen of Magendie
b. The floor is divided into 3 parts vertically, the superior and inferior parts are triangular in shape
c. The floor is divided longitudinally into 2 symmetrical halves by the median sulcus
d. All are true

Ref. Rhoton p455

80. All the following statements about vascular relations of 4th ventricle are true, except:

a. Superior cerebellar artery is intimately related to the superior half of the roof
b. The PICA is related to the inferior half of the roof
c. The AICA is related to the lateral recess and the foramen of Luschka
d. The choroidal branches of AICA supply the choral plexus in the roof of the 4th ventricle

Ref. Rhoton p456

81. Which of the following statements regarding SCA (superior cerebellar artery) are correct?

a. The SCA is divided into 4 segments; anterior pontomesencephalic, lateral pontomesencephalic, cerebellomesencephalic and cortical
b. Anterior pontomesencephalic is located between dorsum sellae and the upper brainstem
c. Lateral pontomesencephalic begins at the anterolateral margin of the brainstem and frequently dips caudally into the lateral side of upper pans
d. Cerebellomesencephalic segment courses within the cerebellomesencephalic fissure
e. All are true

Ref. Rhoton p462

82. All the following statements about tentorial arteries are true, except:

a. the artery of Bernasconi and Cassinari arise from the meningohypophyseal trunk
b. The marginal tentorial artery arise from the inferolateral trunk
c. The marginal tentorial artery passes laterally below the abducens nerves
d. Superior cerebellar artery and posterior cerebellar artery also are sources of tentorial arteries

Ref. Rhoton p575

ANSWERS

76. d. **77.** c. **78.** e. **79.** d. **80.** d. **81.** e. **82.** c.

83. All the following statements about foramen magnum are true, except:

a. The occipital bone surrounds the foramen magnum

b. The foraminal opening is oral shaped and is wider anteriorly than posteriorly

c. The structures located in it are lower cranial and upper spinal nerves, caudal brainstem, rostral spinal cord

d. The most common surgical approach to access the foramen is the posterior route

Ref. Rhoton p587

84. All the following statements regarding dentate ligament of spine are correct, except:

a. The dentate ligament is a white fibrous sheet that is attached to the spinal cord medially and to the dura laterally

b. At the craniocervical junction, the dentate ligament is located between the vertebral artery and the ventral roots of CI anteriorly and the branches of the posterior spinal artery and the spinal accessory nerve posteriorly

c. Its most rostral attachment is located at the level of foramen magnum

d. The first cervical nerve courses along the antero superior surface of the vertebral artery as it pierces the dura

Ref. Rhoton p599

85. All the following statements about the first cervical vertebra are correct, except:

a. It is ring shaped and it lacks a spinous process and vertebral body

b. It consists of two thick lateral masses situated at the anterolateral parts of the ring

c. The lateral masses are connected in front by a long anterior arch and behind by a short posterior arch

d. The position of the usual vertebral body is occupied by the odontoid process of the axis

Ref. Rhoton p589

86. All the following statements regarding posterior inferior-cerebellar-artery are correct, except:

a. The PICA has the most complex, tortuous and variable course and area of supply of the cerebellar arteries

b. The PICA is intimately related to the cerebello medullary fissure, the inferior half of the ventricular roof, the inferior cerebellar peduncle and the suboccipital surface

c. The PICA is divided into 5 segments; anterior medullary, lateral medullary, tonsillomedullay, telovelotonsillar and cortical

d. Most PICA's bifurcate into a larger medial and smaller lateral trunk

Ref. Rhoton p489

87. All the following statements about anterior inferior cerebellar arteries are correct, except:

a. The AICA courses through the central part of the cerebellopontine angle near the facial and vestibulo-cochlear nerve

b. The AICA is intimately related to the pons, lateral recess, foramen of Luschka, cerebellopontine fissure, middle cerebellar peduncle and petrosal cerebellar surface

c. The AICA is divided into 5 segments

d. The AICA originates from the basilar artery as a single vessel but sometimes may arise as duplicate or triplicate

Ref. Rhoton p476

88. All the following statements regarding jugular foramen are true, except:

a. The jugular foramen is divided into 3 compartments; two venous and a neural or intrajugular compartment

b. The jugular foramen is located between the temporal bone and the occipital bone

c. The left foramen is usually larger than the right

d. Sigmoid sinus, jugular bulb, inferior petrosal sinus, meningeal branches of the ascending pharyngeal and occipital arteries, 9, 10, 11th cranial nerves

Ref. Rhoton p699

ANSWERS

83. b. **84.** d. **85.** c. **86.** d. **87.** c. **88.** c.

89. All the following statements regarding cerebellopontine cistern are true, except:

a. It lies between the anterolateral surface of the pons and cerebellum and the arachnoid membrane that rests on the posterior surface of the petrous bone

b. Superiorly this cistern is separated from the ambient cistern by the lateral pontomescencephalic membrane

c. Inferiorly this cistern is separated from the cerebellomedullary cistern by the lateral and pontomedullary membrane

d. Laterally this cistern extends to the edge of the cerebellar surface that wraps around the pons

e. All are true

Ref. Rhoton 722

ANSWERS

89. e

EXPLANATION

1. The AChA originates from the posterior wall of the ICA between origin of posterior communicating artery (PCOM), which is 2-5 mm proximally and the internal carotid termination, which is 2-5 mm distal to the AChA. It measures ~1 mm in diameter.

   The AChA is located lateral to the optic tract, it then curves medially to its inferomedial surface, to curve again laterally to run along the lateral aspect of the optic tract and circumvents the cerebral peduncles to reach the lateral geniculate body. It traverse in the posterolateral direction above the uncus to enter the choroidal fissure. The AChA can be divided into two segments: cisternal segment - extends from its origin until the choroidal fissure; measures ~2.5 cm (range 1.5-3.5 cm) in length, intraventricular segment - after entering the choroidal fissure.

5. The vein of Labbé, also known as inferior anastamotic vein. The vein of Labbé is the largest channel that crosses the temporal lobe between the Sylvian fissure and the transverse sinus and connects the superficial middle cerebral vein and the transverse sinus. There is a relationship between the size of the terminal superficial middle cerebral vein, the anastamotic vein of Trolard and the vein of Labbé. During temporal lobectomies care should be taken not to injure it.

7. Recurrent artery of Heubner, is also known as the medial striate artery or long central artery, is the largest perforating branch from the proximal anterior cerebral artery. Its origin is from the proximal A2 in 90% of cases, and from the distal A1 in 10% of cases. It then curves back sharply on itself, paralleling the A1. It supplies the head of caudate nucleus, anterior portion of the lentiform nucleus and anterior limb of the internal capsule.

9. Vein of Galen, also known as the great cerebral vein or great vein of Galen, is a short trunk formed by the union of the two internal cerebral veins and basal veins of Rosenthal. It lies in the quadrigeminal cistern. It curves backward and upward around the posterior border of the splenium of the corpus callosum to drain into the confluence of the inferior sagittal sinus and the anterior extremity of the straight sinus.

10. The origin of the VA is usually from the posterior superior part of the subclavian artery.

    The vertebral artery is typically divided into 4 segments:

    V1: origin to transverse foramen of C6, V2: from the transverse foramen of C6 to the transverse foramen of C2, V3: from C2 to the dura, V4: from the dura to their confluence to form the basilar artery. The left vertebral artery is dominant in most of the population.

11. The diagnostic criteria for VBD is a basilar artery or vertebral artery diameter >4.5 mm or deviation of any portion of them higher than 10 mm from the shortest expected course, or basilar length >29.5 mm or intracranial vertebral artery length >23.5 mm.

13. The cerebellum originated as a specialized part of the acoustico-lateralis area. The oldest part of the cerebellum—the archicerebellum—is concerned with equilibrium and connected with the inner ear and the lateral-line system. The anterior lobe of the cerebellum represents the paleocerebellum, an area that regulates equilibrium and muscle tone.

20. The hippocampus (named after its resemblance to the seahorse. It belongs to the limbic system and plays important roles in the consolidation of information from short-term memory to long-term memory. It contains two main interlocking parts: Ammon's horn and the dentate gyrus.

25. The mesencephalic nucleus is involved with proprioception of the face, that is, the feeling of position of the muscles. Unlike many nuclei within the central nervous system (CNS), the mesencephalic nucleus contains no chemical synapses but are electrically coupled Neurons of this nucleus are pseudounipolar cells that receive proprioceptive information from the mandible and send projections to the motor trigeminal nucleus to mediate monosynaptic jaw jerk reflexes.

28. The pia mater of the spinal cord has a pair of denticulate ligaments (one on each side of the spinal cord) with 21 attachments per side which attach it to the arachnoid and dura mater. Named for their tooth-like appearance, the denticulate ligaments are traditionally believed to provide stability for the spinal cord against motion within the vertebral column.

30. The anterior longitudinal ligament is a ligament that runs down the anterior surface of the spine. It traverses all of the vertebral bodies and intervertebral discs. The ligament is thick and slightly more narrow over the vertebral bodies and thinner but slightly wider over the intervertebral discs which is much less pronounced than that seen in the posterior longitudinal ligament. The ligament actually has three layers: superficial, intermediate and deep. The superficial layer traverses 3 – 4 vertebrae, the intermediate layer covers 2 – 3 and the deep layer is only between individual vertebrae.

31. The ligamenta flava [*flavum*, Latin for *yellow ligament*] are ligaments of the spine. They connect the laminae of adjacent vertebrae, all the way from the second vertebra, axis, to the first segment of the sacrum. They are best seen from the interior of the vertebral canal; when looked at from the outer surface they appear short, being overlapped by the lamina of the vertebral arch. Each ligament consists of two lateral portions which commence one on either side of the roots of the articular processes, and extend backward to the point where the laminae meet to form the spinous process; the posterior margins of the two portions are in contact and to a certain extent united, slight intervals being left for the passage of small vessels. Each consists of yellow elastic tissue, the fibers of which, almost perpendicular in direction, are attached to the anterior surface of the lamina above, some distance from its inferior margin, and to the posterior surface and upper margin of the lamina below.

32. The posteromedial middle fossa triangle, also known as Kawase's triangle, Kawase-Shiobara's triangle, or the posteromedial triangle, is defined by the porus trigeminus, the cochlea, and the mandibular division of the trigeminal nerve.

The infratrochlear triangle, also known as Parkinson's triangle, is bounded by the trochlear nerve and the ophthalmic division of the trigeminal nerve.

This is a triangular space bounded by –Bony labyrinth anteriorly, Sigmoid sinus posteriorly,

Dura containing superior petrosal sinus superiorly.

33. Arachnoid granulations, also known as a Pacchionian granulation, are projections of the arachnoid membrane into the dural sinuses that allow CSF flow from the subarachnoid space to the venous system. They most frequently occur in a parasagittal location and can cause an osteolytic, sharply circumscribed lucency on skull x-rays, or a filling defect in dural venous sinuses.

35. The medial posterior choroidal artery is a small branch usually arising from the P2 segment of the PCA. It may also arise from one of the PCA branches, e.g. parieto-occiptal, calcarine, splenial artery. It ascends deep to the rest of the PCA and supplies small branches to the tegmentum, midbrain, posterior thalamus and pineal gland as the *cisternal segment*. It then penetrates the velum interpositum, becoming the *plexal segment* and then runs in the roof of the third ventricle supplying the ipsilateral choroid plexus.

43. The area postrema is a small protuberance found at the inferoposterior limit of the fourth ventricle. The area postrema is separated from the vagal triangle by the funiculus separans, a thin semitransparent ridge. The vagal triangle overlies the dorsal vagal nucleus and is situated on the caudal end of the rhomboid fossa or 'floor' of the fourth ventricle. The area postrema is situated just above the obex, the inferior apex of the caudal ventricular floor. Both the funiculus separans and area postrema have a similar thick ependyma-containing tanycyte covering. Ependyma and tanycytes may also participate in chemoreception. The eminence of the area postrema is considered a circumventricular organ because its endothelial cells do not contain tight junctions, which allows for free exchange of molecules between blood and brain tissue.

47. The fundus of the eye is the interior surface of the eye opposite the lens and includes the retina, optic disc, macula, fovea, and posterior pole. The optic disc or optic nerve head is the point of exit for ganglion cell axons leaving the eye. Because there are no rods or cones overlying the optic disc, it corresponds to a small physiological blind spot in each eye. The optic disc is placed 3 to 4 mm to the nasal side of the fovea. A normal optic disc is orange to pink in color. It is a vertical oval, with average dimensions of 1.76mm horizontally by 1.92mm vertically. There is a central depression, of variable size, called the optic cup.

50. The subthalamic nucleus is a small lens-shaped nucleus in the brain where it is, from a functional point of view, part of the basal ganglia system. It is located ventral to the thalamus. It is also dorsal to the substantia nigra and medial to the internal capsule.

51. The bridging veins of the cerebrum do not drain into the SPS, however veins from cerebellum and brainstem do drain.

52. It is directed forwards against the direction of flow as it joins the sinus.

53. The tail extends from the atrium into the roof of the temporal horn and is continues with the amygdaloid nucleus means the tip of the temporal horn.

58. The fimbrae arise in the floor of the temporal horn on the ventricular surface of the hippocampal formation

62. The basilar sinus, the largest and most constant intercavernous connection across the midline passes **posterior** to the dorsum sellae.

65. The posterior root of the trigeminal nerve emerges from the **upper portion** of the mildle cerebellar peduncle just below the anterior angle of the cerebellum

67. The anterior part of the 3rd ventricle projects into the anterior incisural space dividing it into supra and infrachiasmatic portions.

68. It has a base, apex, 3 surfaces and margins. The apex is located in the angle between the greater wing of the sphenoid and the occipital bone and is the site of the carotid canals medial opening.

71. Choroidal branches of AICA supply the choroid plexus in the CP cistern

73. The marginal tentorial artery passes laterally over the abducens nerve, then superiorposteriorly near the trochlear nerve to enter the tentorial edge. If this artery is absent a branch from the meningohypophyseal artery may replace it.

74. The foraminal opening is oval shaped and is wider posteriorly than anteriorly. The wider posterior part transmits the medulla and the narrower anterior part sits about the odontoid process.

76. The anterior part of the 3rd ventricle projects into the anterior incisural space dividing it into supra and infrachiasmatic portions.

77. It has a base, apex, 3 surfaces and margins. The apex is located in the angle between the greater use of the sphenoid and the occipital bone and is the site of the carotid canals medial opening.

80. Choroidal branches of AICA supply the choroids plexus in the CP cistern

82. The marginal tentorial artery passes laterally over the abducens nerve, then superiorposteriorly near the trochlear nerve to enter the tentorial edge. If this artery is absent a branch from the meningohypophyseal artery may replace it.

83. The foraminal opening is oral shaped and is wider posteriorly than anteriorly. The medulla and the narrower anterior part sits about the odontoid process.

84. The first cervical nerve courses along the postero-inferior surface of the vertebral artery as it pierces the dura. The ventral root is located anterior to the dentate ligament and the dorsal root which is infrequently present, passes posterior to the dentate ligament.

85. The lateral masses are connected in front by a short anterior arch and posteriorly by a curved long arch.

86. Most PICAs bifurcate into a similar medial and larger lateral trunk. The smaller medial trunk supplies the vermis and adjacent part of the hemisphere and the larger lateral trunk supplies most of the hemispheric and tonsillar parts of the suboccipital surface

87. AICA is divided into 4 segments antero-pontine, lateral pontine, flocculonodular and cortical. PICA is divided into 5 segments.

CHAPTER 7

Neuroradiology

Nayil Khursheed, Rumana Makhdoomi

MULTIPLE CHOICE QUESTIONS

1. **Unidentified bright objects (UBOs) on MRI are seen in:**
   a. Optic pathway gliomas
   b. Craniopharyngiomas
   c. AVMs
   d. Germinomas
   Ref. Pediatric Radiology 2008;38(3):305-10

2. **Mother-in-law appearance on angiogram is seen in:**
   a. Meningiomas
   b. Gliomas
   c. Choroid plexus papillomas
   d. Ependymomas
   Ref. Al-Mefty, p212

3. **Sunburst appearance on angiogram is seen in:**
   a. Medulloblastomas
   b. Craniopharyngiomas
   c. Meningiomas
   d. Gliosarcoma
   Ref. Al-Mefty, p212

4. **Which vein on angiogram is frog-leg shaped?**
   a. Vein of Rosenthal
   b. Thalamostriate vein
   c. Vein of Galen
   d. Septal vein
   Ref. Osborn Angiography, 1st/e, p343

5. **Venous angle on angiogram is formed by the union of:**
   a. Septal and thalamostriate vein
   b. Internal cerebral veins
   c. The four major sinuses (Torcular Herophil)
   d. None of the above
   Ref. Osborn Angiography, 1st/e, p342

6. **Caput medusae is seen in which of the following vascular malformations?**
   a. Venous angiomas
   b. Cavernomas
   c. Telangiectasia
   d. AV fistulas
   Ref. Greenberg, 4th/e, p873

7. **Hemosiderin ring is usually seen in which of the following lesions:**
   a. Tuberculomas
   b. Cystecercosis
   c. Hydatid cyst
   d. Cavernomas
   Ref. Youmans, 5th/e, p2169

ANSWERS

1. a. **2.** a. **3.** c. **4.** a. **5.** a. **6.** a. **7.** d.

8. Candlebra appearance on angiogram is given by branches of:

a. ACA b. MCA

c. PCA d. None of the above

Ref. Osborn Angiography, 1st/e, p243

9. The classical ice cream cone appearance on MRI brain is seen in which of the following tumors?

a. Olfactory groove meningiomas
b. Vestibular schwannoma
c. Falcine meningioma
d. Intraventricular neurocytoma

Ref. Osborn, 1st/e, p109

10. Truncation of petrous apex is caused by which of the following tumors:

a. Petrous meningiomas
b. Trigeminal nerve schwannomas
c. Vestibular schwannomas
d. Parasellar meningiomas

Ref. Youmans, 5th/e, p1347

11. Mushrooming is seen in which type of tumor?

a. Meningiomas
b. Craniopharyngiomas
c. Choroid plexus papilloma
d. Ependymoma

Ref. Al-Mefty, p94

12. All the following statements about Neurosarcoidosis are true, except:

a. Osteoblastic skull lesions are found
b. About 50% patients have periventricular hyperintenities on T_2W sequence
c. Lacunar infarcts of brainstem or basal ganglia are seen
d. Diffusion weighted MRI distinguishes cytotoxic edema of acute stroke from vasogenic edema of neurosarcoidosis

Ref. Osborn, Section 4, p52

13. All the following statements about vertebral hemangiomas are true, except:

a. Usually seen in elderly females
b. Common level is thoracolumbar
c. Usually posterior elements are involved
d. Most of the patients are asymptomatic

Ref. Greenberg, 4th/e, p346-7

14. Colliculocentral point is where the:

a. precentral cerebellar vein exits from horizontal fissure
b. precentral cerebellar vein (PCV) exits from the precentral cerebellar fissure
c. Vertebral arteries unite to form the basilar artery
d. PICA (Posterior inferior cerebellar artery) loops around the tonsil

Ref. Osborn Angiography, 1st/e, p394

15. All the following are true regarding angiographic signs of hydrocephalus except?

a. Stretching of thalamoperforatoring vessels is seen
b. There is decreased distance between medial and lateral choroidal artery
c. There is decreased distance between choroidal arteries and parieto-occipital artery
d. There is change in venous angle

Ref. Osborn Angiography, 1st/e, p222

16. Which vein on angiogram is antler shaped?

a. Vein of Galen
b. Basal vein of Rosenthal
c. Thalamostriate vein
d. Septal vein

Ref. Osborn Angiography, 1st/e, p346

17. All the following statements regarding hypertensive encephalopathy are true, except:

a. MRI shows cortical and subcortical lesions which are hypo and hyperintense on T_1W and T_2W respectively
b. Diffusion weighted imaging (DWI) shows restricted diffusion
c. Apparent diffusion coefficient (ADC) map shows bright areas
d. Perfusion scan may show hyperdynamic microcirculation

Ref. Osborn, 1st/e, p28-9

Answers

8. b. **9.** b. **10.** b. **11.** a. **12.** a. **13.** c. **14.** b. **15.** c. **16.** c. **17.** b.

18. Meniscus sign on myelogram is seen in:

a. Spinal ependymoma
b. Spinal astrocytoma
c. Spinal neurofibroma
d. Extruded disk

Ref. Greenberg, 4th/e, p342

19. A young man reports with visual disturbances and features of diabetes insipidus. MRI reveals a cystic lesion with peripheral enhancement involving sellar and suprasellar compartments. The most likely diagnosis is:

a. Craniopharyngioma
b. Cystic pituitary adenoma
c. Rathke cleft cyst
d. a and c

Ref. Greenberg, 4th/e, p288-9

20. Which of the following is a radiological differential diagnosis of brain abscess?

a. Resolving hematoma
b. Demyelination
c. Subacute infarct
d. All the above

Ref. Osborn, 1st/e, p25

21. All the following features about tumefactive demyelination are correct, except:

a. It is a form of multiple sclerosis
b. It presents as a mass lesion
c. Magnetic resonance spectroscopy shows reduced glutamine peaks
d. MR perfusion shows reduced regional blood flow of the lesion

Ref. AJNR 2002;23:1378-86 and 2007;28: 272-7

22. Viking helmet ventricles are seen in:

a. Septo-optic dysplasia
b. Cavum vekum interpositum
c. Hydrancephaly
d. None of the above

Ref. AJNR 1998;19:1631-5

23. A 10-year-old girl reports with right hand weakness of acute onset. MRI brain reveals sulcal hyperintensity on FLAIR sequence. Virchow-Robin spaces are more prominent on left side of the brain. Upon contrast administration there is asymmetric diffuse leptomeningeal enhancement. This sign is known as ivy sign and is seen in:

a. Wilson's disease
b. MoyaMoya disease
c. Cerebral palsy
d. Multiple sclerosis

Ref. AJNR, 1999;20:1836-8 and 2009;30: 1709-16

24. The best MRI sequence to diagnose hippocampal sclerosis is:

a. FLAIR sequence
b. T_2-relaxometry
c. Contrast MRI
d. Perfusion MRI

Ref. Youmans, 5th/e, p2487

25. All the following statements about fibrous dysplasia are correct, except:

a. There is ground glass appearance of bone on CT scan
b. Solid variant will have increase signal on T_2W sequence
c. In about 70% of cases, single osseous site is involved
d. Bone scan is used to stage the disease

Ref. Osborn, Section 4, p35-6

26. All the following features are correct about neurodegeneration of brain with iron accumulation, except:

a. Patient presents with mental retardation
b. There is hypointense signal on T_2-weighted MRI sequence in globus pallidus
c. Cerebellum is always normal
d. There is abnormality in PLA_2G_6 gene

Ref. AJNR 2012;33:407-14

ANSWERS

18. c. **19.** d. **20.** d. **21.** c. **22.** b. **23.** b. **24.** b. **25.** b. **26.** c.

27. A 60-year-old male who is suffering from rheumatoid arthritis for last 20-years reports with seizure. His MRI shows a frontal lesion which is subcortical and extending up to the ventricular ependyma. The lesion is hyperintense on both T_1 and T_2-weighted sequences. The lesion enhances on contrast. The most likely diagnosis is:

a. Hallervorden-Spatz disease
b. Astrocytoma
c. Gliomatosis cerebri
d. Amyloidoma

Ref. Ref- AJNR 2003;24:519-22

28. A 30-year-male reports with progressive paraparesis with sphincter disturbances. He is a known case of Cushing's disease also. His MRI spine shows a classical epidural Ysign. The most likely diagnosis is:

a. Hemangiopericytoma
b. Lymphoma
c. Lipomatosis
d. None of the above

Ref. AJNR, case of the week

29. A 60-year-old female presents with dementia. Her MRI brain shows features of periventricular white matter demyelination especially of the temporal lobe white matter. The corpus callosum is spared and so is the cerebellum and the brain-stem. The most likely diagnosis is:

a. Hypertensive leukoencephalopathy
b. Cerebral autosomal dominant arteriopathy with subcortical infarcts and leukoencephalopathy
c. Refsum's disease
d. None of the above

Ref. Greenberg, p32

30. Chordomas most commonly arise from?

a. Clivus
b. Lumbosacral junction
c. S_2 vertebra
d. S_4 and S_5 vertebra

Ref. Pediatric Neurosurgery 2011;47: 22-30

31. An elderly man reports with dementia and ataxia. His MRI shows atrophy of the midbrain especially the superior colliculi. The most likely diagnosis is:

a. Parkinsons disease
b. Ataxiatelangiectasia
c. Progressive supranuclear palsy
d. None of the above

Ref. AJNR, 2004;25:927-32

32. In which of the following conditions MRI shows a hotcross bun appearance of the Pons?

a. Multisystem atrophy
b. Limbic encephalitis
c. Lhermitte-Duclos disease
d. Vermian tumors

Ref. AJNR, March 2009;30:e37

33. A 45-year-old smoker was diagnosed as having small cell carcinoma of lung and was treated for it. After few years he started having dementia and seizures. His MRI brain revealed bilateral medial temporal lobe intensity changes without any mass effect. He is most likely suffering from:

a. Herpes encephalopathy
b. Paraneoplastic limbic encephalitis
c. Medial temporal sclerosis
d. None of the above

Ref. AJNR, 2003;24:507-11

34. In which of the following bony tumors bone scan may be normal?

a. Chordoma
b. Chondrosarcoma
c. Osteosarcoma
d. None of the above

Ref. Journal of Nuclear Medicine 1986;27(5): 627-30

35. In which of the following conditions is Pulvinar sign seen?

a. Fahrs disease
b. Fabrys disease
c. Creutzfeldt-Jacob disease
d. b and c

Ref. AJNR 2003;24:1560-9, 1096-1101

ANSWERS

27. d. **28.** c. **29.** b. **30.** d. **31.** a. **32.** a. **33.** b. **34.** a. **35.** d.

36. In which of the following conditions MRI brain shows signal intensity changes in the brainstem?

a. Posterior reversible encephalopathy
b. Osmotic demyelination syndrome
c. Wernickes encephalopathy
d. All the above

Ref. AJNR 1995;16:1495-7, AJNR 2001;22: 1480-2 and AJNR 2012;33:896-903

37. The commonest artery seen in adults which is reminiscent of fetal carotid basilar communication is:

a. Fetal posterior communicating artery
b. Persistent trigeminal artery
c. Stapedial artery
d. None of the above

Ref. Osborn, 1st/e, p145

38. In which of the following conditions is septo-optic dysplasia an association?

a. Eagles syndrome b. Schizencephaly
c. Band heterotopias d. Occipital encephalocele

Ref. AJNR 2012;33:E16-8

39. In which of the following conditions is Humming bird sign noticed on MRI scan?

a. Sleep disorders
b. Parkinsonism plus syndrome
c. Photogenic epilepsy
d. None of the above

Ref. Movement disorders, p237

40. The eye of the Tiger sign on MRI scan is seen in:

a. Parkinsons disease
b. Hallervorden-Spatz disease
c. Wilsons disease
d. Brain metastasis

Ref. Movement disorders, p237

41. All the following statements about traumatic carotid-cavernous fistula are true, except:

a. It is a high flow fistula
b. Proptosis is a key clinical feature
c. Superior ophthalmic vein is small
d. Cavernous sinus is large

Ref. Osborn, 1st/e, p63

42. All the following statements about chronic brain infarcts are true, except:

a. There are poorly delineated high-attenuation areas on CT scan
b. Adjacent sulci and gyri are prominent
c. There is atrophy of ipsilateral ventricle
d. a and c

Ref. Osborn, 1st/e, p84

43. All the following statements regarding lacunar infarcts are true, except:

a. These infarcts are small and typically located in basal ganglia and thalamus
b. Their size ranges up to 25 mm
c. These are typically round or oval in shape
d. MRI shows hyperintense signal at T_2W_1

Ref. Osborn, 1st/e, p88

44. All the following statements regarding sinus pericranii are true, except:

a. It is a vascular scalp mass which communicates with dural venous sinus via emissary vein
b. There is a well-defined bone defect through which the emissary vein runs
c. The commonest location is parietal
d. Infantile hemangioma is a strong differential diagnosis

Ref. Osborn, 1st/e, p21

45. All the following statements about choroid plexus papilloma are true, except:

a. Cranial sonogram reveals a hypoechoic mass with frond like projections
b. Angiogram shows an enlarged choroidal artery
c. There is prolonged vascular stain
d. Gradient MRI detects blood products and calcium

Ref. Osborn, 1st/e, p61

ANSWERS

36. d. **37.** a. **38.** b. **39.** b. **40.** b. **41.** c. **42.** d. **43.** b. **44.** c. **45.** a.

46. All the following statements regarding dysem bryoplastic neuroepithelial tumor are true, except:

a. It is a well demarcated, wedged shaped lesion
b. Temporal lobe is the commonest site
c. It may cause scalloping of inner table of skull
d. Calcification is always absent

Ref. Osborn, 1st/e, p76

47. All the following statements regarding Virchow-Robin spaces are correct, except:

a. These are usually less than 5 mm in size
b. The commonest location is basal ganglia
c. An adjacent parenchymal hyperintensity is seen usually
d. These spaces are isointense with CSF

Ref. Osborn, 1st/e, p22

48. In which of the orbital tumors is tram-track sign seen?

a. Optic nerve gliomas
b. Optic nerve meningiomas
c. Cavernous hemangioma
d. Peripheral nerve tumor of the orbit

Ref. Youman's, p1372-73

49. The tram-track sign is seen in following conditions, except:

a. Non-specific inflammation of orbit
b. Optic nerve meningiomas
c. Perioptic lymphomas
d. Optic nerve gliomas

Ref. Youman's p1372

50. In which of the following conditions there are no calcifications in the sella/suprasellar region?

a. Pituitary adenoma
b. Pituitary tuberculosis
c. Craniopharyngiomas
d. Rathke cleft cyst

Ref. AJNR, Sept. 18, 2014

51. The temporary disappearance of evidence of infarction in the subacute period is known as:

a. T_2-shine through phenomenon
b. Fogging effect
c. Beam hardening
d. None of the above

Ref. AJNR, March 10, 2014

52. In case of iron overload, the MRI brain reveals increased susceptibility in the following sites, except:

a. Pineal gland
b. Pituitary gland
c. Choroid plexus
d. Hippocampus

Ref. AJNR, Feb. 24, 2014

53. The concentration of Xenon-133 used to measure cerebral blood flow usually is:

a. 10%
b. 20%
c. 33%
d. 45%

Ref. JNS, 1992, vol. 77, p360-8

54. Which modality can be utilized to predict normal-pressure-breakthrough-phenomenon in AVM's?

a. Transcranial Doppler
b. Diamox challenge test
c. CT scan
d. None of the above

Ref. Neurosurgery focus 2011;11(5):1-5

ANSWERS

46. d. **47.** c. **48.** b. **49.** d. **50.** d. **51.** b. **52.** d. **53.** c. **54.** b.

EXPLANATION

1. The histopathological basis of "unidentified bright objects" (UBOs) (hyperintense regions seen on T_2-weighted magnetic resonance (MR) brain scans in neurofibromatosis-1 (NF1)) remains unclear. Such lesions are readily detected on T_2-weighted MRI scans of children and adolescents with the disorder. Such UBOs are typically found in the cerebellum (dentate nuclei, middle cerebellar peduncles, cerebellar deep white matter), brainstem, basal ganglia and thalami. UBOs have been described as hamartomas, regions of abnormal myelination or heterotopias. Although UBOs may be transient and are considered benign, some persist into adulthood and there is increasing evidence correlating their presence with cognitive dysfunction. *Neuroimage Clin. 2014;4:649-658*
2. The mother in law sign is used to describe lesions that enhance early during the arterial phase and remain opacified well after the venous phase. The joke is that a mother in law comes early and stays late. It is most frequently equated with the angiographic appearance of a meningioma.
3. Conventional angiography is invasive, but provides useful information such as location of feeding arteries and draining veins, and degree of tumor vascularity. An angiographic finding of early appearance of the draining vein, suggesting the presence of arterio-venous shunting, is often seen in malignant tumors in various organs. Meningiomas typically show a sunburst appearance on angiogram which represents a central artery which branches off in a radial fashion.
4. The basal veins, also known as the veins of Rosenthal, are paired, paramedian veins which originate on the medial surface of the temporal lobe and run posteriorly and medially. It passes lateral to the midbrain through the ambient cistern to drain into the vein of Galen with the internal cerebral veins. It is closely related to the posterior cerebral artery (PCA). On angiography it is frog-leg shaped.
6. The caput medusae sign, refers to developmental venous anomalies of the brain, where a number of veins drain centrally towards a single drain vein. The appearance is reminiscent of Medusa, a gorgon of Greek mythology, who was encountered and defeated by Perseus. The sign is seen on both CT and MRI when contrast is administered. Angiographically the caput medusa appearance is seen only in the venous phase. The caput medusae sign is also known as a palm tree sign.
7. MRI is the modality of choice, demonstrating a characteristic "popcorn" or "berry" appearance with a rim of signal loss due to hemosiderin, which demonstrates prominent blooming on susceptibility weighted sequences. T_1 and T_2-signal is varied internally depending on the age of the blood products and small fluid-fluid levels may be evident. Gradient echo or T_2 sequences are able to delineate these lesions better than T_1 or T_2-weighted images. In patients with familial or multiple cavernous angiomas GRE T_2 sequences are very important in identifying the number of lesions missed by conventional spin echo sequences. Susceptibility weighted imaging (SWI) may have sensitivity equal to that of GRE in detecting these capillary telangiectasias in brain. SWI is also highly sensitive in detecting calcification as compared to T_1 and T_2 images. If a recent bleed has occurred then surrounding edema may be present. The lesions generally do not enhance, although enhancement is possible.
8. The prefrontal arteries of MCA branch off in a candelobra form around the frontal operculum before coursing to frontal lobe convexity.
10. PACs represent a protrusion of meninges and CSF from the posterolateral portion of Meckel's cave into the petrous apex, which is their characteristic imaging appearance. PACs are usually incidental but may be symptomatic. Similar cysts of the temporal bone lined with fibrous tissue and containing cholesterol-rich fluid have been described in multiple reports as mastoid cysts, epidermoids. mucoceles, and cholesterol granuloma. Truncation of petrous ape x is classically induced by trigeminal schwannomas, vestibular schwannomas increase the diameter of IAC, meningiomas may show calcification along with erosion of the bone.
11. A meningioma that has multiple lobulated outgrowths on its contour is designated as "mushrooming" meningioma. Lobulated or mushrooming appearances of meningiomas noted on preoperative imaging studies correlate with an increased Ki-67 and a higher recurrence rate for these tumors.
12. Neurosarcoidosis may be the first localized manifestation of the disease or may be part of multisystemic disease. The pathologic hallmark of sarcoidosis is the presence of granulomatous non-caseating focal tissue reactions and inflammation. Plain film of the skull reveals multiple punched-out lesions that are characteristic of osseous sarcoidosis. Bone biopsies may be necessary in osseous sarcoidosis to exclude infections or cancers.

13. Hemangiomas are the most common benign spinal neoplasm, present in up to 5 % of elderly patients. They are often an incidental imaging finding, as the majority of vertebral hemangioma are asymptomatic. Vertebral body is more commonly involved than the posterior elements. Imaging of vertebral hemangiomas reveals thick and vertical bony trabeculae, thus preserving the functional ability of the vertebrae to withstand an axial load. This appearance is described on radiographs and CT as "polka-dot", "jail bar", "corduroy cloth", "salt and pepper", and "honeycomb" with reduced overall density of the affected vertebral body secondary to the presence of fatty bone marrow. Fatty tissue present within the hemangiomas can lead to hyperintensity on T_1-weighted MRI while increased water content leads to hyperintensity on T_2-weighted images. The T_2-hyperintensity is often greater than that of fat, thereby differentiating hemangiomas from focal fat deposition. Aggressive hemangiomas characteristically have reduced fat content and more vascular component causing hypointensity on T_1-weighted MRI. This appearance may resemble vertebral metastasis, however, metastatic foci commonly reveal hypointensity on T_1-weighted images and hyperintensity on T_2-weighted images. In addition, the morphology, including the presence of coarsened trabeculae can be used for differentiation. For indeterminate cases, CT is helpful since the modality is more sensitive to the characteristic osseous remodeling. Paget's disease of the spine can have similar appearance but is usually distinguished by expansion of the vertebral body with peripheral cortical thickening which can be observed on CT, with characteristic "picture frame" vertebral body on radiographs. Lymphoma may also have a similar appearance but is usually distinguished by homogeneous enhancement on contrast enhanced MRI. *J Nat Sci Biol Med 2015;6(2):439-42.*

14. The most anterior point of the pre-central cerebellar vein, where the vein lies between the inferior colliculi and precentral lobe, is called the colliculocentral point. The colliculocentral point defines the interface between the ventral limit of the superior vermis and the rostral fourth ventricle, which for practical purposes also approximates the dorsal surface of the pons.

16. The thalamostriate vein drains the posterior frontal and anterior parietal lobes, caudate nucleus and the internal capsule. The thalamostriate (subependymal) veins outline the inferolateral wall of the body of the lateral ventricle. The principle vein draining the lateral subependymal veins is the thalamostriate vein. At the foramen of Monro, the thalamostriate vein empties into the internal cerebral vein, forming an acute angle. Near the posterior edge of the foramen of Monro, the thalamostriate vein turns abruptly and terminates in the internal cerebral vein. The junction of the internal cerebral and thalamostriate veins is called the venous angle. On angiography this vein is antler shaped.

18. In the intradural extramedullary (IDEM) spinal compartment, tumors like meningiomas and neurofibroma maintain a sharp angle with the adjacent dura and neural element, forming a so-called meniscus sign. Paint brush sign is seen in intramedullary tumors and a cut-off on myelogramis seen in extradural lesions, commonest being an extruded disc.

19. The typical symptoms associated with RCCs include headache, endocrine dysfunction, and visual loss. Visual loss has been reported to develop in 35–50% of patients undergoing surgical intervention and may include deficits in visual fields as well as in visual acuity. Hyperprolactinemia and growth hormone deficiency are relatively common endocrinological findings associated with RCCs, followed by hypocortisolemia and hypogonadism. Diabetes insipidus (DI) has been reported as a presenting feature in approximately 7–20% of patients with RCCs. The majority are intrasellar or intra- and suprasellar, although purely suprasellar lesions may occur in a minority of patients. The majority of RCCs are unilobar with a diameter ranging between 5 and 40 mm (mean ~ 17 mm). They are often identified as having an epicenter located between the anterior and posterior pituitary gland in the region of the pars intermedia. Reported rates for anterior pituitary hormone deficits prior to any operative intervention vary from 35 to 95% for growth hormone, 38 to 82% for follicle-stimulating hormone/luteinizing hormone, 21 to 62% for corticotrophin, and 21 to 42% for thyroid-stimulating hormone. Authors of large patient series have reported that between 6 and 38% of patients present with insufficient secretion of antidiuretic hormone. Before surgery and in 70–90% after surgery.

Neurosurg Focus / Volume 31 / July 2011,1-6 and Neurosurg Focus 28(4):E8, 2010.1-10

21. The increase in choline is thought to result from rapid membrane turnover, high mitotic activity, and dense cellularity in PCNSL and from inflammatory cellular infiltration, reactive astrogliosis, and demyelination in tumefactive demyelination.

23. Leptomeningeal enhancement on postcontrast T_1-weighted images has been reported in association with meningitis (3), meningeal carcinomatosis (4), and angitis (5). Common among these diseases is pathologic inflammation or carcinomatous infiltration of the leptomeninges, with or without involvement of the small leptomeningeal vessels. The "ivy sign" refers to diffuse leptomeningeal enhancement found on postcontrast MR images of patients with moyamoya disease in childhood (1). It is considered to represent the diffuse engorgement of the pial vasculature and it is named like as it resembles ivy creeping on stones. *AJNR 1999;20:1836-8*

25. Fibrous dysplasia (FD) is a non-neoplastic tumor-like congenital process, manifested as a localized defect in osteoblastic differentiation and maturation, with replacement of normal bone with large fibrous stroma and islands of immature woven bone.

X-ray: Ground-glass matrix, may be completely lucent (cystic) or sclerotic, well circumscribed lesions, no periosteal reaction.

CT scan: Ground-glass opacities, homogeneously sclerotic, cystic, well-defined borders, expansion of the bone, with intact overlying bone, endosteal scalloping may be seen.

MRI: T_1: Heterogeneous signal, usually intermediate, T_2: hypointense in solid variants sometimes heterogeneous signal, contrast: heterogeneous contrast enhancement.

26. Iron deposition occurs in multiple sclerosis, human immunodeficiency virus dementia, Freidrich ataxia, and Alzheimer and Parkinson diseases, though to a lesser degree than that seen in neurodegeneration of brain in iron accumulation (NBIA). As a neurometabolic disorder, NBIA leads to an approximately symmetric distribution of iron in key gray matter nuclei that are themselves intrinsically enriched in their iron content in healthy individuals (globus pallidus, substantia nigra, red nucleus, dentate nucleus, putamen, and thalamus).

AJNR Am J Neuroradiol 2012;33:407-14

27. Amyloidosis is a disease complex that results in the extracellular deposition of insoluble fibrillar protein with a beta-pleated sheet configuration. The systemic form includes primary amyloidosis related to plasma cell dyscrasias, reactive or secondary amyloidosis, and the familial forms. Localized amyloidosis includes organ-limited forms, focal amyloid deposits, and senile amyloidosis. Amyloid deposition within the brain can take many forms, including cerebral amyloid angiopathy, senile plaques of Alzheimer dementia, and deposits seen in the encephalopathy of Kuru and of Creutzfeldt-Jacob disease. Tumor-like deposition (amyloidoma) is the least common form of the brain involvement by amyloid proteins. Cerebral lobar white matter is most commonly affected, with occasional involvement of the cortex (5, 11). The mass is supratentorial. Amyloidomas are usually hyperintense on T_1 & T_2-weighted images. The increased signal intensity is attributed to the dense amyloid protein deposition. Amyloidomas enhance on contrast. *AJNR Am J Neuroradiol 2003;24:519-522*

28. Epidural lipomatosis refers to excessive accumulation of fat within the spinal epidural space, such that the thecal sac is compressed. On cross sectional imaging, the thecal sac has a striking stellate appearance with three rays emanating from a central core. This produces a trifid shape resembling the letter "Y". Causes are: Obesity, Cushing disease, Cushing syndrome: most frequently due to corticosteroid use.

29. Cerebral Autosomal Dominant Arteriopathy with Subcortical Infarcts and Leukoencephalopathy (CADASIL) is an autosomal dominant microvasculopathy, characterized by recurrent lacunar and subcortical white matter ischemic strokes and vascular dementia in young and middle age patients without known vascular risk factors. There is disproportionate cortical hypometabolism. Presentation is usually with recurrent transient ischemic attacks (TIAs) or strokes in multiple vascular territories. Presenile dementia and migraines develop in the third-to-fourth decades of life. CADASIL results from a mutation on chromosome 19q12 involving the Notch 3 gene. MRI is the investigation of choice, often demonstrating widespread confluent white matter hyperintensities. More circumscribed hyperintense lesions are also seen in the basal ganglia, thalamus and pons. In the initial course of the disease involvement of the anterior temporal lobe and external capsule are classical.

31. Progressive supranuclear palsy (PSP) is a neurodegenerative disease that results in severe disability. It is characterized by supranuclear vertical gaze palsy, pseudobulbar palsy, dystonic rigidity of the neck and upper extremities, and frequent falls. The main neuropathologic characteristics of PSP are neuronal degeneration and loss in the tegmentum of the midbrain, atrophy of the substantia nigra (SN), and changes in the red nucleus and globus pallidus. The clinical diagnosis of PSP, particularly its differential diagnosis with Parkinson disease (PD), can be difficult, especially in early stages. However, the differential diagnosis between PSP and PD is important, because the prognosis of PSP is worse than that of PD. MR imaging investigations of PSP have shown abnormalities mainly involving the midbrain; such changes include abnormal T_2-hyperintensity in the tegmentum, and narrowing of the SN, while as in Parkinsons disease there is atrophy of the superior colliculi.

AJNR 2004;25:927-32

32. The hot cross bun sign refers to the MRI appearance of the pons in a variety of neurodegenerative diseases. T_2-hyperintensity forms a cross on axial images through the pons, representing selective degeneration of pontocerebellar tracts. It has been described in: multiple-system atrophy (MSA), spinocerebellar atrophy types 2 and 3, parkinsonism secondary to vasculitis, variant Creutzfeldt-Jakob disease (vCJD)

33. Paraneoplastic limbic encephalitis is frequently associated with bronchial carcinoma and is considered a particular manifestation of paraneoplastic encephalomyelitis, which includes involvement of other areas in the central (pyriform cortex, frontal orbital surface of the temporal lobe, insula, cerebellum, brain stem) and peripheral nervous system. Patients with paraneoplastic limbic encephalitis present with subacute cognitive dysfunction, severe memory impairment, seizures, and psychiatric features including depression, anxiety, and hallucinations. Other causes of encephalopathy, metastases, drug neurotoxicity, infectious diseases such as herpes encephalitis, and meningeal carcinomatosis must be excluded. Sometimes, antineuronal antibodies such as anti-Hu are found in the CSF in patients with paraneoplastic limbic encephalitis. *AJNR 2003;24:507-11*

35. The pulvinar sign refers to bilateral FLAIR hyperintensities involving the pulvinar thalamic nuclei. It is classically described in variant Creutzfeldt-Jakob disease (vCJD). It is also described in other neurological conditions: Fabry disease (although the hyperintense signal is seen on T_1WI), bilateral thalamic infarcts, ADEM.

37. A fetal PCOM or fetal origin of the posterior cerebral artery is a very common variant in the posterior cerebral circulation. It is estimated to occur in up to 30% individuals. The posterior communicating artery (PCOM) is larger than the P1 segment of the posterior cerebral artery (PCA) and supplies the bulk of the blood to the PCA. If bilateral, the basilar artery is significantly smaller than normal.

38. Septo-optic dysplasia (SOD) is a condition characterized by optic nerve hypoplasia and absence of septum pellucidum and, in two-thirds of patients hypothalamic-pituitary dysfunction. Clinical presentation of septo-optic dysplasia is varied, and mostly dependent of whether or not it is associated with schizencephaly (~ 50% of cases). The abnormality develops during 4th-6th weeks of gestation, during early forebrain development. The etiology of SOD is unknown. MRI is the modality of choice for assessing septo-optic dysplasia. It shows: "point down" appearance of the lateral ventricular frontal horns on coronal images, absent septum pellucidum, hypoplastic pituitary stalk, hypoplastic optic chiasm/optic nerves and globes.

39. The hummingbird sign, also known as the penguin sign, refers to the appearance of the brainstem in patients with progressive supranuclear palsy (PSP). The atrophy of the midbrain results in a profile of the brainstem (in the sagittal plane) in which the preserved pons forms the body of the bird, and the atrophic midbrain the head, with beak extending anteriorly towards the optic chiasm.

40. Hallervorden-Spatz syndrome, now known as pantothenate kinase-associated neurodegeneration (PKAN), is an autosomal recessive disorder causing involuntary spasticity and progressive dementia. It is a subset of neurodegeneration with brain iron accumulation (NBIA). Described features include: rigidity, dysarthria, dystonia, retinitis pigmentosa, progressive mental retardation, cognitive impairment, spasticity, tremors. On MRI: T_2-weighted MRI images often demonstrate hypointense changes in globi pallidi and pars reticulata of substantia nigra and SWI/T_2: shows susceptibility artefact (low signal) in corresponding areas from iron deposition. Cortex is usually spared but caudate atrophy may be seen in more advanced cases. The "eye of the tiger" sign refers to a central T_2 relatively hyperintense spot (line) within the hypointense globi pallidi due to gliosis and vacuolization. MR spectroscopy shows decreased NAA peak due to neuronal loss and may show increased myoinositol.

43. Lacunar infarcts are small (<20 mm) infarcts in the distal distribution of deep penetrating vessels (lenticulostriate, thalamoperforating, and pontine perforating arteries, recurrent artery of Heubner). They result from occlusion of one of the small penetrating end arteries at the base of the brain and are due to fibrinoid degeneration. Pathologically, they are small holes of encephalomalacia and are traversed by a cob-web-like mesh of fibrous strands.

CT / MRI picture: small discrete foci of hypodensity / diffusion restriction, 3–20 mm in diameter, most commonly 10-mm, may enhance in the late acute or early subacute stage, unilateral pontine infarcts have a sharp demarcation at the midline, higher signal intensity than CSF (marginal gliosis).

44. Sinus pericranii (SP) is a cranial venous anomaly in which there is an abnormal communication between intracranial dural sinuses and extracranial venous structures, usually via an emissary trans-osseous vein. It is considered a type of low flow vascular malformation. It occurs in close communication with the cranial vault and most frequently involves the superior sagittal sinus. When suspected on radiological basis, a simple clinical test can be performed. Unless thrombosed, the sinus pericranii will appear more prominent on lying down than when sitting, because of variable venous pressure with gravity. It is comprised of non-muscular venous blood vessels which tightly adhere to the outer calvarium and directly communicate with an intracranial venous sinus through diploic veins. Color Doppler may show communication with superficial veins and dural venous sinuses.

46. Dysembryoplastic neuroepithelial tumors (DNET) are benign (WHO Grade I) slow growing tumors arising from either cortical or deep grey matter. The vast majority are centered in cortical grey matter, arise from secondary germinal layers and are frequently associated with cortical dysplasia (up to 80% of cases). They characteristically cause intractable partial seizures. The temporal lobe is the most common location, but all parts of the CNS containing grey matter are potential locations: temporal lobe (60%), frontal lobe (30%), caudate nucleus, cerebellum.

47. Perivascular spaces (PVS), also known as Virchow-Robin (VR) spaces, are pial lined interstitial fluid filled spaces that surround perforating vessels. They do not have a direct connection with the subarachnoid space and in fact the fluid within them is slightly different. On imaging they appear as smoothly demarcated fluid-filled cysts, typically less than 5 mm in diameter, showing the same CSF attenuation or intensity and often found in the basal ganglia or midbrain.

48,49. Tram-track sign is a linear calcification of optic nerve on CT scan. It is seen in orbital tumors-like optic nerve meningiomas, perioptic lymphomas, and inflammatory conditions like optic neuritis and non-specific inflammation of orbit.

50. Rathke's cleft cysts (RCCs) are thought to originate from Rathke's pouch, an epithelialized rostral invagination of the stomadeum. The Rathke's pouch has an anterior and posterior wall in addition to a central embryonic cleft. The anterior pituitary and the pars tuberalis arise from the anterior wall, while the posterior portion develops into the pars intermedia. The central lumen becomes the Rathke cleft, and normally regresses. However, this structure may persist and enlarge, resulting in the formation of a cyst. Calcification is not a feature of RCC.

51. "Fogging effect" is a well known phenomenon consisting of transient disappearance of a cerebral infarction on CT images. Few case reports have described the same phenomenon on T_2-weighted MRI and DWI, usually occurring in the subacute stages of a cerebral infarction (2–20 days) and mainly involving cortical or posterior cerebral fossa ischemia. In cortical infarction, "fogging effect" mainly consists of a reduction and shading of the ischemic regions, while in posterior cerebral fossa infarction, MRI findings may apparently disappear. The causes of this "imaging effect" are poorly understood. Different hypotheses have been suggested: Reparative processes occurring in subacute stages may "hide" the underlying infarction. Diapedesis of red blood cells containing paramagnetic hemoglobin (deoxy- and metahemoglobin) may account for T_2-susceptibility effects. Mild hemorrhagic transformation may occur and change the signal. In conclusion, attention should be paid when evaluating a patient with infarction involving the brainstem in the 20–30 day period (subacute stage) from the ictus. *AJNR, March 10, 2014*

There are many different types of CT artifacts, including noise, beam hardening, scatter, pseudoenhancement, motion, cone beam, helical, ring, and metal artifacts. Noise can be reduced using iterative reconstruction or by combining data from multiple scans. This enables lower radiation dose and higher resolution scans. Metal artifacts can also be reduced using iterative reconstruction, resulting in more accurate diagnosis. Dual and multi-energy CT can reduce beam hardening and provide better tissue contrast. Methods for reducing noise and out-of-field artifacts may enable ultra-high resolution limited-field-of-view imaging of tumors and other structures. Beam hardening and scatter both produce dark streaks between two high attenuation objects (such as metal or bone), with surrounding bright streaks. These can be reduced using iterative reconstruction.

J Med Imaging (Bellingham). 2014 Oct;1(3):033507

52. Hemochromatosis refers to iron overload, which results from a hereditary/primary cause or from a metabolic/hematologic disorder. Organs commonly affected by hemochromatosis include the liver, heart, and endocrine glands. In the brain, iron deposition is typically seen at sites outside the blood-brain barrier, which include the pituitary gland, choroid plexus, pineal gland, and area postrema. Increased iron load will result in increased susceptibility. This can be seen on T_2WI but still better on gradient-echo or susceptibility-weighted images. Thus, increased susceptibility involving the 4 p's—the pituitary gland, choroid plexus, pineal gland, and area postrema—should suggest hemochromatosis. In the current case, hemochromatosis occurred secondary to iron overload from blood transfusions for thalassemia. *AJNR, Feb. 24, 2014*

53. Acetazolamide is a carbonic anhydrase inhibitor that penetrates the blood-brain barrier slowly and acts as a cerebral vasodilator agent. Inhibition of carbonic anhydrase causes carbonic acidosis, which induces a considerable increase in CBF. Xe-CT combined with ACZ challenge is an established technique, which has been used for >20 years to evaluate chronic cerebral ischemia. It provides quantitative assessment of CBF and CVR. The inhaled xenon gas dissolves in blood rapidly and freely crosses the blood-brain barrier and concentrates in the brain by virtue of its liposolubility. CBF is calculated by measuring the rate of xenon clearance from the brain by using the Kety-Schmidt model, which provides reliable CBF quantization, along with high-resolution imaging. The XeCT technique can be used in the intubated head injury patient to determine the appropriate rate of assisted ventilation that seeks to balance the need to lower intracranial vascular volume while maintaining adequate blood flow. The loss of normal chemoregulation (a 3% lowering of CBF in response to a 1 mm Hg lowering of PCO_2 during a double XeCT study) is a significant indicator of irreversible cerebral injury, and the level and pattern of CBF reduction in the injured tissues have been prognostic of poor outcome. Because of the short cerebral residence time of inhaled xenon, the study can be repeated in the same session. *AJNR 2009;30(5):876-84*

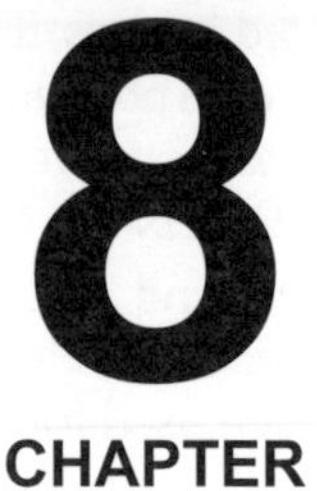

CHAPTER

Neuropathology

Rumana Makhdoomi, Nayil Khursheed

MULTIPLE CHOICE QUESTIONS

1. **Which of the following tumors has a biphasic architecture on histopathology?**
   a. Gliosarcoma
   b. Glioblastoma
   c. Medulloblastoma
   d. Chordoma

   Ref. Rosai and Ackerman, ed. 9th, p2364

2. **The following statements about brain tumors is/are true, except:**
   a. Primary glioblastoma is common in elderly age group
   b. Secondary glioblastoma is common in young adults
   c. Giant cell glioblastoma has better prognosis than classical glioblastoma
   d. Pilocytic astrocytoma has worse prognosis than oligodendrogliomas

   Ref. Kleihues, 2000, p51

3. **Preferred sites of pilocytic astrocytoma are the following, except:**
   a. Optic pathway
   b. Thalamus
   c. Cerebellum
   d. Spinal cord

   Ref. Kleihues, 2000, p45

4. **Rosenthal fibers are seen in all the conditions, except:**
   a. Pilocytic astrocytoma
   b. Pleomorphic xanthoastrocytoma
   c. Reactive gliosis
   d. Glioblastoma multiforme

   Ref. Kleihues, 2000, p47

5. **Oligodendroglioma-like cells are seen in following tumors:**
   a. Pilocytic astrocytoma
   b. DNET's
   c. Both
   d. None of the above

   Ref. Kleihues, 2000, p105

6. **All the following about pleomorphic xanthoastrocytoma are true, except:**
   a. It has relatively favorable prognosis
   b. Characterized by pleomorphic cells
   c. Cells express Glial-Fibrillary-Acidic-Protein (GFAP)
   d. Histologically corresponds to WHO III

   Ref. Kleihues, 2000, p52

7. **Mini-gemistocytes are seen in:**
   a. Pilocytic astrocytoma
   b. Oligodendroglioma
   c. Astrocytoma
   d. Ependymoma

   Ref. Kleihues, 2000, p57

Answers

1. a. **2.** d. **3.** d. **4.** d. **5.** b. **6.** d. **7.** b.

8. Pseudo-palisading necrosis is seen in:

a. Medulloblastoma
b. Ependymoma
c. Glioblastoma multiforme
d. Choroid plexus papilloma

Ref. Kleihues, 2000, p36

9. Tumor associated with tuberous sclerosis is:

a. Subependymal giant cell astrocytoma
b. Glioblastoma
c. Oligodendroglioma
d. Choroid plexus papilloma

Ref. Kleihues, 2000, p229

10. Paragangliomas are positive for following immunohistochemical stains, except:

a. Chromogranin
b. S-100
c. Synaptophysin
d. Actin

Ref. Kleihues, p. 2000, p114

11. Which of the following sub-types of ependymomas commonly involves the conus region?

a. Tanycytic
b. Myxopapillary
c. Cellular
d. Clear cell

Ref. Kleihues, 2000, p78

12. WHO grade I meningiomas include all the following, except:

a. Psammomatous meningioma
b. Angiomatous meningioma
c. Chordoid meningioma
d. Secretory meningioma

Ref. Kleihues, p176

13. 1_p 19_q mutation is found in which of the following tumors?

a. Medulloblastoma
b. Choroid plexus papilloma
c. Secretory meningioma
d. Oligodendroglioma

Ref. Kleihues, p60

14. Choroid plexus papilloma histopathologically qualifies for:

a. WHO grade I
b. WHO grade II
c. WHO grade III
d. WHO grade IV

Ref. Kleihues p84

15. In which of the following tumors "specific glioneural element of Dumas Duport" is seen?

a. DNET [dysembroplastic neuroepithelial tumor]
b. Transitional meningioma
c. SEGA
d. Oligodendroglioma

Ref. Kleihues, p104

16. Central neurocytoma is immunohistochemicallystrongly positive for:

a. Synaptophysin
b. GFAP
c. Cytokeratin
d. EMA

Ref. Kleihues, p106

17. WHO grade II meningiomas are:

a. Grade I meningiomas with brain invasion
b. Mitotic index of >20 hpf
c. Angiomatous meningiomas
d. Secretory meningiomas

Ref. Rosai and Ackerman vol. 2, ed. 10th, p2394

18. The medulloblastoma with the worst prognosis is:

a. Classical medulloblastoma
b. Anaplastic medulloblastoma
c. Medullomyoblastoma
d. Medulloblastoma with extreme nodularity

Ref. Rosai and Ackerman vol. 2, ed. 10th, p2556

19. The nuclei in medulloblastomas are:

a. Carrot shaped
b. Egg shaped
c. Banana shaped
d. Elongated

Ref. Kleihues, p129

ANSWERS

8. c. **9.** a. **10.** d. **11.** b. **12.** c. **13.** d. **14.** a. **15.** a. **16.** a. **17.** a. **18.** b. **19.** a.

20. Schwannomas are positive for:
a. S-100
b. Desmin
c. Cytokeratin
d. None of the above
Ref. Kleihues, p166

21. All the following statements about schwannomas are true, except:
a. Abrogation of merlin function is an essential step in schwannoma tumorigenesis
b. Antoni A and Antoni B are the two patterns seen on histopathology
c. Most common cranial nerve involved is 8th nerve
d. Ancient schwannomas having nuclear pleomorphism and mitotic figures are malignant tumors
Ref. Kleihues, p165

22. Malignant transformation of schwannoma is common in patients with:
a. Neurofibromatosis
b. Diabetes
c. van Hippel Landau syndrome
d. Tuberous sclerosis
Ref. Kleihues, p172

23. The term malignant triton tumor refers to:
a. Malignant melanoma of brain
b. Atypical teratoid rhabdoid tumor
c. Malignant peripheral nerve sheath tumor with rhabdomyosarcomatous differentiation
d. None of the above
Ref. Kleihues, p173

24. For atypical meningiomas, mitotic activity has been defined as:
a. 4 or more mitosis per 10 hpf
b. 2 or more mitosis per 10 hpf
c. 10 or more mitosis per 10 hpf
d. 6 or more mitosis per 10 hpf
Ref. Kleihues, p179

25. Which of the following statements about MIB-1 labeling index is correct?
a. MIB-1 antibody binds to the cytoplasmic antigen
b. The index is not valid for grading meningiomas
c. This index is a cell proliferation index
d. MIB-1 labeling index is valid even if the tissue is autolysed
Ref. Rosai and Ackerman, vol. 2, ed. 8th, p48

26. Lymphocytic hypophysitis occurs commonly in:
a. Men
b. Postmenopausal women
c. Children
d. Women during pregnancy and postpartum period
Ref. Rosai and Ackerman, vol. 2, ed. 8th, p2435

27. Primary CNS lymphoma usually is a:
a. B-cell lymphoma
b. T-cell lymphoma
c. Maltoma
d. Hodgkin's lymphoma
Ref. Kleihues, p200

28. Electron microscopy and immunohistochemistry is helpful in the diagnosis of:
a. Craniopharyngioma
b. Granulomatous hypophysitis
c. Meningioma
d. Pituitary adenoma
Ref. Rosai and Ackerman, vol. 2, ed. 8th, p2428

29. Primary CNS lymphoma is histologically characterized by:
a. Rossette formation
b. Hyaline change
c. Calcification
d. Angiocentric pattern
Ref. Kleihues, p199

30. All the following are synonymous with granular cell tumor of the neurohypophysis, except:
a. Abrikosoff's tumor
b. Pituicytoma
c. Choristoma
d. Xanthogranuloma
Ref. Kleihues, p247

ANSWERS

20. a. **21.** d. **22.** a. **23.** c. **24.** a. **25.** c. **26.** d. **27.** a. **28.** d. **29.** d. **30.** d.

31. Which of the statements is/are true about olfactory neuroblastoma?

a. Is seen usually in elderly
b. Is positive for neuron-specific-enolase (NSE)
c. Has a good prognosis
d. All the above

Ref. Kleihues, p156

32. Following are true about gliosarcoma, except:

a. It is comprised of glial component and a sarcomatous component
b. Histopathology shows microvascular proliferation
c. Necrosis is also common
d. It does not have better prognosis than GBM

Ref. Kleihues, p44

33. After steroid treatment, biopsy may be negative in:

a. Oligodendroglioma
b. Lymphoma
c. Dysembryoplastic neuroepithelial tumor (DNET)
d. Ganglioglioma

Ref. Kleihues, p199

34. Pilomyxoid astrocytoma is usually seen in:

a. Hypothalamus b. Optic chiasm
c. Cerebellum d. All the above

Ref. Rosai and Ackerman, vol. 2, ed. 10th, p2349

35. Liponeurocytoma is characterized by all of the following, except:

a. It is a WHO grade II tumor
b. It is characterized by lipocytic differentiation
c. It has a very bad prognosis
d. It is seen in the cerebellum

Ref. Rosai and Ackerman, vol. 2, ed. 10th, p2372

36. Hemangiopericytoma is a tumor of:

a. Brain parenchyma b. Pituitary gland
c. Pineal gland d. Meninges

Ref. Kleiheus, p190

37. Chordomas are seen in:

a. Sacral region
b. Clivus
c. Spheno-occipital area
d. All the above

Ref. Rosai and Ackerman, vol. 2, ed. 9th, p2183

38. Physalipharous cells are seen in:

a. Oligodendrogliomas b. Central neurocytomas
c. Chondroma d. Chordoma

Ref. Rosai and Ackerman, vol. 2, ed. 9th, p2184

39. Which of the following is/are pathologic markers of cerebral malaria in brain?

a. Ring hemorrhages
b. Petechial hemorrhages
c. Durck's granuloma
d. All the above

Ref. Robbins, p388

40. Which of the following pathological features are seen in amyotrophic lateral sclerosis?

a. Hirano bodies
b. Bunina bodies
c. Lewy-body like hyaline inclusions
d. None of the above

Ref. Robbins, p1324

41. All the following can cause thickening of the nerves, except:

a. Leprosy
b. Amyloidosis
c. Guillian-Barre syndrome
d. Refsum's disease

Ref. Midroni, p153

42. Onion bulb formation in a nerve means:

a. Recurrent demyelination with remyelination
b. Demyelination
c. Remyelination
d. None of the above

Ref. Midroni, p131

ANSWERS

31. b. **32.** d. **33.** b. **34.** d. **35.** c. **36.** d. **37.** d. **38.** d. **39.** d. **40.** d.
41. c. **42.** a.

43. Immunohistochemistry for chordomas will reveal positivity for:

a. EMA and NSE
b. EMA and S-100
c. GFAP and EMA
d. GFAP alone

Ref. Rosai and Ackerman, vol. 2, ed. 9th, p2184

44. Desmoplastic infantile gangliogliomas/desmoplastic infantile astrocytomas, except:

a. The present in first two years of life
b. They have supratentorial location
c. They have collagenized regions dominated by spindly astrocytes
d. They are accorded WHO grade III

Ref. Rosai and Ackerman, vol. 2, ed. 10th, p2370

45. Medulloblastoma may occur in association with:

a. Type 2 Turcot syndrome
b. Gorlin syndrome
c. Both a and b
d. None of the above

Ref. Rosai and Ackerman, vol. 2, ed. 10th, p2377

46. Following are true about atypical teratoid/rhabdoid tumor (AT/RT), except:

a. It is rare in children
b. It possesses complex histology
c. It is a highly aggressive tumor
d. Loss of nuclear INI-1 protein expression on IHC characterizes this entity

Ref. Rosai and Ackerman, vol. 2, ed. 10th, p2385-6

47. Pineoblastoma is:

a. WHO grade IV neoplasm
b. Seen in elderly
c. Not having rosettess
d. Self-limiting

Ref. Rosai and Ackerman, vol 2, ed. 10th, p2386

48. Meningioma containing bone, cartilage or adipocytic elements is:

a. Microcytic meningioma
b. Secretory mengioma
c. Lymphoplasmacyte rich meningioma
d. Metaplastic meningioma

Ref. Rosai and Ackerman, vol. 2, ed. 10th, p2391

49. Clear cell meningiomas are characterized by all, except:

a. Show predilection for young subjects
b. Are characterized by stubborn recurrence
c. Histologically show papillary architecture
d. Composed of glycogen rich water clear cells

Ref. Rosai and Ackerman, vol. 2, ed. 10th, p2392

50. In a toxoplasma abscess:

a. The core is devoid of identifiable organisms
b. The core is rich in the organisms
c. The tachyzoite is not responsible for tissue injury
d. The Bradyzoites are immunologically active

Ref. Rosai and Ackerman, vol. 2, ed. 10th, p2332

51. Following statements about CNS Aspergillosis are true, except:

a. Aspergillus has marked tendency to invade arteries and veins producing necrotizing angitis
b. Patient present with focal neurological deficits that commonly involve areas supplied by anterior and middle cerebral arteries
c. Most cases are due to Aspargillus fumigatus or Aspargillus flavus
d. Aspergillus consist of non-branching non-septate hyphae with hyphal branching at acute angles

Ref. Brain Pathology, p614

ANSWERS

43. b. **44.** d. **45.** c. **46.** a. **47.** a. **48.** d. **49.** c. **50.** a. **51.** d.

52. The following statement about Cryptococcus neoformans is true, except:

a. Cryptococcus neoformans is a spherical budding yeast
b. Cryptococcus neoformans infection is common in immunocompromised patients
c. Cryptococcus neoformans does not involve meninges
d. Cryptococcus neoformans has a polysaccharide capsule which is important for virulence

Ref. Brain Pathology, p621

53. Following statement about Polio virus is correct:

a. It is a member of Picornavirus family
b. It is a DNA virus
c. Infection usually occurs by parenteral route
d. Paralytic polio is very common

Ref. Brain Pathology, p700

54. The following statements about mucormycosis of CNS are true, except:

a. It is seen in patients with diabetic ketoacidosis
b. It is common in patients with intravenous drug abuse
c. It develops secondary to the infection of lungs
d. It has broad, branching, non-septate hyphae

Ref. Brain Pathology, p615

55. Following statements about tetanus are true, except:

a. Tetanus is caused by neurotoxin called tetanospasmin
b. The causative organism is Clostridium tetani
c. It is a Gram-negative anaerobic rod
d. It possesses a terminal spore that has a "drumstick appearance"

Ref. Brain Pathology, p643

56. Which of the following statement is correct?

a. Brucella is a motile, non-capsulated Gram-negative organism
b. Human disease does not follow animal brucellosis
c. Leptomeningeal involvement is common in septicemic phase of brucellosis
d. It does not cause arteritis

Ref. Brain Pathology, p643

57. Following are true of Pineocytoma, except:

a. It is a slow-growing World Health Organization (WHO) grade I lesion
b. It accounts for 14%–60% of pineal parenchymal neoplasms
c. It occurs predominantly in children
d. It is composed of cells resembling Pineocytes

Ref. J Neurooncol 2010 Nov;100(2): 255-260

58. Microscopic variants of chordoma include:

a. Chondroid chordoma
b. Dedifferentiated chordoma
c. both a and b
d. Chondromyxosarcoma

Ref. Turk Neurosurg 2013;23(6):700-6

59. Following statement about MPNST are false:

a. These are malignant tumors arising from a peripheral nerve or in extraneural soft tissue and showing nerve sheath differentiation
b. Malignant spindled tumors in NF1 patients should be considered MPNST until proven otherwise
c. They show Strong S-100 positivity
d. None of the above

Ref. Kleihues, p172

Answers

52. c. **53.** a. **54.** c. **55.** c. **56.** c. **57.** c. **58.** c. **59.** c.

EXPLANATION

1,32. Gliosarcoma is a rare central nervous system (CNS) neoplasm with biphasic glial and non-glial malignant components. The World Health Organization (WHO) classifies gliosarcoma as a high-grade tumor (Grade IV) similar to glioblastoma. Gliosarcomas represent approximately 2% of grade IV glial neoplasms and present a similar age distribution as glioblastoma. Gliosarcoma and glioblastoma also share multiple morphologic, radiologic and clinical characteristics and their definitive differentiation is based only on histopathology. The most common presentation of gliosarcomas is as secondary tumors, frequently arising after cerebral radiotherapy to treat a primary glial neoplasm. At microscopic examination, the gliosarcomas are characterized by biphasic morphology composed of neoplastic astrocytes (pleomorphic and atypical), placed in a fibrillary stroma rich in blood vessels, with endothelial vascular proliferation similar to that seen in glioblastoma multiforme. The neoplastic cells demonstrate positive immune reactivity for GFAP in glial components and vimentin positivity in mesenchymal areas. There is however, little GFAP expression in minimal mesenchymal dedifferentiated areas with complete GFAP loss in areas with complete dedifferentiation into pure sarcoma. Currently, gliosarcomas are considered to be the product of a metaplastic change in a glioblastoma.

3,4. Pilocytic astrocytoma (PA) is a rare, slow-growing glioma, classified as grade I by the World Health Organization (WHO); it typically occurs in children and young adults. PA is the most common glial neoplasm in children. Only one-third of patients are older than 18 years of age and only 17 % are older than 30 years of age. In the pediatric population, two-thirds of lesions are located in the cerebellum; in adults, one-half of tumors are supratentorial. The cerebellum and the region around the third ventricle are the most common sites of origin; however, the entire neuraxis can be affected, with a preference for the optic nerve, optic chiasma, hypothalamus, cerebellum, brainstem, thalamus, basal ganglia, and cerebral hemispheres. PAs usually follow an indolent course, with an extremely high survival rate—over 90% at 10 years of age. The macroscopic appearance of PAs is typically well-circumscribed, cyst-like masses with a discrete mural nodule. The name "pilocytic" (directly translated as "hair cell") is derived from the long, hair-like projections that emanate from the neoplastic astrocytes. Microscopically, this tumor often reveals a biphasic pattern in which more compact areas composed of bipolar areas and brightly eosinophilic Rosenthal fibers alternate with looser, spongier areas with prominent microcysts. A Rosenthal fiber is a thick, elongated, worm-like or "corkscrew" eosinophilic (pink) bundle that is found on H and E staining of the brain in the presence of long-standing gliosis, occasional tumors, and some metabolic disorders. Eosinophilic granular bodies are found in both compact and loose areas. Pleomorphism, infrequent mitosis, or vascular proliferation may be observed; however, unlike other astrocytomas, they are rather degenerative and do not have an ominous prognosis. Hyalinization of the blood vessels is another feature of PAs. Microvascular proliferation of PAs accounts for the contrast enhancement that accompanies these tumors on cross-sectional imaging.

5,15. Dysembryoplastic neuroepithelial tumor (DNET) is a benign brain tumor arising from dysplastic brain development of the subpial granular layer. The tumor affects children and young adults, ranging in age from 9 to 17 years old at the time of diagnosis. Dysembryoplastic neuroepithelial tumor of man has three recognized histological patterns: multinodular, nodular and diffuse, with most of the tumor masses localized to the frontal and temporal lobes and occasional occurrence in the parietal and occipital lobes. Originally described by Daumas-Duport et al. DNET is composed of invariant specific glioneuronal elements (oligodendrocyte-like cells [OLCs], astrocytes and neurons) with the OLCs forming the bulk of the tumor mass. Hallmark histoarchitectural features of DNET are microcystic or alveolar patterns, with intracystic 'floating neurons' in a mucinous matrix and hypercellular background of OLCs. Cortical dysplasia, mitotic figures, nuclear atypia, calcification and necrosis tend to be variable among the histological types of DNET and in many cases are found inconsistently.

6. Astrocytic neoplasm with relatively favorable prognosis, typically in children and young adults. WHO grade II. It has mostly superficial meningocerebral location. 98% arise supratentorially, with preferential temporal lobe involvement. May arise in cerebellum, spinal cord and rarely in retina. Key histopathological features are usually seen in superficial compact component of tumor, including pleomorphic cells (mono- or multinucleated with frequent nuclear inclusion and occasional cytoplasmic xanthomatous change), spindle cells arranged in fascicular pattern. Other features include perivascular lymphocytic cuffing, scattered eosinophilic granular bodies, reticulin rich network. Underlying cortex shows infiltrative astrocytic component. Variable hemorrhage and protein granular degeneration (similar to pilocytic astrocytoma). No necrosis and no mitotic activity, except in tumors "with anaplastic features

7. Minigemistocytes are plasmacytoid, (i.e. have a plasma cell-like appearance) cells seen in oligodendrogliomas. They are usually strong GFAP +ve. In contrast to gemistocytic astrocytoma cells, which demonstrate pleomorphic astrocytic nuclear morphology and ill-defined fibrillary processes emanating from the eosinophilic cytoplasm, the mini gemistocytes demonstrate oligodendroglial type nuclei and well circumscribed almost inclusion-like eosinophilic cytoplasm.
9. Subependymal giant cell astrocytoma (SEGA) is a rare, benign brain tumor developing in patients with tuberous sclerosis complex (TSC). Tuberous sclerosis is a genetic disease with a broad clinical spectrum that has the potential to affect almost every organ system. It involves mutations in certain genes (TSC1 and TSC2) that are responsible for the production of proteins that usually help to regulate cell division and growth in the body. Subependymal giant cell astrocytoma (SEGA) occurs in up to 20% of individuals with tuberous sclerosis complex (TSC) and is more likely to develop during childhood and adolescence. Typically, SEGAs are very slow growing, but occasionally they may begin to grow more rapidly. Typical histopathological findings of this neoplasm are solid sheets and perivascular pseudorosettes of large, gemistocytic, polygonal and occasionally ganglion-like cells within a fibrillated background, accompanied by spindle-shaped cells creating broad fascicles. Rich vascular stroma, and numerous calcifications are common. Mitoses, focal necrosis, and endothelial proliferation are rarely encountered.
10. Paragangliomas are rare neuroendocrine tumors that arise from the extra-adrenal autonomic paraganglia, small organs consisting mainly of neuroendocrine cells that are derived from the embryonic neural crest and have the ability to secrete catecholamines. These tumors histologically are characterized by discrete small nests of cells (alveolar pattern or "Zellballen"). A broad anastamosing or trabecular pattern is more characteristic in these tumors. They are positive immunohistochemically for chromogranin, synaptophysin and the cells in between the nests called sustentacular cells are positive for S-100.
11. Ependymal tumors affect the whole neuraxis; however, their anatomical distribution varies according to the age of the patient. Those arising from below the occipital foramen most frequently affect adults, and are observed either in the spinal cord or in the filum terminale. The latter location is also common with children. Posterior fossa ependymomas occur more frequently in infants and children whereas supratentorial locations are more often seen in older children and adults. Although ependymal tumors are closely related to the ventricular system and the central canal, they can exceptionally be observed extradurally in the sacral region, in the cerebrum at distance from the ventricular system and in the subarachnoidal space. Histological hallmarks that allow recognition of ependymomas include: Perivascular rosettes, Ependymal rosettes. At an immunohistochemical level, ependymal tumors are always positively labeled for GFAP. Histologically there are many types of ependymomas i.e. Papillary ependymomas, Clear cell ependymomas, Tanycytic ependymomas, Myxopapillary ependymomas and Cellular ependymoma. Cellular ependymomas are highly cellular lesions presenting a monotonous appearance, and devoid of anaplastic feature. Papillary ependymomas are characterized by a papillary architecture in which the central vascular core is surrounded by cylindrical cells. Clear cell ependymoma is a variant observed predominantly in the supratentorial compartment, and, less frequently, in the posterior fossa and spinal cord. It mostly affects teenagers and young adults. Histologically, it resembles the classic 1p/19q-deleted oligodendroglioma, with cells that are regularly distributed, arranged back-to-back, with clear cytoplasms. The similarity with oligodendrogliomas extends to the blood vessels, which show chicken-wire architecture. Perivascular rosettes may be inconspicuous, and GFAP may be needed to highlight them. When areas of endothelial cell proliferation and mitosis are encountered in these tumors, they are graded as WHO grade III. When absent, the lesion is graded as II. Tanycytic ependymoma is a rare variant occurring more frequently in the spinal cord than in the brain. Tumor cells are typically elongated and arranged in fascicles requiring a differential diagnosis with schwannoma or pilocytic astrocytoma are also slow-growing lesions classically located in the conus/filum terminale. Although they affect patients of all ages, they are most frequent in young adults. Clinically, they are revealed by back pain of long duration. Like all ependymomas, they can give rise to CSF dissemination, reported to be more frequent in children than in adults.

12. The WHO grading of CNS tumors establishes a malignancy scale based on histologic features of the tumor. The histologic grades are as follows:

WHO grade I includes lesions with low proliferative potential, a frequently discrete nature, and the possibility of cure following surgical resection alone.

WHO grade II includes lesions that are generally infiltrating and low in mitotic activity but recur more frequently than do grade I malignant tumors after local therapy. Some tumor types tend to progress to higher grades of malignancy.

WHO grade III includes lesions with histologic evidence of malignancy, including nuclear atypia and increased mitotic activity. These lesions have anaplastic histology and infiltrative capacity. They are usually treated with aggressive adjuvant therapy.

WHO grade IV includes lesions that are mitotically active, necrosis prone, and generally associated with a rapid preoperative and postoperative progression and fatal outcomes. The lesions are usually treated with aggressive adjuvant therapy.

13. Deletion of chromosomes 1p and 19q occurs through a translocation event and is common in oligodendrogliomas. 1p/19q codeletion is a powerful prognostic factor and may predict for response to chemotherapy

14. Most intraventricular papillary neoplasms derived from choroid plexus epithelium are benign in nature and can be cured by surgery (choroid plexus papilloma, WHO Grade I, ICD-O 9390/0). At the other side of the spectrum is the choroid plexus carcinoma (WHO Grade III,) with frank signs of malignancy, including brisk mitotic activity, increased cellularity, blurring of the papillary pattern, necrosis and frequent invasion of brain parenchyma. The WHO Working group proposes to introduce an additional entity with intermediate features, designated 'atypical choroid plexus papilloma' which is primarily distinguished from the choroid plexus papilloma by increased mitotic activity.

12,17, 24.

In the current WHO edition (2007) grade I meningiomas (benign) are recognized by their histologic subtype and lack of anaplastic features. Grade II meningiomas (atypical) are defined by one or more of the following four criteria: 1) chordoid or clear cell histologic subtype, 2) four to 19 mitoses per ten high-power field (HPFs), 3) brain infiltration, and 4) three or more of the following five histologic features: small cell change, increased cellularity, prominent nucleoli, sheet-like growth, or necrosis. Grade III meningiomas (anaplastic/malignant) are defined by rhabdoid or papillary subtypes, a histological picture of frank malignancy resembling that of carcinomas, melanomas, or high grade sarcomas, or 20 or more mitosis per ten HPFs. The only change between the WHO 2007 and 2000 edition is that brain-infiltrative and otherwise benign meningiomas are classified as grade II.

18,19.

Anaplastic medulloblastoma- is characterized histologically by marked nuclear pleomorphism, nuclear moulding, cell–cell wrapping, and high mitotic activity, often with atypical forms. Although all medulloblastomas show some degree of atypia, these changes are particularly pronounced and widespread in the anaplastic variant. Histological progression from classic to anaplastic medulloblastomas may be observed, even within the same biopsy. The highly malignant large cell medulloblastomas and anaplastic medulloblastomas have considerable cytological overlap. The large cell variant features often spherical cells with round nuclei, open chromatin and prominent central nucleoli. The patterns may coexist. The nuclei of classical medulloblastoma are otherwise carrot shaped.

20,21,22,23.

Peripheral nerve sheath tumors encompass a spectrum of well defined clinicopathologic entities ranging from benign tumors, such as schwannoma, to high grade malignant neoplasms termed malignant peripheral nerve sheath tumors (MPNST) which are often resistant to conventional treatments. Schwannomas are benign neoplasms of Schwann cell origin. The gross appearance is characteristic, in the form of well circumscribed masses with degenerative changes and variable admixture of compact spindled (Antoni A) areas and hypocellular, microcystic (Antoni B) areas rich in macrophages and collagen fibers. A well formed collagenous capsule is a consistent finding (as well as hyalinized vessels. By immunohistochemistry, schwannomas typically show diffuse, strong expression of S100 protein and abundant pericellular collagen type IV consistent with the presence of a continuous pericellular basal lamina. Glial fibrillary acid protein (GFAP) is expressed in a subset of schwannomas.

Malignant triton tumor (MTT) is a rare aggressive subtype of malignant peripheral nerve sheath tumor (MPNST characterized histopathologically by focal rhabdomyoblastic differentiation. Incidence of malignant triton tumors is not known. MTT accounts for about 5% of all MPNSTs. The sex distribution is equal. Most cases are reported in adults, but reports have concerned patients of all ages. It is estimated that between 40 and 70% of cases occur in patients with neurofibromatosis type 1 (NF1; see this term), with an earlier age of onset and predominantly male subjects. The remaining cases are sporadic and occur at a later age. MTT generally arises from a peripheral nerve in the head, neck, extremities and trunk. Rare localizations include the brain, buttock, viscera, mediastinum and retroperitoneum. Exceedingly rare intracranial MTT not associated with a cranial nerve has been reported. MTT is defined histologically as malignant peripheral nerve sheath tumor with additional rhabdomyoblastic differentiation. Prognosis is generally very poorer than classical MPNST, and is often difficult to completely resect. Local recurrence and distant metastases are common. 5-year survival for MTT is reported to be about 10–14%.

27,29.

Primary central nervous system are defined as the presence of non-Hodgkin's lymphoma in the brain or spinal cord in the absence of lymph node, bone marrow, or other organ involvement at the time of diagnosis. It is relatively uncommon, accounting for only 2.7% of all central nervous system malignancies and 1–2% of all lymphomas. Immunodeficient patients, including acquired immune deficiency syndrome (AIDS) patients and organ transplant recipients, are at an increased risk of developing primary central nervous system lymphomas. However, even in immunocompetent individuals, the incidence of primary central nervous system lymphoma is increasing. The most common type of primary central nervous system lymphoma is the diffuse large B-cell type. Primary central nervous system lymphoma carries a poor prognosis. Median survival is 17–45 months in immunocompetent patients, and only 13.5 months in those with AIDS. Although several clinical factors, including age, performance status, and extent of disease, have been found to be prognostically significant in some studies, a validated method of predicting prognosis in these patients remains to be elucidated. Primary CNS lymphomas are characterized by a dismal prognosis relative to other extranodal lymphomas. Approximately 98% of primary central nervous system lymphomas are of B-cell origin, and most belong to the diffuse large B-cell type. Recently, diffuse large B-cell lymphomas have been subcategorized into germinal center and non-germinal center types based on gene expression profiles and immunohistochemical expression of CD10, Bcl-6, and MUM1. Studies have shown that the overall survival rate of the germinal center group is better than that of the non-germinal center lymphomas. On histopathology primary CNS lymphomas display an angiocentric pattern.

28. Pituitary adenomas are classified clinically into 2 groups—clinically functioning adenomas and clinically nonfunctioning adenomas—according to whether an endocrine syndrome is present or absent. Most adenomas are functioning tumors; these include prolactin (PRL)–producing, growth hormone (GH)–producing, adrenocorticotropic hormone (ACTH)–producing, and thyroid-stimulating hormone (TSH)–producing adenomas. Pituitary adenomas are also classified according to the hormone content of the tumor cells as determined by immunohistochemistry (IHC). This classification provides significant information for clinical practice. [17] In a few tumors, however, analysis of the adenoma's ultrastructural aspects is necessary.

30. Granular cell tumors are glial tumors that arise either in the pituitary stalk or posterior pituitary—they are usually incidental tumors found in adults at autopsies and only rarely present as symptomatic masses (there are about 60 reported cases in the literature; granular cell tumors of the sella are also known as choristoma of the neurohypophysis, granular cell pituicytoma, granular cell myoblastoma, and granular cell tumorette.

34. Pilomyxoid astrocytoma (PMA) occurs typically in the hypothalamic/chiasmatic region, sites that are also affected by classical pilocytic astrocytomas. PMA is histologically characterized by a prominent myxoid matrix and angiocentric arrangement of monomorphous, bipolar tumor cells. The close relationship to pilocytic astrocytoma is underscored by a report of two cases that occurred in the setting of neurofibromatosis type 1 (NF1). PMA affects predominantly infants and children (median age, 10 months) and appears to have a less favorable prognosis. Local recurrences and cerebrospinal spread are more likely to occur in pilomyxoid than in pilocytic astrocytomas. The Working Group therefore recommended an assignment to WHO grade II.

35. Liponeurocytomas occur generally in the cerebellum and are characterized by many lipidized cells found in clusters or scattered between small neoplastic cells. Immunohistochemical staining has demonstrated that both neuronal and glial differentiation is present. Mitotic activity is generally low in these lesions. This rare tumor is WHO grade I–II, generally with an accordingly indolent behavior.

37,38,43,58.

Chordoma is a slow growing malignant bone tumor arising from the notochord remnants. The tumor causes local destruction of the bone and may extend into the surrounding soft tissue. 50% arise from sacrococcygeal area. 35% in the spheno-occipital area (base of skull). 15% cervico- thoraco-lumbar (mobile) spine. Symptoms depend on the location and are usually present for a long time. The tumor usually occurs between 55 and 65 years. Spheno-occipital tumors may occur in children. Soft, blue gray, lobulated tumor with gelatinous appearance. Focal areas of hemorrhage and areas of cystic degeneration may be present. The tumor is composed of lobules separated by fibrous tissue. The tumor cells are arranged in cords, columns or trabeculae. The tumor cells are set in a basophilic to metachromatic mucinous or myxoid stroma. There are two types of cell - small, uniform, non-vacuolated cells with ovoid nuclei and larger cells with multivacuolated or bubble like cytoplasm and vesicular nuclei. These large cells are known as "Physaliphorous cells" (Greek word for bubble or drop) and are diagnostic of chordomas. Occasional mitotic figures may be identified. Some cellular pleomorphism may be present which is of no prognostic significance. The physaliphorous cells are PAS positive. The matrix is alcian blue and mucicarmine positive.

Immunohistochemistry:

The tumor cells are positive for cytokeratins, epithelial membrane antigen (EMA), S100 protein and are rarely positive for CEA. Microscopic variants of chordoma: Chondroid chordoma- Shows prominent chondroid differentiation. Has a better prognosis. Commonly located in the spheno-occipital region. Some authors consider these tumors to be chondrosarcoma. EMA and CEA positivity is less common in this variant. Dedifferentiated chordoma- Highly malignant biphasic tumor composed of areas of high grade sarcoma and areas of typical chordoma. Indicates poor prognosis.

Differential diagnosis: Myxoid tumors of soft tissue

Chondrosarcoma: Epithelial markers are negative. There are no fibrous bands separating lobules.

42. "Onion bulb" formations are concentric layers of Schwann cell processes and collagen around an axon. This proliferation is caused by repetitive segmental demyelination and regeneration of myelin and can cause gross thickening of peripheral nerves (hypertrophic neuropathy). The central axon is often demyelinated or has a thin layer of myelin. Onion bulb formations are the histological hallmark of Charcot-Marie-Tooth disease, but are also seen in other hereditary neuropathies (Dejerine-Sottas disease, Refsum disease), in diabetic neuropathy, and in chronic inflammatory demyelinative neuropathy.

44. Desmoplastic infantile ganglioglioma (DIG) is a rare supratentorial brain tumor occurring mostly before the age of 2 years. It has a good prognosis and total excision of the tumor is curative, necessitating no further treatment. An accurate pathologic diagnosis is crucial. this tumor is recognized as a distinct entity and is included in the World Health Organization (WHO) classification under the category of neural and mixed glioneuronal tumors, and is in the grade I of the WHO classification. They are massive, firmly attached to the dura, extensively infiltrate the subarachnoid space but do not involve the ventricular system. Most commonly, CT scan and magnetic resonance imaging show a large superficial large cerebral mass with solid and cystic areas. Histologically, the most prominent feature of DIG is desmoplasia and spindle cells with a storiform pattern of arrangement. There is also a ganglion cell component, which is present as single cells or clusters. The first component can be shown to be GFAP positive, but the latter component is of neuroepithelial origin and reactive with markers such as synaptophysin. The main histologic differential diagnoses are reticulin-rich desmoplastic tumors such as pleomorphic xanthoastrocytoma, which can be differentiated by age of the patient, prominent lipidization of the cells and absence of neural component.

46. Atypical teratoid/rhabdoid tumors (AT/RTs) are highly malignant central nervous system (CNS) tumors that primarily affect young children, and characterized by varying numbers of distinctive rhabdoid cells. The majority of the tumor cells demonstrate a rhabdoid phenotype, characterized by an eccentrically placed vesicular nucleus, a prominent nucleolus, and an eosinophilic inclusion-like cytoplasm. Areas of the tumor show a primitive neuroectodermal tumor (PNET)-like, blue-colored small-cell appearance. Mitoses were frequently observed. Immunostaining reveals a lack of integrase interactor-1 (INI-1) protein expression in the tumor cells, and fluorescence in situ hybridization (FISH) reveals a hemizygous deletion of the INI-1 gene region on 22q11.2. The tumor cells are either entirely or partially positive for glial fibrillary acidic protein, epithelial membrane antigen (EMA), vimentin, oligodendrocyte transcription factor 2, nestin, and actin, but are negative for desmin, S100 protein, and SRY-related HMG-box gene 10 (SOX-10). The most important differential diagnosis of AT/RT is medulloblastoma of the posterior fossa in a young child. Other important differential diagnoses are other embryonal tumors, choroid plexus carcinoma and anaplastic ependymoma. Indeed, in a child <3 years of age, any tumor with a high proliferation index is potentially an AT/RT. Ancillary diagnostic studies are critical in the determination of the distinction of these embryonal tumors. Approximately 5% of AT/RTs that contain ependymoblastic rosettes result in a considerable number of cases with a differential diagnosis of embryonal tumor with abundant neuropils and true rosettes; this tumor type can be distinguished based on a high level of focal amplification of chromosome 19q13.41. The loss of INI-1 expression may play a key role in the ability to distinguish AT/RT from the aforementioned tumors.

47. Pineblastoma is a poorly differentiated malignant embryonal neoplasm arising in the pineal gland. It usually occurs in children and is histologically characterized by the presence of small immature neuroepithelial cells. Pineoblastomas tend to spread via cerebrospinal fluid (CSF) pathways and often follows an aggressive clinical course Pineoblastomas are highly malignant WHO grade IV lesions that represent the most primitive form of pineal parenchymal tumors and account for 40% of pineal parenchymal tumors They are embryonal tumors described as a primitive neuroectodermal tumor of the pineal gland They most commonly occur in the first 2 decades but can occur at any age, and there is no gender predilection. The 5-year survival is 58%. Pineoblastomas are highly cellular embryonal neoplasms that resemble other primitive neuroectodermal neoplasms of the central nervous system. Cells have scant cytoplasm and are arranged in diffuse sheets (Homer-Wright rosettes (neuroblastic differentiation) or Flexner-Wintersteiner rosettes (retinoblastic differentiation) may be seen, and hemorrhage or necrosis may be present. Infiltration into adjacent structures and craniospinal dissemination commonly occurs.

51. Aspergillus is branching septate hyphae, varying from 4–12 micrometer in width. Multiple septa are seen at regular intervals and hyphal branching from acute angles in the same direction as the main hyphae.

52. Cryptococcus neoformans usually causes basal meningitis which may be subacute or chronic.

53. Polio virus is a single stranded RNA virus of picornavirus family. Paralytic polio is exceedingly rare. Infection occurs by feco-oral route.

54. Unlike most other mycoses in which cerebral involvement is secondary to a primary focus in lungs, this mycoses develops most frequently from an infection of the skin of face or in the mucosa of nose or nasopharynx and spreads to adjacent regions and to arteries with orbit and internal carotid arteries.

56. Brucella is a non-motile organism and the human disease follows animal brucellosis and it causes arteritis.

57. It is a WHO grade I tumor. It occurs throughout life but predominantly in adults (mean age, 38 years) No gender predilection is reported. The 5-year survival is 86–100%, and there are no reported relapses after gross total resection Cerebrospinal fluid (CSF) dissemination rarely occurs. Pineocytomas are composed of relatively small, uniform, mature cells that resemble pineocytes. Lobular architecture and pineocytomatous rosettes are common features.

59. These are malignant tumors arising from a peripheral nerve or in extraneural soft tissue and showing nerve sheath differentiation. Arguably, the diagnosis of MPNST has historically suffered from a lack of entirely specific morphological criteria and/or ancillary immunohistochemical or molecular tests. It is thus likely that a variety of non-nerve sheath sarcomas have been placed incorrectly into this category over the years. Most authors would agree that any sarcoma with intrinsic involvement of a major nerve, without a specific diagnosis reflecting an alternative line of differentiation (e.g., intraneural synovial sarcoma, angiosarcoma), or clearly arising from a pre-existing benign nerve sheath tumor should qualify Similarly, malignant spindled tumors in NF1 patients should be considered MPNST until proven otherwise. More difficult to classify are those tumors that are unrelated to a major nerve, and in these instances a combination of morphologic findings, immunohistochemistry (e.g. partial S100 expression) or ultrastructural features of Schwann cell or perineural differentiation, must be present. Frequent histologic findings, although not entirely specific, include fascicles of alternating cellularity, whorls, palisades or rosette-like arrangements, perineural/intraneural spread when associated with nerve, subendothelial accentuation of tumor cells, and large areas of geographic-like necrosis. Heterologous differentiation in the form of cartilage and bone, or less commonly skeletal muscle (so called malignant triton tumor smooth muscle, angiosarcoma, and even well formed glands occur on occasion particularly in patients with NF.